The American Opioid Epidemic

From Patient Care to Public Health

The American Opioid Epidemic

From Patient Care to Public Health

Edited by
Michael T. Compton, M.D., M.P.H.
Marc W. Manseau, M.D., M.P.H.

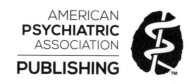

AMERICAN
PSYCHIATRIC
ASSOCIATION
PUBLISHING

Copyright © 2019 American Psychiatric Association Publishing

ALL RIGHTS RESERVED

First Edition

Manufactured in the United States of America on acid-free paper
23 22 21 20 19   5 4 3 2 1

American Psychiatric Association Publishing
800 Maine Avenue SW
Suite 900
Washington, DC 20024-2812
www.appi.org

Library of Congress Cataloging-in-Publication Data
Names: Compton, Michael T., editor. | Manseau, Marc W., editor. | American Psychiatric Association Publishing, issuing body.
Title: The American opioid epidemic : from patient care to public health / edited by Michael T. Compton, Marc W. Manseau.
Description: First edition. | Washington, D.C : American Psychiatric Association Publishing, [2019] | Includes bibliographical references and index.
Identifiers: LCCN 2018037457 (print) | LCCN 2018038487 (ebook) | ISBN 9781615372140 (ebook) | ISBN 9781615371570 (pbk. : alk. paper)
Subjects: | MESH: Opioid-Related Disorders | Analgesics, Opioid—adverse effects | Naloxone—therapeutic use | Drug Overdose | United States
Classification: LCC RC568.O45 (ebook) | LCC RC568.O45 (print) | NLM WM 284 | DDC 615.7/822—dc23
LC record available at https://lccn.loc.gov/2018037457

British Library Cataloguing in Publication Data
A CIP record is available from the British Library.

Contents

Contributors

Kavita Babu, M.D.
Professor of Emergency Medicine and Chief of Division of Medical Toxicology, University of Massachusetts Medical School, Worcester, Massachusetts

Leo Beletsky, J.D., M.P.H.
Associate Professor of Law and Health Sciences, School of Law and Bouvé College of Health Sciences, Northeastern University, Boston, Massachusetts; Adjunct Professor, University of California, San Diego School of Medicine, San Diego, California

Snehal Bhatt, M.D.
Associate Professor, Department of Psychiatry and Behavioral Sciences, and Chief, Addiction Psychiatry, University of New Mexico, Albuquerque, New Mexico

Adam Bisaga, M.D.
Professor of Psychiatry, Division on Substance Use Disorders, Columbia University Department of Psychiatry; Research Scientist, New York State Psychiatric Institute, New York, New York

Edward W. Boyer, M.D., Ph.D.
Director of Research and Academic Development, Brigham and Women's Hospital, and Associate Professor of Emergency Medicine, Harvard Medical School, Boston, Massachusetts

S. Brook Burkley, M.S.W.
Senior Project Manager, Treatment Research Institute Center on Addiction, Public Health Management Corporation, Philadelphia, Pennsylvania

Michael T. Compton, M.D., M.P.H.
Professor of Clinical Psychiatry, Columbia University College of Physicians and Surgeons; New York State Psychiatric Institute, New York, New York

Katherine Devin, M.D.
Assistant Professor of Emergency Medicine, University of Connecticut Medical School, Farmington, Connecticut

Karen L. Dugosh, Ph.D.
Senior Research Scientist, Treatment Research Institute Center on Addiction, Public Health Management Corporation, Philadelphia, Pennsylvania

David S. Festinger, Ph.D.
Senior Research Scientist, Treatment Research Institute Center on Addiction, Public Health Management Corporation; Professor and Director of Substance Abuse Research and Education, Department of Psychology, Philadelphia College of Osteopathic Medicine, Philadelphia, Pennsylvania

Carl E. Fisher, M.D.
Assistant Professor of Clinical Psychiatry, Department of Psychiatry, Columbia University College of Physicians and Surgeons; New York State Psychiatric Institute, New York, New York

Bellelizabeth Foster, M.D.
Assistant Professor, Department of Psychiatry and Behavioral Sciences, and Medical Director, Services and Treatments for Adolescents in Recovery (STAR), University of New Mexico, Albuquerque, New Mexico

Aaron Fox, M.D., M.S.
Associate Professor of Medicine, Division of General Internal Medicine, Montefiore Medical Center, Bronx, New York

Helena Hansen, M.D., Ph.D.
Assistant Professor, Departments of Psychiatry and Anthropology, New York University, New York, New York

Benjamin Hayes, M.D., M.P.H., M.S.W.
Resident Physician, Division of General Internal Medicine, Montefiore Medical Center, Bronx, New York

Keith A. Hermanstyne, M.D., M.P.H., M.S.H.P.M.
Attending, Traditions Behavioral Health, San Francisco, California

Vanessa Jacobsohn, M.D.
Assistant Professor, Department of Psychiatry and Behavioral Sciences, and Medical Director, ASAP Primary Care and Hepatitis C Treatment Program, University of New Mexico, Albuquerque, New Mexico

Abhishek Jain, M.D.
Forensic Psychiatry Research Fellow, Department of Psychiatry, Columbia University College of Physicians and Surgeons; New York State Psychiatric Institute, New York, New York

Samuel Kolander, M.D.
PGY-2 Resident, Department of Psychiatry, Columbia University Medical Center, New York State Psychiatric Institute, New York, New York

Nathan M. Kunzler, M.D.
Clinical Fellow in Emergency Medicine, Division of Medical Toxicology, Department of Emergency Medicine, Brigham and Women's Hospital, Harvard Medical School, Boston, Massachusetts

Marc W. Manseau, M.D., M.P.H.
Clinical Assistant Professor of Psychiatry, New York University School of Medicine, New York, New York

Leslie Marino, M.D., M.P.H.
Assistant Professor, Department of Psychiatry, Columbia University Medical Center, New York State Psychiatric Institute, New York, New York

Silvia S. Martins, M.D., Ph.D.
Associate Professor, Department of Epidemiology, Mailman School of Public Health, Columbia University, New York, New York

William Mathews, R.P.A.-C.
Physician Assistant, Harm Reduction Coalition, New York, New York

Bethany Medley, M.S.W.
Opioid Program Manager, Harm Reduction Coalition, New York, New York

Julie Netherland, Ph.D.
Director, Office of Academic Engagement, Drug Policy Alliance, New York, New York

Sarah Oreck, M.D., M.S.
Addiction Psychiatry Fellow, University of California, Los Angeles

Paul Romo, M.D.
Assistant Professor, Department of Psychiatry and Behavioral Sciences, and Medical Director, Addiction and Substance Abuse Programs, University of New Mexico, Albuquerque, New Mexico

Roxanne Russell, M.D.
Resident Physician, Psychiatry, University of New Mexico, Albuquerque, New Mexico

Julian Santaella-Tenorio, M.P.H.
Doctoral candidate, Department of Epidemiology, Mailman School of Public Health, Columbia University, New York, New York

Lloyd I. Sederer, M.D.
Chief Medical Officer, New York State Office of Mental Health; Adjunct Professor, Columbia/Mailman School of Public Health, New York, New York

Luis E. Segura, M.D., M.P.H.
Doctoral student, Department of Epidemiology, Mailman School of Public Health, Columbia University, New York, New York

Tyler Seybert, M.D.
Resident Physician, Psychiatry and Behavioral Sciences, University of New Mexico, Albuquerque, New Mexico

Matisyahu Shulman, M.D.
Addiction Psychiatry Fellow, Division on Substance Use Disorders, Columbia University Department of Psychiatry, New York State Psychiatric Institute, New York, New York

Sharon Stancliff, M.D.
Medical Director, Harm Reduction Coalition, New York, New York

Vitor S. Tardelli, M.D., M.P.H.
Research Assistant, Department of Epidemiology, Mailman School of Public Health, Columbia University, New York, New York

Leila M. Vaezazizi, M.D.
Fellow, Division on Substance Abuse, Department of Psychiatry, New York State Psychiatric Institute, Columbia University Medical Center, New York, New York

Arthur Robin Williams, M.D., M.B.E.
Assistant Professor of Clinical Psychiatry, Division on Substance Use Disorders, Columbia University Department of Psychiatry; Research Scientist, New York State Psychiatric Institute, New York, New York

Tauheed Zaman, M.D.
Assistant Clinical Professor, University of California, San Francisco, School of Medicine, San Francisco, California

Disclosure of Competing Interests

The following contributors to this book have indicated a financial interest in or other affiliation with a commercial supporter, a manufacturer of a commercial product, a provider of a commercial service, a nongovernmental organization, and/or a government agency, as listed below:

Adam Bisaga, M.D.—*Research funding*: Alkermes; *Site investigator*: Alkermes-funded multisite trial

Lloyd I. Sederer, M.D.—*Book royalties*: Scribner, W.W. Norton, Cognella, American Psychiatric Association Publishing

The following contributors to this book have indicated no competing interests to disclose:

Kavita Babu, M.D.
Snehal Bhatt, M.D.
Leo Beletsky, J.D., M.P.H.
Edward W. Boyer, M.D., Ph.D.
S. Brook Burkley, M.S.W.
Michael T. Compton, M.D.,
   M.P.H.
Katherine Devin, M.D.
Karen L. Dugosh, Ph.D.
David S. Festinger, Ph.D.
Carl E. Fisher, M.D.
Bellelizabeth Foster, M.D.
Aaron Fox, M.D., M.S.
Helena Hansen, M.D., Ph.D.
Benjamin Hayes, M.D., M.P.H.,
   M.S.W.
Keith A. Hermanstyne, M.D.,
   M.P.H., M.S.H.P.M.
Vanessa Jacobsohn, M.D.
Abhishek Jain, M.D.
Samuel Kolander, M.D.

Nathan M. Kunzler, M.D.
Marc W. Manseau, M.D.,
   M.P.H.
Leslie Marino, M.D., M.P.H.
Silvia S. Martins, M.D., Ph.D.
William Mathews, R.P.A.-C.
Bethany Medley, M.S.W.
Julie Netherland, Ph.D.
Sarah Oreck, M.D., M.S.
Paul Romo, M.D.
Roxanne Russell, M.D.
Julian Santaella-Tenorio, M.P.H.
Luis E. Segura, M.D., M.P.H.
Tyler Seybert, M.D.
Matisyahu Shulman, M.D.
Sharon Stancliff, M.D.
Vitor S. Tardelli, M.D., M.P.H.
Leila M. Vaezazizi, M.D.
Arthur Robin Williams, M.D.,
   M.B.E.
Tauheed Zaman, M.D.

Foreword

The problems brought about by opioids are now surpassing their medicinal utility. Opioids have become a corrosive and deadly cluster of natural and synthetic drugs doing great damage to our society. Their path to this dubious distinction is largely the product of their huge effectiveness in relieving (acute) pain and psychic distress and in transporting our minds from the everyday discomfort and general ennui of human existence. Their utility is coupled with well-intentioned physicians' prescribing too much for too long, a (now defunct) policy to make pain the "fifth vital sign," and pharmaceutical manufacturers' unbridled misrepresentation and greed in promoting opioid analgesic pills (most notably, OxyContin).

The annual death toll from overdoses in the United States surpasses the total American death count from the Vietnam War. The price, each year, for our communities in terms of medical, social welfare, and correctional services, as well as to the operations of American businesses, is approaching $1 trillion, not to mention the incalculable suffering and grief that individuals and families endure.

This brief foreword is no call for the elimination of (legal) opioids, at least not until scientists discover and deliver highly effective nonopioid analgesics and nervous system stimulation techniques—which are not around the corner. It is certainly not a call for arresting and incarcerating people who use or are addicted to opioids—a profoundly uninformed, ineffective, and very expensive approach of which segments of this country and its elected and appointed governmental leaders remain enamored. It is, however, a call for changing the patterns of prescribing and use: the supply and demand side of medical care.

As doctors, along with other health and mental health (including addiction) professionals, we must join and help lead a national campaign to curtail the opioid epidemic. Our efforts need to begin with relearning what we know about these drugs because much of our training has become outdated or was laced with attitudes that stigmatized the individuals who use these substances. We must appreciate the benefits and risks of these drugs; their actions on the brain, mind, and body; the neuroscience of addiction; and effective means of prevention, early detection, and treatment. Nothing less than comprehensive, uninterrupted treatment, with its additive effects when biological, psychological, and social approaches are all applied, is needed; yet, we are far from achieving this level of care.

In this carefully constructed and engaging book, clinical readers will find the best of science and practice to inform both work and public policy endeavors. The book gives us as readers the chance to take a deep dive into the public health approaches to this epidemic, from both psychiatric and medical perspectives. We learn about prescription and illicit opioids, including the growing menace of fentanyl, which is 50–100 times more powerful than morphine, and its readily made derivatives that today flood our borders and the brains of those who (often unknowingly) use them. Overdoses, now ubiquitous, can be prevented and treated, but we need to know how to access and use naloxone, which is a key topic of this book, as are a variety of harm reduction techniques that need far wider adoption than we have seen to date. The editors and chapter authors provide us with comprehensive, useful treatment and prevention strategies, which can and do work.

Too many lives have been lost. Too much misdirection has been perpetrated by those who have yet to adopt a public mental health approach to addictions. The road is made by walking it, to paraphrase the Spanish poet Antonio Machado. This book is a necessary traveling companion for our journey in overcoming the epidemic of opioid addiction and overdose.

Lloyd I. Sederer, M.D.
Chief Medical Officer, New York State Office of Mental Health;
Adjunct Professor, Columbia/Mailman School of Public Health;
contributing writer for *U.S. News & World Report* and *Psychology Today*

Preface

Opioid misuse, addiction, and overdoses have evolved into public health crises with iatrogenic, sociocultural, and policy/regulatory underpinnings. American psychiatrists and other mental health professionals have a role to play in addressing this crisis. In this book, we hope to provide this audience of mental health clinicians, and indeed an even broader one, with a comprehensive but concise and clinically relevant resource, containing the very latest information on the complex issues surrounding the American opioid crisis.

In the first chapter, we provide a brief overview of the opium poppy, opium production, and the three key analgesic alkaloids within opium: morphine, codeine, and thebaine. We describe how morphine is derived from opium and heroin from morphine and discuss opium derivatives for medical use. We give an overview of the current crisis; federal, state, and local responses; and actions that mental health professionals can take to contribute to solutions.

In Chapter 2, Mr. Santaella-Tenorio and Drs. Segura, Tardelli, Vaezazizi, and Martins give a thorough overview of prescription opioids. They describe the agents and their physiological effects, give details on the origins of the prescription opioid use and misuse epidemic, and present national trends in the nonmedical use of these prescription medications. They also cover the consequences of the long-term use of prescription opioids, including the risk of initiating use of heroin and other illegal opioids.

Then, in Chapter 3, Drs. Jain and Fisher give an overview of the remarkable history and global impact of opium over the past thousands of years. They describe modern-day use and production of opium and its derivatives, with a focus on heroin use and its history, pharmacology, administration, street terminology, and the "cutting" of heroin with various adulterants. The authors cover heroin addiction and its epidemiology, heroin tolerance and withdrawal, and heroin use comorbidities, as well as heroin overdose and its morbidity and mortality, risk factors, and considerations for recognizing, treating, and preventing it.

In Chapter 4, Drs. Kunzler, Devin, Babu, and Boyer provide a comprehensive examination of the opioid overdose epidemic. They cover the epidemiology, pathophysiology, and toxicology of opioid-related overdose and guide clinicians in key principles of overdose management, from evaluation to treatment to prevention. Readers will learn about the pharmacology and clinical use of naloxone, the main opioid overdose reversal agent, as well as the toxic profiles of the most common opioids implicated in overdose deaths. Drs. Vaezazizi, Netherland, and Hansen describe the social determinants of the opioid epidemic, and associated health inequities, in Chapter 5. They outline historical perspectives and current trends in the epidemic in terms of race, gender, and urban versus rural differences. The authors also detail pharmaceutical marketing and regulatory considerations, as well as local, state, and national policies that shape health disparities and inequities around opioid addiction, and their consequences.

Chapters 6 and 7 cover medical and psychiatric comorbidities with opioid use disorder (OUD), respectively. In Chapter 6, Drs. Fox and Hayes describe the most common and important medical problems that co-occur with OUD, carefully breaking down the physical health effects related to the routes of drug administration (i.e., injection, intranasal insufflation, inhalation), co-occurring behaviors (e.g., co-occurring substance use, sexual behaviors), and the direct physiological effects of opioids. They detail the impact of medical comorbidities on overdose risk and point clinicians and public health practitioners toward best practices for the treatment and prevention of medical problems in individuals with OUD. In Chapter 7, we address mental illnesses and nonopioid substance use disorders (SUDs) that co-occur with OUD. Alerting readers to recent signs that psychiatric comorbidity might be a silent driver of the opioid addiction and overdose epidemic, we review the epidemiological and clinical literature on the psychiatric disorders and SUDs that most commonly accompany opioid addiction. Separately addressing the older problem of heroin-related OUD and newer trends related to nonmedical prescription opioid use, we explore underlying explanations for the close association between psychiatric illness and opioid addiction and overdose death. We also discuss important considerations for integrated treatment of individuals with co-occurring disorders involving OUD.

In Chapter 8, Drs. Bhatt, Foster, Jacobsohn, Romo, Seybert, and Russell provide a thorough review of screening, assessment, and treatment planning for patients with OUD. The authors describe how to engage patients in a collaborative, empathetic, and nonjudgmental manner that instills hope and acknowledges the highly personal and profound individual experience of living with addiction. They lay out the effects of stigma, and they describe the process of recovery, around which all clinical encounters should be centered. Drs. Shulman, Williams, and Bisaga give readers a comprehensive overview of opioid withdrawal management and transition to treatment in Chapter 9. They begin by describing the pathophysiology and clinical signs of acute opioid withdrawal. Next, they outline principles of acute withdrawal management (i.e., detoxification). Finally, they discuss detailed clinical strategies for transitioning patients from problematic opioid use to effective treatment. In Chapter 10, Drs. Marino, Oreck, and Kolander provide a detailed summary of medication-assisted treatment (MAT), the key component of effective treatment for OUD. They present evidence demonstrating that MAT improves and saves lives by mitigating intense cravings and agonizing withdrawal; reducing or eliminating opioid misuse; and preventing harms associated with opioid abuse, including medical problems and overdose death. They also take readers through a careful review of the pharmacology, clinical use, and challenges of each MAT agent, specifically methadone, buprenorphine, and injectable extended-release naltrexone. They end with a discussion of MAT in special populations.

Drs. Dugosh and Festinger and Ms. Burkley provide a review in Chapter 11 of psychosocial interventions, including motivational approaches, cognitive-behavioral approaches, contingency management, family-based approaches, and mutual-help groups such as Narcotics Anonymous. They point out that research demonstrates that many of these interventions can be effective when used in combination with MAT. The authors also present the various levels of care for OUD, ranging from psychoeducational early intervention approaches to medically managed inpatient services. In Chapter 12, Dr. Stancliff, Ms. Medley, and Mr. Mathews present the harm reduction philosophy and related strategies as powerful tools to combat the opioid epidemic. They define *harm reduction* as "a public health approach that aims to reduce the negative consequences associated with drug use on both individuals and communities," as well as a clinical stance that is forcefully person centered and social justice oriented. They show how clinicians can embrace the harm reduction philosophy in general and how they can apply it specifically to the treatment of OUD, including opioid agonist treatment. The authors then describe an array of innovative harm reduction strategies, such as dispensing naloxone kits in the community to prevent overdose death and making drug injection safer.

Chapter 13 provides a critical look at prevention-oriented strategies and policies designed to mitigate the opioid crisis. In this chapter, Dr. Zaman, Mr. Beletsky, and Dr. Hermanstyne not only review strengths and limitations of mainstream preventive measures, such as prescription drug monitoring programs and clinical opioid prescribing guidance, but they also argue that in order to successfully manage the opioid epidemic, we will need public health strategies that directly address the social and political roots of the problem. Finally, in Chapter 14, Dr. Williams brings the discussion of the opioid crisis to a higher level by bridging the clinical and policy domains. He begins the chapter with a critical look at the epidemic's scale by evaluating advantages and limitations of available systems-level data. He then identifies gaps in current quality measures that are relevant to OUD treatment, with the rationale that addressing these deficiencies would allow treatment providers and policy makers to identify areas for improvement and guide efficient resource allocation. Lastly, he proposes an innovative cascade of care model for OUD, based on previous successful frameworks such as the HIV cascade of care. He cogently argues that this type of well-coordinated, systems-level transformative approach is our best chance at ending the opioid epidemic and saving numerous lives.

In coordinating and compiling this book, we have tried to provide psychiatrists and other mental health professionals with everything they need to know in order to confidently take part in addressing the current opioid crisis. In several instances, there is some intended overlap because we want each chapter to be a stand-alone review of the topic at hand, and the repetition serves to emphasize important themes for readers who read the book from cover to cover (as we encourage). Finally, we hope that this book will be one key tool, among many others that will be useful, to assist our colleagues in helping their patients and advocating for necessary policy change.

Michael T. Compton, M.D., M.P.H.
Marc W. Manseau, M.D., M.P.H.

Acknowledgments

Managing the compilation of 14 chapters on a critical issue facing American public health and health care is a complex and time-consuming task. We thank Kendrick Hogan and Brian Faas for forgiving us for the late evenings and long weekends required for each of us to meet our deadlines and accomplish our shared goal. We appreciate the team at American Psychiatric Association Publishing, including John McDuffie, Laura Roberts, Bessie Jones, and others, for entrusting us with this important work. We offer deep gratitude to the more than 30 authors, from all across the country, who contributed to this work. Their commitment to this project, as well as their daily dedication to addressing the opioid crisis, is heartening. They provided scholarly yet accessible, and comprehensive yet concise, reviews of all of the key topics readers need to know about in order to take part in solutions to the crisis. And they did this despite having major responsibilities in busy clinical and academic posts. We are also thankful for, and wish to acknowledge, the excellent education and training during our residencies and fellowships a number of years ago. Our fellowship training in community and public psychiatry and our training in public health in addition to medicine and psychiatry taught us that addressing an addiction-related public health crisis does not necessarily require specialty training in addictionology; it does, however, require community, public health, and policy perspectives. Perhaps most importantly, we are grateful for having been able to serve many patients through the years who have taught us about struggling with addiction in a very personal way. They have inspired us, and it is for them that we endeavor to work toward solutions and improved health and happiness.

Michael T. Compton, M.D., M.P.H.
Marc W. Manseau, M.D., M.P.H.

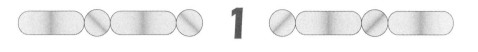

From Fields of Poppies to a National Crisis

Michael T. Compton, M.D., M.P.H.
Marc W. Manseau, M.D., M.P.H.

Introduction

From the innocent and beautiful *Papaver somniferum* flower has evolved a fascinating global saga over the course of centuries. Thousands of fields have been cultivated. Wars have been fought. Medical advances have been hailed. Now, our country finds itself in a crisis of devastating scale, with countless lives being lost. America finds itself here because of a confluence of many events and contexts. The pharmaceutical industry heavily promoted opioids for the treatment of pain while minimizing their addictive potential. The medical community embraced the need to more effectively assess and treat both acute and chronic pain. The availability, distribution, and purity of heroin have evolved in recent years. New synthetic opioids have made their way into the black market.

Meanwhile, many Americans have been experiencing stressors that increase the risk for addiction. The American people have faced major uncertainties in the world (e.g., terrorism, wars, natural disasters), as

1

well as uncertainties in our homeland (e.g., factory closures, unemployment, lack of affordable housing, other economic strains such as an expanding income and wealth inequality). Opioids offer a fast and effective, albeit temporary, salve for the emotional distress caused by many of these miseries. In fact, it has been shown that as a county's unemployment rate increases by 1%, the opioid death rate per 100,000 rises by 0.19 (3.6%) and the opioid overdose–related emergency department visit rate per 100,000 increases by 0.95 (7.0%) (Hollingsworth et al. 2017). Loss of opportunity and hope undoubtedly puts entire communities at risk when combined with easy access to powerful opioids.

Despite the convergence of multiple factors setting the stage for a public health crisis, governments and health systems have been too slow to respond. The stigma around substance abuse has also delayed progress. All of these contexts, and more, have led to the current epidemic of opioid use disorder (OUD), overdoses, and overdose deaths.

The Opium Poppy

How can a plant with beautiful flowers in an array of pinks, reds, oranges, purples, and blues—a plant that graces both formal and rustic gardens in many parts of the world and all across the United States—spark wars, destroy lives, and lead to an American public health crisis with staggering death statistics? People have been growing the poppy for centuries, perhaps as far back as 3400 B.C. in lower Mesopotamia. The ancient Sumerians called it the "joy plant." While the plant's flower itself has always been and remains joyous—the subject of songs, poetry, and paintings by Vincent van Gogh, Claude Monet, and Georgia O'Keeffe—the milky sap that oozes from its seedpod when scratched has the power to transform medicine and devastate entire families and communities.

Intoxicating Alkaloids

The plant kingdom not only nourishes us and provides us with breathtaking beauty throughout our world, but it also includes a number of species that induce calming, a sense of well-being, and maybe even euphoria, by producing alkaloid compounds that can quite literally captivate the mind. Alkaloids are naturally occurring, usually plant-based, compounds that often have physiological effects. From a chemical perspective, alkaloids contain nitrogen from amino acids within their carbon ring structure.

There are several well-known alkaloids. The alkaloid caffeine comes from coffee "beans," the seeds within the small "cherry" fruit of the tropical shrub *Coffea arabica*, part of the Rubiaceae family. *Nicotiana tabacum*, or cultivated tobacco, is an annually grown herbaceous plant of the Solanaceae, or nightshades, family of flowering plants (which also includes potatoes, many vines, tomatoes, peppers, many weeds, and various ornamentals). The alkaloid nicotine is found within the plant's broad leaves. The coca plant (*Erythroxylum coca* and *Erythroxylum novogranatense*) is a tropical shrub of the Erythroxylaceae family of flowering trees and shrubs. Its leaves contain the alkaloid cocaine. *Cannabis sativa*, or marijuana, is a member of the Cannabaceae or hemp family of trees and herbaceous plants. Its flowers/buds are dried and then smoked, conferring the "high" primarily caused by tetrahydrocannabinol (which is technically not an alkaloid, because its structure does not contain nitrogen; it is a terpenophenolic compound). Among the mind-altering plant-based alkaloids that have transformed humanity—in addition to caffeine, nicotine, cocaine, and the not-technically-an-alkaloid tetrahydrocannabinol—is one with perhaps the most storied past and most rapidly evolving present: morphine.

From Flower to Raw Opium

The opium poppy (*Papaver somniferum*), of the Papaveraceae family, is a flower known worldwide for its beauty. Native to Turkey, it grows up to 3 feet tall and is topped with brightly colored flowers that bloom at the tips of long green stems about 3 months after seeds are sown. The growing of a variety of poppies is perfectly legal in the United States. However, the *Papaver somniferum* poppy, whose seeds are sold legally, can only be legally grown for culinary or aesthetic purposes; because the plant contains opium, it cannot be grown with the intent to produce opium (despite it being a relatively simple process).

After the poppy blooms, an attractive green pod remains on the stem. The pods, when dried, are often used in floral arrangements, and also contain the seeds that are used for culinary purposes (e.g., poppy seed bagels, pastries). But our interest here is the green pod, on the stem, before it is left to dry and brown. When the flower petals fall away, the pod remains behind, about the size of a brussels sprout. The immature green seedpods can be shallowly scratched or "scored," allowing an exudate of white "poppy tears" to leak out. That substance dries as a sticky yellowish-brown residue, called latex, that can then be scraped off the pod—this is raw opium. The six opium alkaloids that occur naturally in the largest amounts in raw opium are morphine, narcotine, codeine, thebaine, papaverine, and narceine. Of these, morphine, codeine, and thebaine are under international control.

From Opium to Morphine

The sticky raw opium contains approximately 12% *morphine* (the principal alkaloid opiate of interest here, which, as a medication, is a Schedule II drug under the Controlled Substances Act of 1970 [P.L. 91-513], meaning that it has a high potential for abuse but has a currently accepted medical use); the alkaloids *codeine* and *thebaine* are also Schedule II drugs. As has occurred with the other plants mentioned above (e.g., *Cannabis sativa*), selective breeding of the *Papaver somniferum* poppy has greatly increased the content of these analgesic alkaloids. In 1803, morphine was first extracted from opium resin, and physicians began to widely prescribe it in the mid-1800s. Morphine is still the standard against which new pain relievers are measured. Codeine has weaker analgesic properties (e.g., the combination of codeine and acetaminophen is a Schedule III drug, deemed to have low to moderate potential for physical and psychological dependence) and is also used for cough suppression (e.g., cough syrup with codeine is a Schedule V drug, considered to have very low potential for abuse, although physical or psychological dependence could develop). Thebaine is used to produce oxycodone (which, like morphine, is a Schedule II drug).

Outside the United States, opium production is on the rise. Opium poppies are grown mainly by impoverished farmers on small plots of land in rarely visited, dry, warm parts of the world. Afghanistan, currently the primary producer of opium for illegal trade, has many thousands of acres under poppy cultivation. Some production also takes place in Pakistan, Myanmar (Burma), Colombia, Guatemala, and Mexico. For farmers, poppy cultivation can be up to 10 times more profitable than growing wheat. For the illegal drug trade, a morphine base is extracted from the opium, reducing the bulk weight of opium by nearly 90%, and making it easier to transport and smuggle (in fact, opium in its smokable form is nearly impossible to obtain today because morphine and heroin are much easier and more lucrative to smuggle). Thus, for efficiency, most traffickers do the refining of opium to morphine close to the poppy fields, making compact, claylike morphine "bricks" that are easier to transport and smuggle than bundles of pungent, jelly-like opium would be.

From Morphine to Heroin

Heroin, or diacetylmorphine, was first synthesized from morphine in 1874 by Charles Romley Alder Wright, an English chemistry researcher. He is said to have unwittingly synthesized heroin while boiling morphine and acetic anhydride over a stove for several hours. Bayer, a German company, introduced heroin for medical use in 1898. Physicians remained largely unaware of its addictive potential for years; however, by the early 1900s, heroin addiction was clearly on the rise in the United States. All use of heroin was made illegal by federal law in 1924.

Morphine is converted to heroin through a simple chemical reaction with acetic anhydride, followed by varying degrees of purification. Heroin is 2–4 times more potent than morphine, increasing its value by the same degree. A growing fraction of opium is processed into morphine base and heroin in rural drug labs in Afghanistan, despite international efforts to restrict availability of acetic anhydride. Heroin is classified as a Schedule I drug, meaning that it has a high potential for abuse, and no current accepted medical uses in the United States.

When heroin emerges from laboratories in Asia, it enters a multilayered chain of distribution (Frontline 1998). Top brokers usually deal in bulk shipments of 20–100 kg (kilos). A broker in New York, for example, might divide a bulk shipment into wholesale lots of 1–10 kilos for sale to underlings. By the time heroin is peddled on city streets in small "bags" costing $5 to $100 (e.g., a "dime bag" for $10), its value has ballooned more than 10-fold since its arrival in the United States (Frontline 1998). In addition to the selective breeding of the poppy plant noted above, the purity of heroin has risen remarkably, from rarely more than 10% pure only several decades ago, to 50%–60% pure nowadays, but with great variability from batch to batch and from bag to bag. This improved purity, in addition to giving those who are addicted a more powerful effect, allows dealers to expand their markets to reach users preferring to smoke or sniff it rather than inject it (although the natural course of tolerance and withdrawal with heroin addiction often leads to intravenous drug use). Being able to use the drug in these ways is thought to have contributed to the spread of heroin use to younger, white users in suburban areas, beginning in the 1990s (Keilman 2017).

Opium Derivatives for Medical Use

Narcotics have benefited humanity through their effectiveness in treating pain, suppressing cough, alleviating diarrhea, and inducing anesthesia. Legal opium production is allowed under the United Nations Single Convention on Narcotic Drugs of 1961, as well as other international drug treaties, subject to strict supervision by the law enforcement agencies of individual countries. A number of pharmaceutical companies legally import opium to the United States from India and Turkey; other countries import and export as well. About 2,000 tons of opium are produced each year to supply the world with the raw material needed to make medicinal opioids. Countries must submit annual reports to the International Narcotics Control Board, stating the year's actual consumption as well as projected quantities for the next year, which allows for production quotas to be allotted. Commercial opium is standardized to contain 10% morphine. In the United States, a small percentage of the morphine obtained from opium is used directly (about 15 tons); the rest is converted to semisynthetic derivatives (about 120 tons) (Drug Enforcement Administration 2017).

The term *opiate* indicates a naturally occurring alkaloid that comes from opium (e.g., morphine, codeine). *Opioids* are either semisynthetic derivatives or fully synthetic compounds that act on the same opioid receptors (μ, κ, and δ). Thus, *semisynthetic opioids* are synthesized from naturally occurring opiates (morphine, codeine, and thebaine) and include heroin, oxycodone, hydrocodone, and hydromorphone. *Synthetic opioids* are made entirely in a lab and include meperidine, fentanyl, and methadone, among others (Drug Enforcement Administration 2017). Whether a person uses a naturally occurring opiate or a semisynthetic or synthetic opioid, tolerance develops quickly, leading to escalation in use and risk of overdose, especially if the usual dose is resumed after a period of abstinence or detoxification.

Current Crisis

Prescription Opioids

According to the Centers for Disease Control and Prevention, the amount of prescription opioids sold to pharmacies, hospitals, and doctors' offices nearly quadrupled from 1999 to 2010; yet, there had not been an overall change in the amount of physical pain experienced by Americans

(Centers for Disease Control and Prevention 2018). Approximately one in five patients with noncancer pain or pain-related diagnoses are prescribed opioids in office-based settings. Prescribing rates are highest among providers in pain medicine (49%), surgery (37%), and physical medicine/rehabilitation (36%) specialties; however, primary care providers account for about half of opioid pain relievers dispensed (Centers for Disease Control and Prevention 2018). Americans consume more opioids than people in any other country in the world, and in 2015, the amount of opioids prescribed was enough for every American to be medicated around the clock for 3 weeks (White House 2017). Rates of prescribing opioids vary widely across the U.S. states: prescribers in the highest-prescribing states write almost 3 times as many opioid prescriptions per person as those in the lowest-prescribing states. Although many people who misuse opioid medications obtain them from one or more physicians, many also obtain them from friends or relatives or by buying them from a drug dealer.

As many as one in four people who receive prescription opioids long term for noncancer pain in primary care settings struggle with addiction. In 2014, almost 2 million Americans abused or were dependent on prescription opioids (Centers for Disease Control and Prevention 2018). Every day, over 1,000 people are treated in emergency departments for misusing prescription opioids, making OUD expensive from diverse perspectives, including that of the health care system. There is some evidence, however, that opioid prescribing guidelines and policies have slowed the growth of prescribing. Despite a plateau or initial decline in opioid prescribing, overdose deaths continue to rise. Deaths from heroin and synthetic opioids are increasing, which may be due in part to the fact that addicted individuals who are cut off from prescription opioids transition to illicit opioids like heroin (Weeks and Goertz 2017), which are increasingly contaminated with very high-potency fentanyl and related compounds. Four out of every five new heroin users begin with nonmedical use of prescription opioids (White House 2017).

Heroin Use and Opioid Overdoses

Overdoses from prescription opioids are a driving factor in a 18-year increase in opioid overdose deaths, up to the year 2017. Deaths from prescription opioids—drugs like oxycodone, hydrocodone, and methadone—have more than quadrupled since 1999 (Centers for Disease Control and

Prevention 2018). Heroin overdose deaths are similarly on the rise. In 2017, the number of overdose deaths involving opioids (including both prescription opioids and heroin) was 5 times higher than just a decade and a half before. From 1999 to 2017, more than 630,000 people died from drug overdoses. On average, 115 Americans die each day from an opioid overdose (Centers for Disease Control and Prevention 2018). Opioids (including prescription opioids, heroin, and fentanyl) killed more than 60,000 people in 2017, which is more than any year on record (see Figure 1–1). Figure 1–2 shows deaths per 100,000 population.

Fentanyl and Related Analogues

Of drug overdose deaths in 2017, the sharpest increase occurred among deaths related to fentanyl and fentanyl analogues (synthetic opioids), with approximately 30,000 overdose deaths (Figure 1–1). Fentanyl is a synthetic (man-made) opioid that is 50 times more potent than heroin and 100 times more potent than morphine. Carfentanil, another synthetic derivative, is about 5,000 times more potent than heroin. Most of the increases in fentanyl deaths over the last 3 years reported (Centers for Disease Control and Prevention 2018) do not involve prescription fentanyl but are related to illicitly made fentanyl that is being mixed with or sold as heroin—with or without the users' knowledge and increasingly as counterfeit pills. From 2015 to 2016 alone, the age-adjusted rate of drug overdose deaths involving synthetic opioids other than methadone (including fentanyl, fentanyl analogues, and tramadol) doubled (Hedegaard et al. 2017).

Scope of the Crisis

The crisis is not affecting all U.S. states equally; major variation exists. In 2016, for example, the states with the highest age-adjusted drug overdose death rates were West Virginia, Ohio, New Hampshire, and Pennsylvania (52.0, 39.1, 39.0, and 37.9 per 100,000 population, respectively). The states with the lowest rates were Nebraska (6.4), South Dakota (8.4), Texas (10.1), Iowa (10.6), and North Dakota (10.6) (Hedegaard et al. 2017). It has been reported that West Virginia not only has the highest rate of opioid-related deaths in the United States but, along with several other states, has had a higher total of opioid prescriptions than residents. Geographic variation at the county level is also

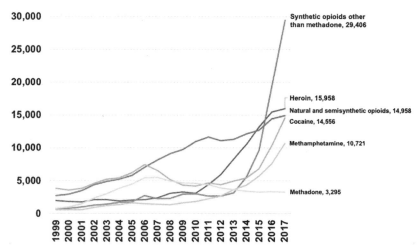

FIGURE 1–1. Drugs involved in U.S. overdose deaths, 1999–2017.

Source. Reprinted from National Institute on Drug Abuse: Overdose Death Rates. September 2017. Available at: www.drugabuse.gov/related-topics/trends-statistics/overdose-death-rates. Accessed September 2018.

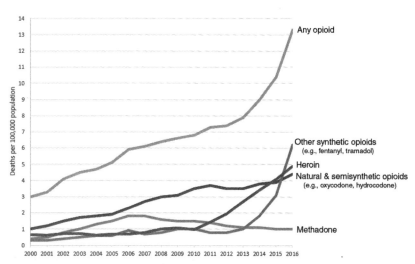

FIGURE 1–2. Overdose deaths involving opioids, by type of opioid, United States, 2000–2016.

Source. Reprinted from Centers for Disease Control and Prevention: Opioid Overdose: Opioid Data Analysis. February 9, 2017. Available at: www.cdc.gov/drugoverdose/data/analysis.html. Accessed March 27, 2018.

substantial. Across both states and counties, geographic variation also exists in terms of whether prescription opioids or heroin predominates.

The current crisis is not only about addiction and overdose. It is also about long-term social adversities among those affected, as well as long-term physical health consequences. For example, hepatitis C virus infection is on the rise, especially among young people who share needles (Bartolone 2017); the highest number of new infections is occurring in people in their 20s. Additionally, the opioid epidemic is causing great pain for the many family members of those with addiction or those who die by overdose, perhaps especially for the children of addicted parents, many of whom find themselves removed from their homes and placed into care elsewhere.

Federal, State, and Local Responses

Congress has passed legislation in recent years to enhance the response to the opioid crisis, including the Comprehensive Addiction and Recovery Act of 2016 (P.L. 114-198) and the 21st Century Cures Act of 2016 (P.L. 114-255), both signed into law by President Barack Obama. The former act was the first piece of major federal legislation pertaining to addiction in 40 years, authorizing over $181 million each year in new funding to fight the opioid epidemic, although moneys must be appropriated every year through the regular appropriations process. The latter designated $1 billion in grants for states over 2 years to fight the opioid epidemic (e.g., by improving prescription drug monitoring programs, making treatment programs more accessible, training health care professionals in addiction treatment, and funding research on the most effective approaches to prevent addiction), among many other provisions.

Many have argued, however, that the federal response has been too slow, uncoordinated, and overly concerned with supply-side interventions (e.g., law enforcement) rather than a unified national push to increase access to treatment services. On October 26, 2017, President Donald Trump declared the opioid crisis a "public health emergency," as opposed to a "national emergency"; the latter would have allowed for use of federal disaster relief funds. On November 1, 2017, "The President's Commission on Combating Drug Addiction and the Opioid Crisis," a 138-page report with 56 recommendations, was issued (White House 2017). Some argue that the federal response has been too restrained and has provided inadequate funding to actually carry out most of the commission's many recommendations (Blake 2017). The commission report highlights such concerns as lack of health insurance coverage and lack of access to substance use treatment, given that the vast majority of people who would benefit from treatment are not receiving it.

Despite criticism of the federal response, many states and local governments are, nonetheless, addressing the crisis (Ghandnoosh 2017). Their efforts entail removing hurdles to receiving medication-assisted treatment (MAT), which include inadequate health insurance coverage; continuing efforts to discourage the overprescribing of narcotic analgesics (e.g., through education for health professionals and enhanced use of and communication between prescription drug monitoring programs); placing limits on the number of opioids that can be sold by pharmaceutical companies; increasing the availability of naloxone; embracing harm reduction approaches, even those that are controversial; working with law enforcement to divert those in need of treatment to treatment, rather than jail; expanding drug courts; and improving professional treatment (including MAT) for those already in the criminal justice system.

A Multipronged Response Strategy

Given the extent of the opioid crisis, major strides are needed in a number of areas. There has been insufficient uptake of evidence-based approaches—including harm reduction programs (e.g., needle exchanges, safe injection facilities), MAT, and naloxone. Most clinicians have been insufficiently engaged in addressing the problem, as exemplified by too few of them receiving buprenorphine training; among those who do, too few obtain the Drug Addiction Treatment Act of 2000 (DATA 2000) waiver, and among those who do obtain the waiver, too few prescribe buprenorphine.

The New York Times Editorial Board (2017) published "America's 8-Step Program for Opioid Addiction," which provides a concise blueprint for what needs to be done. It includes 1) saving lives by enhancing supplies of naloxone and spending more on needle exchange and clean syringe programs so that those actively using will have a chance to seek treatment; 2) engaging law enforcement to refer to treatment rather than arresting; 3) funding treatment (e.g., by not repealing the Patient Protection and Affordable Care Act of 2010 [P.L. 111-148] and by urging more states to adopt Medicaid expansion); 4) combating stigma (e.g., through mass mailings of educational brochures and tuition incentives for medical students to enter addiction-related specialties); 5) supporting MAT through a number of policy approaches; 6) strictly enforcing mental health parity laws and educating Americans about their legal right to treatment; 7) improving education around pain management for health professionals and continuing to pursue legal action against pharmaceutical manufacturers whose irresponsible policies laid the foundation for the crisis; and 8) expanding prevention programs for children and adolescents, especially programs that emphasize life skills as opposed to traditional anti–drug abuse lectures.

An additional consideration pertains to the demography of the opioid epidemic. The recent discourse in the media has focused almost entirely on white users in suburban and rural areas, who are often cast as sympathetic victims deserving of treatment. At the same time, however, people of color living in urban neighborhoods struggle with the same addiction but often are portrayed as criminals deserving of punishment (Keilman 2017). They have less access to the most effective treatments, such as buprenorphine. Innovative approaches to eradicating health care inequities related to the opioid crisis must be an objective in ongoing and future efforts.

In a report titled "Pain Management and the Opioid Epidemic: Balancing Societal and Individual Benefits and Risks of Prescription Opioid Use," the National Academies of Sciences, Engineering, and Medicine (2017) noted that the opioid epidemic will not be controlled without deploying multiple policy tools. Committee members emphasized the need to increase access to treatment for individuals with OUD and to expand research on new, nonaddictive treatments for pain. They urged the U.S. Food and Drug Administration (FDA) to reshape and monitor the legal market for opioids and to facilitate use of safe and effective agents for treating OUD and reducing overdose deaths. They also called on professional societies, insurers, health care organizations, pharmaceutical manufacturers, and state and federal agencies to address multiple weaknesses in the health system that led to the epidemic.

A number of innovations may ultimately be beneficial in addressing the crisis. For example, abuse-deterrent medications are being improved, research is under way on the development of vaccines that would make antibodies to capture drugs of abuse, the FDA recently approved a once-monthly injectable form of buprenorphine and the buprenorphine implant, and the FDA also recently approved the NSS-2 Bridge neurostimulator (which is placed behind the ear and emits electrical pulses that stimulate cranial and occipital nerves) to treat symptoms of opioid withdrawal for up to 5 days. In addition, health care providers are increasingly embracing complementary and alternative treatments for pain, including acupuncture, which has been used by the military and the U.S. Department of Veterans Affairs for several years and which some insurance companies and state Medicaid programs are starting to cover.

What Mental Health Professionals Can Do

Some experts have suggested that because the opioid crisis was in part fostered by well-intentioned practices to improve pain management, then, as with other iatrogenic processes, physicians should "feel a sense of angst and trepidation and work actively with patients to correct this mishap" (Weeks and Goertz 2017, p. 974). Psychiatrists and other mental health professionals have substantial training in substance use disorders and their treatments, compared with other medical professionals; as such, psychiatry and allied fields can play a major role. Additionally, psychiatrists and other mental health professionals have a role to play because adults with mental illnesses receive more than 50% of opioid prescriptions in the United States (with 18.7% of adults with a mental illness receiving opioids, compared with 5.0% of adults in the general population), indicating a need for improved pain management for individuals with mental illnesses (Davis et al. 2017). In addition to providing proper treatment for pain, mental health professionals must screen for, assess, and treat OUD among patients and assist in the dissemination and implementation of evidence-based practices to address OUD and overdose. Additionally, outside the clinic's walls, psychiatrists and mental health professionals can advocate for more vigorous treatment and prevention efforts, as well as the pursuit of equity within all such efforts, to address the epidemic.

Key Chapter Points

▶ The opioid crisis is underpinned by marketing of opioids by the pharmaceutical industry, heavy prescribing of opioids by the medical community, increased availability and purity of heroin, new synthetic opioids in the black market, and economic stressors that have affected some communities more heavily than others.

▶ The opium poppy produces the analgesic alkaloids morphine, codeine, and thebaine. Morphine is used for analgesia and is the standard to which other analgesics are compared; it can also be converted to heroin. Codeine is used as a less potent analgesic and cough suppressant. Thebaine is used to produce oxycodone. Synthetic opioids are made entirely in a laboratory, and include meperidine, fentanyl, and methadone.

▶ The current crisis pertains to prescription opioids and heroin, as well as synthetic analogues. Rates of OUD and overdose deaths vary remarkably across the states, and the nature of the epidemic (e.g., whether prescription opioids or heroin predominates) also varies across counties within states. Entire communities and many families have been devastated.

▶ The Comprehensive Addiction and Recovery Act and the 21st Century Cures Act, both passed in 2016, provided federal funding to address the opioid epidemic; yet, some have argued that the federal response has been slow, uncoordinated, and insufficient.

▶ The many facets of a robust response to the crisis will include enhancing supplies of naloxone, expanding needle exchange and clean syringe programs, improving access to treatment rather than arrest and incarceration, combating stigma, supporting medication-assisted treatment through a number of policy approaches, enforcing mental health parity laws, improving education around pain management, and expanding prevention programs for children and adolescents that emphasize life skills. Health care inequities must also be addressed.

▶ Psychiatrists and other mental health professionals must be equipped to screen for, assess, and treat OUD, especially given that adults with mental illnesses receive more than 50% of opioid prescriptions in the United States. Psychiatrists and other mental health professionals can assist in the dissemination and implementation of evidence-based practices to address OUD and overdose, which include advocating for more vigorous treatment and prevention efforts, as well as pursuing equity within all such efforts to address the epidemic.

References

Bartolone P: Treating the new Hep C generation on their turf. Kaiser Health News, December 7, 2017

Blake J: White House opioid commission targets trouble spots, misses some. Psychiatric News, December 1, 2017

Centers for Disease Control and Prevention: Opioid overdose. Available at: https://www.cdc.gov/drugoverdose/index.html. Accessed February 11, 2018.

Davis MA, Lin LA, Liu H, et al: Prescription opioid use among adults with mental health disorders in the United States. J Am Board Fam Med 30(4):407–417, 2017 28720623

Drug Enforcement Administration: Drugs of abuse: a DEA resource guide, 2017 Edition. 2017. Available at: https://www.dea.gov/pr/multimedia-library/publications/drug_of_abuse.pdf. Accessed February 10, 2018.

Frontline: Transforming opium poppies into heroin. 1998. Available at: https://www.pbs.org/wgbh/pages/frontline/shows/heroin/transform. Accessed February 10, 2018.

Ghandnoosh N: Trump's opioid crisis failures mean states must lead the way. Newsweek, December 14, 2017

Hedegaard H, Warner M, Minino AM: Drug overdose deaths in the United States, 1999–2016. NCHS Data Brief No 294, December 2017. Available at: https://www.cdc.gov/nchs/products/databriefs/db294.htm. Accessed March 27, 2018.

Hollingsworth A, Ruhm CJ, Simon K: Macroeconomic conditions and opioid use. National Bureau of Economic Research Working Paper No 23192. 2017. Available at: http://www.nber.org/papers/w23192. Accessed February 12, 2018.

Keilman J: Black victims of heroin, opioid crisis "whitewashed" out of picture, report finds. Chicago Tribune, December 26, 2017

National Academies of Sciences, Engineering, and Medicine: Pain Management and the Opioid Epidemic: Balancing Societal and Individual Benefits and Risks of Prescription Opioid Use. Washington, DC, National Academies Press, 2017

New York Times Editorial Board: America's 8-step program for opioid addiction. The New York Times, October 2, 2017

Weeks WB, Goertz CM: Ineffective policies to address the opioid epidemic. JAMA Psychiatry 74(9):974, 2017 28793131

White House: The President's Commission on Combating Drug Addiction and the Opioid Crisis. 2017. Available at: https://www.whitehouse.gov/sites/whitehouse.gov/files/images/Final_Report_Draft_11-1-2017.pdf. Accessed February 17, 2018.

2

Prescription Opioids

Julian Santaella–Tenorio, M.P.H.
Luis E. Segura, M.D., M.P.H.
Vitor S. Tardelli, M.D., M.P.H.
Leila M. Vaezazizi, M.D.
Silvia S. Martins, M.D., Ph.D.

Clinical Vignette: Glenda's Back Pain

Glenda is a 49-year-old divorced woman who lives with her elderly mother in a medium-sized city in the northeastern United States. She worked for many years as a secretary at a local public school but no longer works and has been receiving Social Security Disability Insurance (SSDI) because of back pain. She has a 19-year-old son who lives about an hour away and who attends a local community college.

About 10 years ago, Glenda was in a car accident and suffered a back injury: a herniated disc at lumbar segments 4 and 5 (L4–L5). She underwent back surgery but continued to have pain and limited mobility. Her pain management doctor started prescribing Percocet 10/325 (oxycodone 10 mg and acetaminophen 325 mg), to be taken up to 4 times a day, a treatment that Glenda reported provided only partial pain relief. She frequently had difficulty getting out of bed and was missing multiple days of work; she eventually stopped working and began receiving SSDI. She developed depressive symptoms and started to see an outpatient psychiatrist, who prescribed sertraline 100 mg/day and clonazepam 0.5 mg twice daily. Over the course of a year, Glenda's prescription opioid use escalated, and she began running out of her monthly prescriptions after only 1 or 2 weeks. She frequently presented to emergency departments (EDs) complaining of exacerbations of back pain and received short-term prescriptions for various opioids such as hydromorphone. She also took prescription opioid medications from her elderly mother's supply and purchased more illicitly from a local dealer.

After several years of treating Glenda, the pain clinic she had been attending started to enforce more strict treatment guidelines because of increased state and federal oversight of opioid prescribing. Glenda was eventually discharged from the pain clinic because of disruptive behaviors, such as yelling at the staff and doctors when they refused to provide certain prescriptions or increase her opioid dose, and repeated breaches of her treatment contract, including asking for early refills and getting opioid prescriptions from outside providers. Without her regular prescriptions, the cost of buying opioid medications off the street became exceedingly high for Glenda, and she was unable to afford much else with her limited monthly income. When she ran out of medication, the opioid withdrawal symptoms she experienced were intolerable. She experienced nausea, diarrhea, tremors, severe back pain, and anxiety. Glenda eventually tried heroin from her dealer, who told her that the effect would be better for a much cheaper price. She quickly transitioned to heroin and started using 6–10 bags daily. She tried intravenous heroin a few times, but generally preferred intranasal heroin use, believing it to be less addictive.

Six months after she started using heroin regularly, she was found by her son at home, unconscious, unarousable, and breathing irregularly. He called 911, and when the emergency medical service arrived, Glenda's overdose was reversed with naloxone. She was then taken by ambulance to the ED at a local hospital. Her urine toxicology test was positive for oxycodone, morphine, and benzodiazepines. She was stabilized and subsequently discharged after refusing services, referrals, and further care.

Two months after her overdose, Glenda walked into a local outpatient substance abuse treatment center accompanied by her son, who had been urging her to seek treatment. She met with addiction psychiatrist Dr. Lamar, and told him that since her overdose 2 months earlier, she had been increasingly worried about her heroin use and had been trying unsuccessfully to taper herself off it. She said she was using up to 3 mg of clonazepam daily to self-medicate her opioid withdrawal symptoms. At the time of her evaluation, she was showing signs and symptoms of opioid withdrawal. She was afebrile, her heart rate was 96 beats per minute, and her blood pressure was 156/102. She had mildly dilated pupils and appeared anxious, tremulous, and unable to sit still. She stated that she wanted to stop using heroin and benzodiazepines, but she was worried about how she would tolerate the withdrawal symptoms, as well as how she would manage her back pain and insomnia. Dr. Lamar recommended that she be admitted to the hospital's detoxification unit, and Glenda agreed.

Later that day, Glenda was admitted to an inpatient detoxification unit for treatment of opioid and sedative/hypnotic use disorders. Her admission labs were significant for a new diagnosis of hepatitis C virus infection. The inpatient doctor explained to Glenda the different medication-assisted treatment options for opioid use disorder (OUD), including buprenorphine, methadone, and long-acting injectable extended-release naltrexone (XR-naltrexone). Glenda opted for buprenorphine. She was inducted and stabilized on Suboxone (buprenorphine 8 mg and naloxone 2 mg) twice daily. Upon discharge, she was given follow-up appointments with an intensive outpatient program for substance use, an addiction psychiatrist, a primary care physician, and a hepatologist. Her back pain became manageable with the combination of buprenorphine/naloxone, nonsteroidal anti-inflammatory medications, and physical therapy.

Glenda's case illustrates the processes that many patients in the United States encounter while being treated for chronic pain, including an escalation in opioid use and a transition to more potent opioids. Her case also brings up important questions that will lead to a better understanding of the opioid use epidemic in the United States, which we explore in depth in this chapter. Is there a risk of transitioning from medical to nonmedical use of opioids? Has there been an increase in the nonmedical use of prescription opioids over time in the United States? What accounts for this increase? What prescription opioids exist, and what are their physiological effects? What are the long-term effects of prescription opioid use? Which sociodemographic groups have been most affected by the opioid epidemic? What factors lead to and characterize transitions from nonmedical use of prescription opioids to other opioids, such as heroin or fentanyl? Of note, the term *nonmedical use* refers to the use of a prescription drug 1) without a doctor's prescription; 2) in greater amounts, more often, or longer than prescribed; or 3) for a reason other than the doctor's reason for prescribing.

Introduction

During the past two decades, the United States has experienced an opioid addiction and overdose epidemic with devastating outcomes. The opioid epidemic has been linked to a 200% increase in the rate of overdose deaths involving opioids from 2000 to 2014, including prescription opioids and heroin (from 3 per 100,000 persons in 2000 to 9 per 100,000 in 2014) (Rudd et al. 2016a). Since 2000, more than 600,000 persons have died from drug overdoses in the United States; in 2014 alone, there were 47,055 drug overdose deaths, of which 61% (28,647 deaths) were opioid related (Rudd et al. 2016a). More recent reports from the Centers for Disease Control and Prevention (CDC) show that in 2016, there were around 64,000 fatal overdoses, with more than 50,000 of these being opioid related, including 14,400 due primarily to prescription opioids. The epidemic has also been linked to a 99.4% increase in the rate of opioid-related ED visits from 2005 to 2014 (from 89.1 visits per 100,000 in 2005 to 177.7 visits per 100,000 in 2014). An estimated 4.7 million persons used prescription opioids nonmedically in the past month at any given time in 2008. It is estimated that 1.9 million individuals had a prescription-related OUD in 2014 (Center for Behavioral Health Statistics and Quality 2015).

The opioid epidemic has affected communities in ways beyond the impact of fatal and nonfatal overdoses, including the deterioration of the social fabric due to higher levels of crime, distrust, and isolation. Additionally, because those abusing opioids often inject prescription opioids, sharing drug injection equipment is believed to be in part responsible for a tripling of hepatitis C virus infections between 2010 and 2015. Furthermore, it is estimated that in 2012, around 21,700 infants were born with neonatal abstinence syndrome due to opioids, equating to one neonate born with opioid withdrawal symptoms every 25 minutes. Newborns with neonatal abstinence syndrome are more likely to have low birth weight, respiratory and central nervous system complications, and longer hospital stays, costing hospitals an estimated $1.5 billion in 2012 alone, with more than 80% of this cost being paid by state Medicaid programs (Patrick et al. 2015).

The total economic burden of the opioid epidemic in the United States for 2013, based on the incidence of overdose deaths and the prevalence of prescription opioid abuse and dependence for that year, was estimated to be around $78.5 billion. Of this total, 36.8% was estimated to be due to increased health care and substance abuse treatment costs ($28.9 billion), 9.75% due to criminal justice costs ($7.65 billion), and 26% due to lost productivity ($20.4 billion) (Florence et al. 2016).

Prescription Opioid Compounds and Their Physiological Effects

Prescription opioids are drugs that are chemically similar to endogenous opioids, the neurotransmitters and neuromodulators that the human body makes to reduce the intensity of pain signal perception by interacting with opioid receptors in both the spinal cord and the brain. Various opiate medications derived from the opium poppy have been used for centuries to treat pain, cough, and diarrhea. Opioids can be classified into the following categories according to how they are manufactured: 1) natural opiates, which are made from the opium poppy (morphine and codeine are the only two used as narcotic opiate analgesics); 2) semisynthetic opiates (derived from the naturally occurring opium alkaloids, such as hydromorphone from morphine, hydrocodone from codeine, and buprenorphine from thebaine); and 3) fully synthetic opioids, such as fentanyl, methadone, and meperidine (synthesized from chemicals different from the alkaloids found in opium). Because of their influence on brain areas controlling emotions, opioid medications can produce euphoria and pleasant experiences that can cause a person to begin or continue misusing these drugs and to develop abuse and dependence symptoms when taking them for long periods or at high doses.

Prescription opioid medications include hydrocodone, oxycodone, oxymorphone, morphine, codeine, and fentanyl, among others (a list of generic and commercial names is provided in Table 2–1). Hydrocodone and extended- and immediate-release oxycodone are by far the most prescribed opioids in the United States. Although the distribution of both opioids to U.S. pharmacies increased from 2002 to 2010, oxycodone showed the steepest increase (287%) in its distribution (Kenan et al. 2012).

Both opioid medications and endogenous opioids (β-endorphin, dynorphins, and enkephalins) interact with μ, κ, and δ opioid receptors on neuronal membranes distributed throughout the spinal cord, peripheral nerves, and many supraspinal sites (Garland et al. 2013). Endogenous and exogenous opioids modulate the pain transmission pathway by activating μ receptors in the superficial layers of the dorsal horn in the spinal cord, reducing excitatory neurotransmitter release from primary afferent terminals and depolarizing second-order dorsal-horn neurons. The activation of μ receptors in supraspinal sites also contributes to the

TABLE 2–1. Generic and brand names of opioids

Generic name	Brand name	Brand name of combination formulations (e.g., with acetaminophen)
Natural opioids/opiates		
Morphine	Astramorph, Avinza, Duramorph, Kadian, MorphaBond ER, MS Contin, Oramorph, Roxanol-T	Embeda
Codeine		Fioricet with codeine, Fiorinal with codeine, Promethazine VC with codeine, Soma Compound with codeine, Tuzistra XR, Tylenol #3 and #4
Semisynthetic opioids		
Hydromorphone	Dilaudid, Palladone	Exalgo
Hydrocodone	Hysingla, Zohydro ER	Anexsia, Co-Gesic, Hycet, Hycodan, Hycofenix, Hydromet, Ibudone, Liquicet, Lorcet, Lortab, Maxidone, Norco, Obredon, Reprexain, Rezira, TussiCaps, Tussionex, Vicodin, Vicoprofen, Vituz, Xodol, Zolvit, Zutripro, Zydone
Oxycodone	OxyContin, Oxaydo, Roxicodone, Xtampza ER	Oxycet, Percocet, Percodan, Roxicet, Targiniq ER, Xartemis XR
Oxymorphone	Opana	

TABLE 2–1. Generic and brand names of opioids *(continued)*

Generic name	Brand name	Brand name of combination formulations (e.g., with acetaminophen)
Semisynthetic opioids (continued)		
Buprenorphine	Belbuca, Buprenex, Buttrans	Suboxone
Heroin		
Fully synthetic opioids		
Tapentadol	Nucynta ER	
Tramadol	Conzip, Ultram	Ultracet
Fentanyl	Abstral, Actiq, Alfenta (Alfentanil for injection), Duragesic, Fentora, Ionsys, Lazanda, Onsolis, Sublimaze, Subsys	
Meperidine	Demerol	
Methadone	Dolophine, Methadose	
Propoxyphene	Darvon	
Diphenoxylate		Lomotil

Note.   ER=extended release; MS=morphine sulfate; T=tinted/flavored; VC=addition of decongestant; XR=extended release.

analgesic effect of opioids. Opioids activate the descending system that controls nociceptive transmission via a pain modulatory circuit including frontal lobe cortical regions; the hypothalamus; amygdala and projections to the periaqueductal gray; and the rostral ventromedial medulla (Garland et al. 2013).

Opioids also provide pain relief by reducing affective dimensions of pain. The analgesic opioid effect occurs in part through the modulation of the central autonomic network, including the cingulate cortex, the anterior insula, and the hypothalamus (Garland et al. 2013), which regulates attention, emotion, and neurovisceral integration processes. Also, by activating the mesolimbic dopaminergic reward system, opioids can enhance positive mood and reward, which in turn can contribute to reductions in pain perceptions. By also inhibiting the action of the neurotransmitter γ-aminobutyric acid (GABA) in the nucleus accumbens, opioids contribute to the liberation of dopamine and activation of the reward system. In addition, opioid intake can reduce neural activity in the brain stem and medial thalamic nuclei, as well as in brain regions involved in executive function, resulting in cognitive and psychomotor impairments (Garland et al. 2013). The transient activation of the reward system and cognitive impairment are believed to contribute to the initiation of addiction patterns among certain individuals who use opioids.

Because of the diversion of prescription opioids and their misuse and abuse potential (as noted in the introduction to this chapter, an estimated 4.7 million persons used prescription opioids nonmedically in the past month at any given time in 2008), some pharmaceutical companies have developed new abuse-deterrent and tamper-resistant opioid formulations (e.g., OxyContin OP, Oxycodone DETERx). New formulations aim to prevent alteration of the tablet, capsule, or patch by rendering it inactive during attempted use via snorting or injection. However, some evidence suggests that these new products have been successfully altered for misuse (Cicero and Ellis 2015).

Origins of the Prescription Opioid Epidemic

Opioids were often prescribed to treat cancer and postsurgery pain before the 1990s, but it was not until 1996, when Purdue Pharma conducted an extensive marketing campaign to promote extended-release oxycodone (OxyContin), that opioids became widely available and prescribed for chronic noncancer pain conditions (U.S. General Accounting Office

2003). OxyContin, a product whose active ingredient, oxycodone, is twice as potent as morphine, was marketed using strategies that included the support of the American Pain Society (APS), the American Academy of Pain Medicine (AAPM), and the Federation of State Medical Boards. These organizations publicly claimed that prescription opioids could be used to treat chronic pain with a low risk for addiction or overdose (U.S. General Accounting Office 2003). Purdue also promoted OxyContin by expanding its physician speaker bureau, conducting over 40 pain management conferences, and sponsoring more than 20,000 pain-related educational programs to promote the long-term use of prescription opioids for noncancer pain (U.S. General Accounting Office 2003).

In addition, Purdue funded programs to educate hospital physicians and staff on how to comply with the pain standards of the Joint Commission on Accreditation of Healthcare Organizations, now called the Joint Commission; issued free limited-time OxyContin prescription starter coupons (from 1998 to 2002); and distributed marketing materials to health care professionals (U.S. General Accounting Office 2003). Purdue also used a promotional video that included a statement that opioids cause addiction in less than 1% of patients and that encouraged patients to talk about their pain, in order to reduce patients' concerns about opioid use (U.S. General Accounting Office 2003). The company also marked OxyContin as a safe drug that would not make individuals addicted to opioids if "taken as prescribed." This statement allowed Purdue to claim that once patients started taking OxyContin in greater amounts, more often, or for longer periods than prescribed, they could be considered addicts because they were not taking the drug "as prescribed" (Temple 2015).

Part of the marketing success of OxyContin also included the launch of a campaign called "Pain Is the Fifth Vital Sign" by the APS in 1995, which encouraged health care professionals to improve the identification of pain and called for wider use of opioids to treat chronic noncancer pain (Kolodny et al. 2015). The AAPM and the APS also issued a consensus statement endorsing the use of opioids for noncancer pain, which indicated that the risk of opioid addiction was low, that respiratory depression tended to be a short-lived phenomenon, that there was not an arbitrary upper dosage limit for most opioids, and that efforts to stop diversion of opioids should not interfere with opioid prescribing (Haddox et al. 1997). The evidence cited to support opioids' low risk of addiction came from an 11-line letter published in 1980 in the *New England Journal of Medicine*, based on hospitalized patients with no history of addiction (Porter and Jick 1980) and a study of 38 patients treated with opioids for noncancer pain (Portenoy and Foley 1986). Today, it is widely accepted, even by one of the authors of the latter study, that this evidence by no means supported the "low-risk" statements that were aggressively promoted before and during the first decade of the opioid epidemic.

Other pharmaceutical companies followed Purdue Pharma's lead in developing (lucrative) opioid pain killers: Cephalon produced fentanyl lollipops (Actiq) for noncancer pain; Janssen Pharmaceuticals developed tramadol-acetaminophen combination pills (Ultracet); Endo developed oxymorphone formulations (Opana), oxycodone-acetaminophen combination pills (Percocet), and oxycodone-aspirin combination pills (Percodan); and Mallinckrodt Pharmaceuticals produced Roxicodone, a generic form of OxyContin. These companies followed similar marketing strategies, promoting the benefits of prescription opioids to treat noncancer pain while minimizing the risks of addiction and overdose.

Manufacturers and pain organizations also promoted a message exaggerating the efficacy of long-term use of opioids to treat chronic pain, despite the lack of quality studies demonstrating their efficacy and safety, as well as evidence suggesting that most patients under long-term treatment with opioids continue experiencing pain that interferes with functioning and activities (Kolodny et al. 2015).

As a result of the successful marketing strategy, by 2003, primary care physicians, without adequate training in pain management, were prescribing almost half of all OxyContin prescribed in the United States (U.S. General Accounting Office 2003). During this time, Purdue was selling almost $1.5 billion worth of the drug per year (Temple 2015). Marketing strategies were successful in reducing physicians' fear of prescribing opioids for noncancer or postsurgical pain; rates of long-term use of opioids to treat noncancer pain doubled from 1997 to 2005 (from 23.9 to 46.8 per 1,000) (Boudreau et al. 2009), and prescription opioid sales increased fourfold from 1999 to 2010 (from 1.8 kg to 7.1 kg per 10,000) (Paulozzi et al. 2011). Parallel to the rise in opioid sales, there was a fourfold increase in opioid-related fatal overdoses from 1999 to 2008 and an almost sixfold increase in prescription opioid abuse treatment admissions from 1999 to 2009 (Paulozzi et al. 2011) (Figure 2–1).

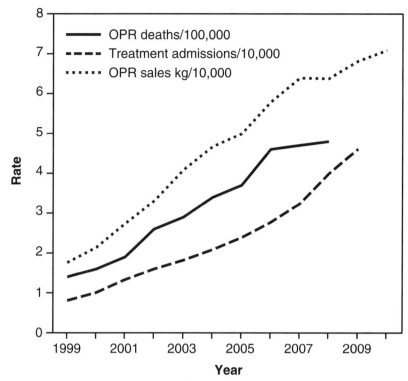

FIGURE 2–1. Trends in rates of opioid pain reliever (OPR) overdose deaths, treatment admissions, and kilograms sold, United States, 1999–2010.

Source. Reprinted from Centers for Disease Control and Prevention. Available at: www.cdc.gov/mmwr/preview/mmwrhtml/mm6043a4.htm. Accessed March 28, 2108.

The Drug Enforcement Administration (DEA) quota system, created to reduce diversion from legitimate channels of trade by restricting the quantities of controlled substances being manufactured, was not used to confront the alarming exponential rise in fatal opioid overdoses since the late 1990s. Moreover, the DEA continued to raise the total amount of oxycodone allowable for manufacture by pharmaceutical companies, from 3,520 kg of oxycodone in 1993 to 70,000 kg in 2007 (an almost 20-fold increase), and later to 153,750 kg in 2013. Although the oxycodone manufacturing quota has gone down since 2014, in 2017 the quota was 108,510 kg (Temple 2015; Drug Enforcement Administration 2017). Similar increases in DEA manufacturing quotas have been observed for hydrocodone, hydromorphone, and fentanyl during this period (Temple 2015; Drug Enforcement Administration 2017).

An additional factor fueling the opioid epidemic around 2007–2008 was the proliferation of pain clinics, which frequently hired physicians willing to deliver prescription opioids to hundreds of patients per week and to provide monthly refills without evaluating patients in detail or asking questions about opioid misuse (Temple 2015). Although some states like West Virginia and Kentucky had implemented prescription drug monitoring programs (PDMPs) to control the diversion of pain-killers and other drugs, by 2008 the number of pain clinics in Florida in particular had increased exponentially, in part due to the state's limited regulations (Temple 2015). Three regulatory loopholes facilitated the rise in pain clinics in Florida (Alvarez 2011; Temple 2015). First, the lack of a statewide prescription database limited the ability to identify individuals visiting multiple treatment providers to procure prescription drugs illicitly and to identify their doctors. Second, a state license was not required to open a pain clinic, meaning that anyone could open one, and although doctors could be prosecuted for malpractice, there was no clear legislation to incriminate clinic owners for this activity. Third, Florida law allowed clinics to sell prescription drugs, securing a closed business that removed pharmacies, an important potential control point, from the distribution chain (Temple 2015).

As a result of weak regulations and an explosion of pain clinics, during the first 6 months of 2010, doctors in Florida were purchasing 9 times more oxycodone units than were doctors from all other 49 states combined (Holske 2013). Pain clinics in Florida not only supplied the local state demand but also provided prescription opioids to people flying to Florida airports or driving from other states on Interstate 75, a route colloquially named the "Oxy Express." During the 2008–2010 period, a single trip to Florida could garner a supply of opioids worth $6,000–$8,000 in the illegal market in Kentucky (Temple 2015).

Because of the damage OxyContin brought to families and communities, many tried to fight Purdue Pharma in court. In response, Purdue hired corporate defense law firms that cost $3 million a month in legal fees. However, in 2007 the company pleaded guilty to federal criminal charges that they had misled regulators, doctors, and the public about OxyContin's risk of addiction (Meier 2007). The company paid $600 million in fines and other payments ($470 million to federal and state agencies and \$130 million to settle civil litigation brought by patients and other complainants), one of the largest amounts ever paid by a drug company. Also, three top executives personally paid \$34.5 million in fines (Meier 2007).

In summary, the origin and escalation of the opioid epidemic was underpinned by a combination of factors that included a successful marketing strategy to promote the use of prescription opioids for non-cancer pain, the generation of misinformed messages to promote the idea that opioids carry a low risk of addiction and overdose and to exaggerate the efficacy of opioids to treat chronic pain, the steep increase in DEA opioid production quotas, and the weak regulations in some states to control the diversion of opioids for nonmedical purposes. Beyond these factors, other elements, including rising unemployment and declining local economies, changes in social dynamics, and poor access to behavioral health treatment, may have contributed to the growing epidemic.

Trends in Nonmedical Use of Prescription Opioids

Trends by Age Group

Recent increases in nonmedical prescription opioid use, particularly among youth, are a significant concern due to an associated increased risk of developing OUD and initiation of heroin use (Martins et al. 2017a). Between 1991–1992 and 2001–2002, nonmedical prescription opioid use increased across all age groups but more prominently among 18- to 34-year-olds in the National Longitudinal Alcohol Epidemiology Survey and the National Epidemiologic Survey on Alcohol and Related Conditions (NESARC)—from 2.6% to 3.5% (Blanco et al. 2007), respectively. Similarly, data from the Monitoring the Future (MTF) survey showed that use of hydrocodone-acetaminophen (Vicodin) and OxyContin increased among twelfth graders, college students, and young adults between 1992 and 2001 (Johnston et al. 2016). However, evidence suggests that from 2002 to 2014, there was an overall reduction, mainly occurring after 2007, in the prevalence of nonmedical use of prescription opioids in those ages 12–17 years (from 7.51% in 2002 to 4.82% in 2014) and those ages 18–25 years (from 11.43% to 7.59%) (Martins et al. 2017b). Among those ages 26–34 years, the prevalence of nonmedical prescription opioid use slightly increased until 2012 (from 6.18% in 2002 to 7.73% in 2012), with a subsequent reduction in 2014 (6.08%). Data from MTF showed similar decreasing trends in the prevalence of Vicodin use between 2002 and 2015 (from 2.8% to 2.5% among eighth graders; from 7.2% to 0.9% among tenth graders; from 10.5% to 4.4% among twelfth graders; from 7.5% to 1.6% among college students; and from 8.6% to 3.8% among young adults) (Johnston et al. 2016). However, the prevalence of OxyContin use reported in the MTF among twelfth graders showed a slight increase from 2003 to 2011, and a declining trend between 2011 and 2015 (Johnston et al. 2016).

Among all adults (age 18 and older), NESARC and NESARC-III data showed that the prevalence rates of past-year and lifetime nonmedical use of prescription opioids significantly increased from 1.8% and 4.7%, respectively, in 2001–2002, to 4.1% and 11.3% in 2012–2013 (these prevalence rates in 2012–2013 represent about 9.7 and 26.6 million American adults) (Saha et al. 2016).

Regarding OUD, there was an increase in prevalence rates from 2002 to 2014 among opioid users ages 18–25 (from 11.98% to 15.11%) and ages 26–34 (from 11.27% to 23.52%) (Martins et al. 2017b). Although there was a sharp increase in the prevalence of OUD among adolescents from 2002 to 2004 (from 12.1% to 18.5%), this prevalence rate followed an overall downward trend thereafter until 2014 (Martins et al. 2017b) (Figure 2–2). Among all adults (age 18 and older), NESARC and NESARC-III data showed that rates of past-year and lifetime *Diagnostic and Statistical Manual of Mental Disorders*, Fourth Edition (DSM-IV; American Psychiatric Association 1994), opioid-related disorders increased from 0.4% and 1.4%, respectively, in 2001–2002, to 0.8% and 2.9% in 2012–2013 (Saha et al. 2016).

Opioid-related death rates in the United States have also changed over time among youth. Data from the CDC and the National Vital Statistics System (NVSS) showed an increasing trend in opioid-related mortality, from 0.7 deaths per 100,000 in 1999 to 3.6 per 100,000 in 2011 among those ages 15–24, and from 1.9 in 1999 to 8.5 per 100,000 in 2011 among those ages 25–34 (Chen et al. 2014). More recently, overdose deaths attributed to synthetic opioids other than methadone have increased between 2014 and 2015 among those ages 15–24 (from 1.2 to 2.3 per 100,000), as well as among those ages 25–34 (from 3.4 to 6.6 per 100,000) (Rudd et al. 2016b).

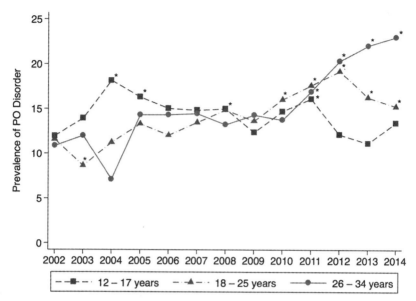

FIGURE 2–2. Adjusted prevalence (from models adjusted by sex and race/ethnicity) of opioid use disorder among those using prescription opioids nonmedically in the past year, stratified by age in the U.S. household population (2002–2014).

*Year prevalence is significantly different ($P<0.05$) from 2002 prevalence.
PO = prescription opioid.
Source.   Reprinted from Martins SS, Segura LE, Santaella-Tenorio J, et al.: "Prescription Opioid Use Disorder and Heroin Use Among 12–34 Year-Olds in the United States From 2002 to 2014." *Addictive Behaviors* 65:236–241, 2017. Copyright 2017, with permission from Elsevier.

Among older adults, NVSS multiple cause of death data show that in those aged 55 and older, the age-adjusted rate of fatal overdoses due to opioids increased from 0.7 per 100,000 in 1999 to 6.3 per 100,000 in 2015 (Centers for Disease Control and Prevention 2017c). Over this same period, the rate of opioid-related fatal overdoses in those ages 35–54 increased from 4.3 per 100,000 in 1999 to 17.3 per 100,000 in 2015 (Centers for Disease Control and Prevention 2017c). (These rates were calculated with CDC Wide-ranging ONline Data for Epidemiologic Research [WONDER] multiple cause of death data, using the ICD-10 underlying cause of death codes X40–44 [unintentional], X60–64 [suicide], and Y10–14 [undetermined intent], and using the ICD-10 multiple cause of death codes for type of opioid involved: opium [T40.0], heroin [T40.1], other opioids [T40.2], methadone [T40.3], and other synthetic opioids [T40.4].)

Regarding opioid-related inpatient hospital stays, although over the 2005–2014 period rates were higher for those ages 25–44 and 45–64, the steepest increase in inpatient stay rates was for those age 65 and older (85% increase). In addition, although all age groups experienced increases in ED visits, these more than doubled for those in the age groups 25–44, 45–64, and 65 and older over the 2005–2014 period (Weiss et al. 2017a).

This evidence suggests that the opioid epidemic has affected all age groups, with fatal overdoses and ED visits increasing among adolescents, young adults, and older adults. Although the trend in the prevalence of nonmedical use of prescription opioids shifted downward after 2007 across age groups, probably because of the implementation of PDMPs and other efforts to curb the epidemic, the past-year prevalence of OUD among young adult and older adult prescription opioid users has continued to increase since 2002. Inadequate access to appropriate treatment for OUD is likely one of the factors behind these findings.

Trends by Racial/Ethnic Group

Data from the National Survey on Drug Use and Health (NSDUH) showed that between 2010 and 2014, non-Hispanic white and American Indian/Alaska Native populations had a higher prevalence of nonmedical use of prescription opioids (4.6% and 7.1%, respectively) compared with non-Hispanic blacks (4.1%) and a higher prevalence of prescription opioid–related disorders (0.8% and 1.8%, respectively) compared with non-Hispanic blacks (0.6%) (authors' analysis of data).

Non-Hispanic whites and American Indians/Alaskan Natives have also been the most affected by opioid-related fatal overdoses. From 1999 to 2015, the rate of opioid-related fatal overdoses increased from 2.0 to 13.3 per 100,000 among non-Hispanic whites and from 1.6 to 7.5 per 100,000 among American Indians/Alaskan Natives (Centers for Disease Control and Prevention 2017c). Although opioid-related fatal overdoses increased from 2.1 to 13.4 per 100,000 among non-Hispanic whites and from 1.9 to 11.6 per 100,000 among American Indians/Alaskan Natives (Centers for Disease Control and Prevention 2017c). Opioid-related fatal overdose rates also increased in non-Hispanic blacks and Hispanics, especially after 2010 (increasing from 2.9 in 2010 to 6.3 in 2015 per

100,000 for non-Hispanic blacks and from 2.5 to 4.3 per 100,000 for Hispanics).[1]

Differences Between Regions and by Socioeconomic Status

Urban Versus Rural

Although the entire nation has been impacted by the opioid epidemic, during the first years of the epidemic, nonmetropolitan counties were particularly affected. From 1999 to 2004, prescription opioid overdose mortality rates increased 371% (from 0.82 to 3.85 per 100,000) in non-metropolitan, noncore counties (defined as not adjacent to a metropolitan area and having a population of 20,000–49,999 or having a population <20,000) and 52% in large central metropolitan counties (from 1.82 to 2.76 per 100,000) (Paulozzi and Xi 2008). Increases in opioid-related inpatient stays and ED visit rates were also greater in small metropolitan and rural areas. Over the 2005–2014 period, inpatient stays increased by 121.6% and 99.1% in small metropolitan and rural areas, respectively (in large metropolitan areas, inpatient stays increased by 28%); ED visits also increased by 121.3% and 103.8% in small metropolitan and rural areas, respectively (in large metropolitan areas, ED visits increased by 92.3%). Over time, metropolitan areas have been increasingly affected, as evidenced by spreading of opioid-related overdose hospital discharges from rural and suburban/exurban "hot spots" to urban areas (Cerdá et al. 2017) and increases in the rate of opioid-related fatal overdoses in medium/large metropolitan areas; in metropolitan areas, heroin and fentanyl fatal overdoses have sharply increased in recent years (Centers for Disease Control and Prevention 2017c).

U.S. Regions

To date, the Central Appalachia region (West Virginia and Kentucky) has been one of the regions most severely impacted by the opioid epi-

---

[1]Rates are calculated with CDC WONDER multiple cause of death data, using ICD-10 underlying cause-of-death codes X40–X44 (unintentional), X60–X64 (suicide), or Y10–Y14 (undetermined intent); and using the ICD-10 multiple cause-of-death codes for type of opioid involved: opium (T40.0), heroin (T40.1), other opioids (T40.2), methadone (T40.3), other synthetic opioids (T40.4).

demic. Prescription opioids were aggressively marketed in the 1990s and 2000s in this region, where coal mining, agriculture, and timbering jobs demanded high levels of physical work and involved significant risk of injury, and pain relief options were in demand. Prescription opioids are believed to be responsible for the observed increases in fatal drug-related overdose rates (over 10 per 100,000) during the first years of the twenty-first century in many counties in Kentucky and West Virginia. However, other regions in the country have also been disproportionately affected by the epidemic. Counties in New Mexico, Nevada, Arizona, and Northern California also experienced high rates (above 8 per 100,000) of fatal overdoses in the initial years of the epidemic (Popovich 2016). By 2015, the rate of overdoses remained very high—over 15 per 100,000—in counties in the Central Appalachia region, but overdose rates had also become high in many counties in Florida, Oklahoma, Missouri, and Alaska, as well as counties in states in the New England region and in states in the West Pacific and Mountain regions (Centers for Disease Control and Prevention 2017b; see www.cdc.gov/nchs/data-visualization/drug-poisoning-mortality/index.htm for a map showing the rate of drug overdose deaths per 100,000 in 2016). The top 10 states with the highest overdose rates are West Virginia, New Hampshire, Kentucky, Ohio, Rhode Island, Pennsylvania, Massachusetts, New Mexico, Utah, and Tennessee (Centers for Disease Control and Prevention 2017a).

Socioeconomic Status

According to 2009–2013 data from the MTF study, among high school seniors in the United States, moderate parental education (compared with low parental education) was found to be a risk factor for reporting lifetime opioid use. In this sample, higher weekly income for students ($\geq$\$51 compared with $\leq$\$10) was also associated with higher risk of lifetime opioid use and lifetime frequent opioid use ($\geq$40 times) (Palamar et al. 2016). These results suggest that students with higher family income may be at higher risk of initiating opioid use than those with lower income.

Among U.S. adults, however, risk of opioid use is greater among those with lower socioeconomic status. Data from the NSDUH 2008–2013, which surveyed individuals ages 12 and older, suggest that those using prescription opioids nonmedically and living in nonmetropolitan areas, compared with nonusers in these areas, were more likely to have less than high school educational attainment (21.6% vs. 17.9%), have a low family income of less than $20,000 (29.3% vs. 22.6%), lack medical insurance (29.1% vs. 15.4%), be unmarried (68.6% vs. 45.3%), and be male (54.9% vs. 48%) (Lenardson et al. 2016). NESARC-III data (2012–2013) also show that in the U.S. population of adults age 18 and older, those reporting past-year use of prescription opioids or meeting *Diagnostic and Statistical Manual of Mental Disorders*, Fifth Edition (DSM-5; American Psychiatric Association 2013) criteria for OUD were more likely to have less than a high school education and to have a family income below $20,000 (Kerridge et al. 2015).

Regarding opioid-related inpatient stays and ED visits, those in the lowest income quartiles had the highest rates but also showed the steepest increases in inpatient stays (65.2% and 73.8% increases for the lowest and second-lowest income quartiles, respectively) and ED visits (121.1% and 95.6% increases, respectively) over the 2005–2014 period (Weiss et al. 2017b).

This epidemiological evidence suggests that adults from lower socio-economic backgrounds are at higher risk of opioid misuse, OUD, and opioid-related problems (e.g., overdosing). Lack of resources and limited access to appropriate treatment (Substance Abuse and Mental Health Services Administration 2014) are likely factors exacerbating the risks associated with opioid use and may in part explain the high rates of fatal opioid-related overdoses observed in certain regions of the United States.

Long-Term Use of Prescription Opioids and Consequences

Chronic prescription opioid use is a meaningful and emerging cause for concern for health care providers in the United States. According to a meta-analysis involving 13 publications, 35.5% of the American population suffers from chronic pain of some kind, while 11% suffer from severe chronic pain (Ospina and Harstall 2002). As described earlier (see "Origins of the Prescription Opioid Epidemic"), prescribing of opioid medications such as OxyContin was aggressively promoted to treat noncancer chronic pain with marketing strategies and educational programs to overcome "myths and prejudices" related to opioid medications, including introducing pain as the fifth vital sign.

Chronic pain is a result of the interaction of an initial painful stimulus, pain processing in the central nervous system, and dysregulation in the cognitive-affective system (Apkarian et al. 2005), which involves brain processes that regulate the sensation of pain through the descending pain modulatory system. Understanding the interaction between the cognitive appraisal and the emotional modulation of pain can help in ascertaining the multiple dimensions of chronic pain. Feelings such as anger and fear might occur during pain episodes and can lead to pain catastrophizing, characterized by interpretation of unpleasant sensations as severe threats (Garland et al. 2013); this leads to a precognitive mental set that is associated with an intensification of pain sensation and functional impairment. Fear of pain can result in pain hypervigilance, which also contributes to functional deficits and diminishes an individual's ability to cope with pain (Garland et al. 2013). Subsequent dysphoria and distress are known to predict craving among chronic opioid users, as well as initiation of and continued misuse of such drugs.

As chronic pain and distress continue and the use of opioids escalates, patients enter a downward spiral of increasing pain and tolerance to opioids that can result in hyperalgesia, pain hypervigilance, and escalating loss of control over opioid use (Garland et al. 2013). Repeated use of prescription opioids is believed to alter the homeostatic process by which the brain maintains reward within a given set point, leading to tolerance and the need for higher opioid doses to achieve pain relief, experience pleasure, and have a sense of psychological well-being (Garland et al. 2013). As opioid use increases, the individual becomes gradually less sensitive to naturally rewarding experiences and progressively more sensitive to pain (Koob and Le Moal 2008). Increasing levels of distress and dysphoria can lead to allostatic overload with activation of the hypothalamic-pituitary-adrenal axis and dysregulation of the noradrenergic system, resulting in increased levels of corticotropin-releasing factor and dynorphins, neuropeptides involved in stress and depressive states (Striebel and Kalapatapu 2014). As this downward spiral progresses, the use of opioid medications becomes routine, regardless of diminished efficacy in pain control due to tolerance (Garland et al. 2015). The sensation of pain and external drug-related cues trigger the habit of taking the medication, with perceived need for escalating doses (Wood and Neal 2007).

In this way, OUD can emerge from alteration of normal reward-learning mechanisms due to repeated exposure to opioids, which leads to adaptations and neuroplasticity in brain circuits (Garland et al. 2015). OUD is often manifested, among other criteria, by unsuccessful efforts to control opioid consumption, which leads to a loss of functioning and failure to fulfill professional and personal role obligations.

The cycle described above—worsening pain, lessened reward response, and escalating opioid doses—is often associated with long-term prescription opioid use and can have serious consequences. Recent evidence indicates that of patients taking opioids for chronic noncancer pain, one in 550 died from an opioid overdose (median of 2.6 years from first opioid prescription), and one in 32 with opioid dosages above 200 morphine milligram equivalents (MME) died from an opioid overdose (Dowell et al. 2016). In primary care settings, opioid dependence (DSM-IV criteria) may be as high as 26% among patients using opioids for chronic noncancer pain (Dowell et al. 2016).

Given the risks associated with opioid use, the CDC guidelines for prescribing opioids for chronic pain (Dowell et al. 2016) offer recommendations that include the following: 1) the preferred use of nonpharmacological therapy and nonopioid pharmacological therapy for chronic pain; 2) establishment of realistic treatment goals with the patient before starting opioid therapy, and consideration of how therapy will be discontinued if benefits do not outweigh risks to patient safety; 3) beginning opioid therapy with immediate-release opioids instead of extended-release/long-acting formulations, using the lowest effective dosage, and avoiding increasing the dosage to ≥90 MME/day; 4) continuous evaluation of benefits and harms with patients initiating long-term opioid use and optimization of other therapies in order to taper opioids to lower dosages or discontinue their use; 5) inclusion of strategies to mitigate risk in the management plan, including prescribing naloxone if there is a history of overdose, substance use disorder, high opioid dosage (≥50 MME/day), or concurrent benzodiazepine use; 6) examination of a patient's history of controlled substance prescriptions using PDMP databases, before starting opioid therapy for chronic pain and periodically during therapy and use of urine drug testing before starting opioid therapy and at least once annually to assess for prescribed medications and other prescribed and illegal substances; 7) avoiding prescribing opioids and benzodiazepines concurrently whenever possible; and 8) offering evidence-based treatment (e.g., medication-assisted treatment with buprenorphine or methadone along with behavioral therapies) for patients with OUD.

Prescription Opioid Use and Risk of Initiating Use of Heroin and Other Illegal Opioids

Heroin

Heroin is a recreational drug derived from morphine (an analgesic alkaloid in opium) and is 3 times more potent than morphine. In the United States, heroin is used illegally and is considered a Schedule I drug under the Controlled Substances Act of 1970 (P.L. 91-513), which means that it has no accepted medical use and a high potential for abuse. Pharmacologically, heroin is similar to prescription opioids and produces its "high" effect through activation of μ, δ, and κ receptors.

Historically, heroin users have been characterized as young members of minority groups who are living in low-income urban areas (Cicero et al. 2014). However, demographic characteristics of heroin users have changed in the past decade to include more older white males and females living in nonurban areas (Cicero et al. 2014) who used prescription opioids prior to heroin (Compton et al. 2016; Martins et al. 2017a). The causes of these changes in the demographic characteristics of heroin users are complex but to a large extent are related to shifts by more recent users from nonmedical use of prescription opioids to heroin.

Prior nonmedical use of prescription opioids is linked to heroin initiation (Martins et al. 2017a). Evidence from a recent nationally representative U.S. sample showed that 76% of heroin users reported prior nonmedical use of prescription opioids (Cerdá et al. 2015). Moreover, heroin use and heroin-related OUD were up to 40 times more likely among those reporting prescription opioid abuse or dependence (Becker et al. 2008; Jones 2013). Despite incurring great risk of heroin initiation by using prescription opioids nonmedically, however, it is estimated that the proportion of those using prescription opioids nonmedically who transition to heroin is small—between 3.6% and 4.3% (Compton et al. 2016).

Among adolescents, those with no heroin experience but with prior nonmedical use of prescription opioids have 13 times higher risk of heroin initiation compared with those who have not used prescription opioids nonmedically (Cerdá et al. 2015). Increased risk of heroin initiation in those using prescription opioids nonmedically has been observed across all racial/ethnic categories and was highest in those initially exposed to nonmedical use of prescription opioids at ages 10–12 years (Cerdá et al. 2015).

An important risk factor for heroin initiation in those using prescription opioids nonmedically is a higher frequency of prescription opioid use. Among individuals age 12 years and older, frequent users (those using prescription opioids nonmedically 100–365 days in the past year) were 4 times more likely than nonfrequent users to inject heroin in the past year and almost 8 times more likely to report heroin abuse or dependence (Jones 2013).

Regarding heroin use and heroin-related OUD trends, there is evidence for increases in both starting around 2006–2007 (Dart et al. 2015). Using NSDUH data, Martins et al. (2017b) showed that from 2002 to 2014, heroin use increased among those using prescription opioids nonmedically in the age groups 18–25 years (from 2.11% to 7.35%) and 26–34 years (from 1.62% to 12.29%) but not among adolescents. In addition, results from NESARC in 2001–2002 and NESARC-III in 2012–2013 showed that between the two survey periods, the prevalence of heroin use increased from 0.33% to 1.6% and the prevalence of heroin-related OUD increased from 0.21% to 0.69% (Martins et al. 2017a). This analysis also showed that between 2001–2002 and 2012–2013, the proportion of people using prescription opioids nonmedically before initiating heroin use also increased, from 35.8% to 52.8% (Martins et al. 2017a). Results consistent with these were observed in NSDUH data, specifically among those using both heroin and prescription opioids nonmedically 100–365 days in the past year; whereas in the 2002–2004 period 64.1% used prescription opioids before heroin, in the 2008–2010 period the proportion increased to 82.6% (Jones 2013).

It is possible that interventions aimed at reducing prescription opioid misuse have had the unintended consequence of fueling heroin use. This is because the implementation of these interventions, while reducing access to prescription opioids, can shift the population already addicted to opioids to heroin, a cheaper, more potent, and more accessible option (Cicero et al. 2014). There is also evidence that for some prescription opioid users, heroin became an option after the introduction of abuse-deterrent opioid formulations (Cicero and Ellis 2015; Dart et al. 2015). However, it is likely that other factors—such as heroin market forces, including the cheaper price, the increasing purity, and the increased availability of heroin—are key contributors to the rise in heroin use during the past decade in the United States (Cicero and Ellis 2015).

Fentanyl and Related Analogues

Fentanyl is a synthetic opioid first developed in the 1960s. It has features that make it ideal for both clinical and illegal nonmedical use, such as high affinity for opioid receptors, rapid onset of pharmacological effects (analgesia, anesthesia, control of breakthrough pain), and availability in forms that can be taken in different routes of administration (Raffa et al. 2018). In the United States, fentanyl is classified as a Schedule II drug, which means that it has an accepted medical use with severe restrictions, it has high potential for abuse, and it may lead to severe physical or psychological dependence. Fentanyl is 50–100 times more potent than morphine.

In recent years, illegal fentanyl, mainly imported into the United States from China and Mexico (Ciccarone 2017), is believed to be the main factor increasing overdose death rates (O'Donnell et al. 2017a; Drug Enforcement Administration 2016). For example, in the eastern region of the United States, opioid-related fatal overdoses have tripled since 2011, with screening indicating 75% of recent deaths as positive for fentanyl (Ciccarone et al. 2017). National trends also show an overall increase in fatal overdoses in recent years mostly attributable to fentanyl; from 2014 to 2015, there was a 72.2% increase in fatal overdoses involving synthetic opioids other than methadone, such as fentanyl (Rudd et al. 2016b). A CDC weekly report from October 27, 2017—examining fatal opioid-related overdoses during July–December 2016 in 10 states—showed that fentanyl was detected in 56.3% of more than 5,000 overdoses, with Maine, Massachusetts, New Hampshire, Rhode Island, and Missouri having the highest percentages (60%–90%) of fatal opioid-related overdoses involving fentanyl (O'Donnell et al. 2017b).

Most fentanyl-related overdoses are believed to be the result of the adulteration of heroin with fentanyl, with heroin users unaware that the heroin was contaminated (O'Donnell et al. 2017a). Adulteration of heroin with carfentanil, a fentanyl analogue 10,000 times more potent than morphine, as well as with other fentanyl analogues, is also believed to be the cause of many recent fatal overdoses in the United States (O'Donnell et al. 2017b). Fentanyl's relative resistance to naloxone rescue treatment is one feature that makes it a particularly worrisome public health concern and an important driver of the current trends in fatal overdoses (Ciccarone 2017).

Future Directions for Research

As indicated in the CDC guidelines for prescribing opioids for chronic pain (Dowell et al. 2016), there is a need to better understand the effectiveness of nonopioid therapies for patients with chronic pain and those at risk of adverse opioid-related outcomes such as addiction and overdose. Future research should focus on the identification of alternatives, including nonpharmacological and nonopioid pharmacological therapies, that can improve treatment for patients with chronic pain. These may include cognitive-behavioral therapy, alternative medications, and new physical therapy approaches. Additional research should examine the effectiveness and limitations of medication-assisted treatment (i.e., buprenorphine, methadone, extended-release naltrexone) to treat OUD specifically related to prescription opioids. This research should include evaluation of multidisciplinary pain interventions, as well as cost-benefit analyses. Furthermore, research is needed to better understand factors associated with treatment access and reasons for treatment dropout in order to improve treatment engagement and retention among patients with OUD.

At the population level, new research should examine the effects of PDMPs in preventing the diversion of opioids for recreational use and identify the specific components of these programs that are more likely to be effective in reducing opioid-related adverse outcomes. Research using a systems science approach can also be useful to better understand the effects of PDMPs, including the unintended consequences of these programs on different population outcomes, such as whether they are driving widespread transitioning to heroin and other illicit opioids.

Finally, future research should continue to examine trends in opioid use and overdose rates related to prescription opioids, heroin, and fentanyl and its analogues in the U.S. population, while tracking the sources of these substances. Researchers should examine trends across an array of groups, including racial/ethnic and age groups, and populations at high risk of opioid-related adverse outcomes. These analyses should include the identification of geographic clusters of opioid overdoses in order to identify areas where additional treatment and prevention efforts are needed and target resources efficiently and appropriately.

Key Chapter Points

▶ The prescription opioid epidemic in the United States, as well as its extension to heroin and fentanyl epidemics, is characterized by a sharp increase in the prevalence of OUD, rates of opioid-related hospital and emergency department visits, and numbers of opioid-related fatal overdoses. These epidemics are also believed to be responsible for the recent increase in rates of hepatitis C virus infections and of babies born with neonatal abstinence syndrome.

▶ The prescription opioid epidemic originated with the aggressive marketing of OxyContin by Purdue Pharma to treat chronic pain during the 1990s, using misinformed messages to support the idea that opioids carry low risk of addiction and to exaggerate the efficacy of opioids to treat chronic pain. Factors that likely fueled the epidemic include the promotion of aggressive pain treatment by regulatory bodies and professional societies, steady increases in Drug Enforcement Administration opioid production quotas, and weak regulations in some states to control the diversion of opioids for nonmedical use.

▶ The binding of exogenous and endogenous opioids to opioid receptors induces analgesia by limiting the efficiency of neurons in transmitting pain signals and also by modulating activity in areas of the brain related to affective pain processing (the psychological component of pain). Opioids also inhibit the action of the neurotransmitter γ-aminobutyric acid (GABA) in the nucleus accumbens, liberating dopaminergic transmission in this area, which results in activation of the reward system, causing pleasurable and euphoric states.

▶ Long-term use of opioids can result in a downward spiral of increasing pain and escalating opioid use, which results in hyperalgesia, pain hypervigilance, distress, dysphoria, and loss of control over opioid use. Repeated use of prescription opioids is believed to alter the homeostatic set point for pain, leading to tolerance and the need to use higher doses of opioids to reach previous levels of reward and analgesia.

▶ The groups most affected by the recent opioid epidemic are non-Hispanic white and American Indian/Alaskan Native populations. These groups have had greater prevalence rates of prescription opioid misuse and OUD and higher rates of opioid-related overdoses. The epidemic has affected all age groups: rates of OUD, opioid-related emergency department visits, and fatal overdoses increased greatly across all age categories. Individuals from lower socioeconomic backgrounds have experienced a higher risk of opioid misuse, OUD, and opioid-related problems.

▶ Demographic characteristics of heroin users have changed in the past decade from younger nonwhite individuals living in more urban areas to older white individuals living in nonurban areas, many of whom used prescription opioids prior to heroin. Efforts to reduce diversion, misuse, and overdoses related to prescription opioids may have contributed to a shift to heroin. Those frequently using prescription opioids nonmedically are at increased risk of using heroin. Over the past 15 years, the prevalence of heroin use has increased greatly, as has the proportion of people using prescription opioids nonmedically before initiating heroin.

▶ In recent years, the often surreptitious adulteration of heroin with fentanyl and fentanyl analogues has been a main driver of the sharp increase in fatal overdoses across the United States.

References

Alvarez L: Florida shutting "pill mill" clinics. The New York Times, August 31, 2011. Available at: http://www.nytimes.com/2011/09/01/us/01drugs.html. Accessed December 20, 2017.

American Psychiatric Association: Diagnostic and Statistical Manual of Mental Disorders, 4th Edition. Washington, DC, American Psychiatric Association, 1994

American Psychiatric Association: Diagnostic and Statistical Manual of Mental Disorders, 5th Edition. Arlington, VA, American Psychiatric Association, 2013

Apkarian AV, Bushnell MC, Treede RD, et al: Human brain mechanisms of pain perception and regulation in health and disease. Eur J Pain 9(4):463–484, 2005 15979027

Becker WC, Sullivan LE, Tetrault JM, et al: Non-medical use, abuse and dependence on prescription opioids among U.S. adults: psychiatric, medical and substance use correlates. Drug Alcohol Depend 94(1–3):38–47, 2008 18063321

Blanco C, Alderson D, Ogburn E, et al: Changes in the prevalence of non-medical prescription drug use and drug use disorders in the United States: 1991–1992 and 2001–2002. Drug Alcohol Depend 90(2–3):252–260, 2007 17513069

Boudreau D, Von Korff M, Rutter CM, et al: Trends in long-term opioid therapy for chronic non-cancer pain. Pharmacoepidemiol Drug Saf 18(12):1166–1175, 2009 19718704

Center for Behavioral Health Statistics and Quality: Behavioral Health Trends in the United States: Results From the 2014 National Survey on Drug Use and Health (NSDUH Series H-50, HHS Publ No SMA-15-4927). Rockville, MD, Center for Behavioral Health Statistics and Quality, 2015. Available at: https://www.samhsa.gov/data/sites/default/files/NSDUH-FRR1-2014/NSDUH-FRR1-2014.pdf. Accessed November 12, 2016.

Centers for Disease Control and Prevention: Drug Overdose Death Data. December 19, 2017a. Available at: https://www.cdc.gov/drugoverdose/data/statedeaths.html. Accessed December 21, 2017.

Centers for Disease Control and Prevention: Drug Poisoning Mortality in the United States, 1999–2016. Data Visualization Gallery. National Center for Health Statistics, 2017b. Available at: https://www.cdc.gov/nchs/data-visualization/drug-poisoning-mortality/index.htm. Accessed July 5, 2018.

Centers for Disease Control and Prevention: Multiple Cause of Death, 1999–2016. CDC WONDER (Wide-ranging ONline Data for Epidemiologic Research), December 20, 2017c. Available at: https://wonder.cdc.gov/mcd.html. Accessed October 30, 2017.

Cerdá M, Santaella J, Marshall BD, et al: Nonmedical prescription opioid use in childhood and early adolescence predicts transitions to heroin use in young adulthood: a national study. J Pediatr 167(3):605.e1-2–612.e1-2, 2015 26054942

Cerdá M, Gaidus A, Keyes KM, et al: Prescription opioid poisoning across urban and rural areas: identifying vulnerable groups and geographic areas. Addiction 112(1):103–112, 2017 27470224

Chen LH, Hedegaard H, Warner M: Drug-poisoning deaths involving opioid analgesics: United States, 1999–2011. NCHS Data Brief Sep(166):1–8, 2014 25228059

Ciccarone D: Fentanyl in the U.S. heroin supply: a rapidly changing risk environment. Int J Drug Policy 46:107–111, 2017 28735776

Ciccarone D, Ondocsin J, Mars SG: Heroin uncertainties: exploring users' perceptions of fentanyl-adulterated and -substituted "heroin." Int J Drug Policy 46:146–155, 2017 28735775

Cicero TJ, Ellis MS: Abuse-deterrent formulations and the prescription opioid abuse epidemic in the United States: lessons learned from OxyContin. JAMA Psychiatry 72(5):424–430, 2015 25760692

Cicero TJ, Ellis MS, Surratt HL, et al: The changing face of heroin use in the United States: a retrospective analysis of the past 50 years. JAMA Psychiatry 71(7):821–826, 2014 24871348

Compton WM, Jones CM, Baldwin GT: Relationship between nonmedical prescription-opioid use and heroin use. N Engl J Med 374(2):154–163, 2016 26760086

Dart RC, Surratt HL, Cicero TJ, et al: Trends in opioid analgesic abuse and mortality in the United States. N Engl J Med 372(3):241–248, 2015 25587948

Dowell D, Haegerich TM, Chou R: CDC guideline for prescribing opioids for chronic pain—United States, 2016. MMWR Recomm Rep 65(No. RR-1):1–49, 2016 26987082

Drug Enforcement Administration: 2016 National Drug Threat Assessment Summary (DEA-DCT-DIR-001-17). November 2016. Available at: https://www.dea.gov/sites/default/files/2018-07/DIR-001-17_2016_NDTA_Summary.pdf. Accessed March 28, 2018.

Drug Enforcement Administration: Federal Register Notices. 2017. Available at: https://www.deadiversion.usdoj.gov/fed_regs/index.html. Accessed September 30, 2017.

Florence CS, Zhou C, Luo F, et al: The economic burden of prescription opioid overdose, abuse, and dependence in the United States, 2013. Med Care 54(10):901–906, 2016 27623005

Garland EL, Froeliger B, Zeidan F, et al: The downward spiral of chronic pain, prescription opioid misuse, and addiction: cognitive, affective, and neuropsychopharmacologic pathways. Neurosci Biobehav Rev 37(10 Pt 2):2597–2607, 2013 23988582

Garland EL, Hanley AW, Thomas EA, et al: Low dispositional mindfulness predicts self-medication of negative emotion with prescription opioids. J Addict Med 9(1):61–67, 2015 25469652

Haddox J, Joranson D, Angarola R, et al: The use of opioids for the treatment of chronic pain. A consensus statement from the American Academy of Pain Medicine and the American Pain Society. Clin J Pain 13(1):6–8, 1997 9084947

Holske R: Prescription drug trafficking and abuse trends. U.S. Drug Enforcement Administration. Slide presentation at EU-US Dialogue on Drugs, Brussels,

Belgium, May 15, 2013. Available at: https://www.deadiversion.usdoj.gov/pubs/presentations/euus2013.pdf. Accessed September 29, 2017.

Johnston LD, O'Malley PM, Miech RA, et al: Monitoring the Future National Survey Results on Drug Use, 1975–2015: Overview, Key Findings on Adolescent Drug Use. Ann Arbor, MI, Institute for Social Research, University of Michigan, 2016

Jones CM: Heroin use and heroin use risk behaviors among nonmedical users of prescription opioid pain relievers—United States, 2002–2004 and 2008–2010. Drug Alcohol Depend 132(1–2):95–100, 2013 23410617

Kenan K, Mack K, Paulozzi L: Trends in prescriptions for oxycodone and other commonly used opioids in the United States, 2000–2010. Open Med 6(2):e41–e47, 2012 23696768

Kerridge BT, Saha TD, Chou SP, et al: Gender and nonmedical prescription opioid use and DSM-5 nonmedical prescription opioid use disorder: results from the National Epidemiologic Survey on Alcohol and Related Conditions—III. Drug Alcohol Depend 156:47–56, 2015 26374990

Kolodny A, Courtwright DT, Hwang CS, et al: The prescription opioid and heroin crisis: a public health approach to an epidemic of addiction. Annu Rev Public Health 36:559–574, 2015 25581144

Koob GF, Le Moal M: Addiction and the brain antireward system. Annu Rev Psychol 59:29–53, 2008 18154498

Lenardson J, Gale J, Ziller E: Rural Opioid Abuse: Prevalence and User Characteristics. Portland, University of Southern Maine, Muskie School of Public Service, Maine Rural Health Research Center, 2016

Martins SS, Sarvet A, Santaella-Tenorio J, et al: Changes in U.S. lifetime heroin use and heroin use disorder: prevalence from the 2001–2002 to 2012–2013 National Epidemiologic Survey on Alcohol and Related Conditions. JAMA Psychiatry 74(5):445–455, 2017a 28355458

Martins SS, Segura LE, Santaella-Tenorio J, et al: Prescription opioid use disorder and heroin use among 12–34 year-olds in the United States from 2002 to 2014. Addict Behav 65:236–241, 2017b 27614657

Meier B: In guilty plea, OxyContin maker to pay $600 million. The New York Times, May 10, 2007

O'Donnell JK, Gladden RM, Seth P: Trends in deaths involving heroin and synthetic opioids excluding methadone, and law enforcement drug product reports, by census region—United States, 2006–2015. MMWR Morb Mortal Wkly Rep 66(34):897–903, 2017a 28859052

O'Donnell J, Halpin J, Mattson C, et al: Deaths involving fentanyl, fentanyl analogs, and U-47700—10 states, July–December 2016. MMWR Morb Mortal Wkly Rep 66(43):1197–1202, 2017b 29095804

Ospina M, Harstall C: Prevalence of chronic pain: an overview. HTA 29, Health Technology Assessment. December 2002. Available at: http://citeseerx.ist.psu.edu/viewdoc/download?doi=10.1.1.510.5502&rep=rep1&type=pdf. Accessed March 29, 2018.

Palamar JJ, Shearston JA, Dawson EW, et al: Nonmedical opioid use and heroin use in a nationally representative sample of U.S. high school seniors. Drug Alcohol Depend 158:132–138, 2016 26653341

Patrick SW, Davis MM, Lehman CU, et al: Increasing incidence and geographic distribution of neonatal abstinence syndrome: United States 2009 to 2012 (erratum). J Perinatol 35(8):667, 2015 26219703

Paulozzi L, Xi Y: Recent changes in drug poisoning mortality in the United States by urban-rural status and by drug type. Pharmacoepidemiol Drug Saf 17(10):997–1005, 2008 18512264

Paulozzi L, Jones C, Rudd R; Centers for Disease Control and Prevention: Vital signs: overdoses of prescription opioid pain relievers—United States, 1999–2008. MMWR Morb Mortal Wkly Rep 60(43):1487–1492, 2011 22048730

Popovich N: A deadly crisis: mapping the spread of America's drug overdose epidemic. The Guardian, 2016. Available at: https://www.theguardian.com/society/ng-interactive/2016/may/25/opioid-epidemic-overdose-deaths-map. Accessed October 24, 2017.

Portenoy RK, Foley KM: Chronic use of opioid analgesics in non-malignant pain: report of 38 cases. Pain 25(2):171–186, 1986 2873550

Porter J, Jick H: Addiction rare in patients treated with narcotics (letter). N Engl J Med 302(2):123, 1980 7350425

Raffa RB, Pergolizzi JV Jr, LeQuang JA, et al: The fentanyl family: a distinguished medical history tainted by abuse. J Clin Pharm Ther 43(1):154–158, 2018 28980330

Rudd RA, Aleshire N, Zibbell JE, et al: Increases in drug and opioid overdose deaths—United States, 2000–2014. MMWR Morb Mortal Wkly Rep 64(50–51):1378–1382, 2016a 26720857

Rudd RA, Seth P, David F, et al: Increases in drug and opioid-involved overdose deaths—United States, 2010–2015. MMWR Morb Mortal Wkly Rep 65(5051):1445–1452, 2016b 28033313

Saha TD, Kerridge BT, Goldstein RB, et al: Nonmedical prescription opioid use and DSM-5 nonmedical prescription opioid use disorder in the United States. J Clin Psychiatry 77(6):772–780, 2016 27337416

Striebel JM, Kalapatapu RK: The anti-suicidal potential of buprenorphine: a case report. Int J Psychiatry Med 47(2):169–174, 2014 25084802

Substance Abuse and Mental Health Services Administration: Results From the 2013 National Survey on Drug Use and Health: Summary of National

Findings (NSDUH Series H-48, HHS Publ No SMA-14-4863), Rockville, MD, Substance Abuse and Mental Health Services Administration, 2014. Available at: https://www.samhsa.gov/data/sites/default/files/ NSDUHresultsPDFWHTML2013/Web/NSDUHresults2013.pdf. Accessed March 29, 2018.

Temple J: American Pain: How a Young Felon and His Ring of Doctors Unleashed America's Deadliest Drug Epidemic. Guilford, CT, Lyons Press, 2015

U.S. General Accounting Office: Prescription Drugs: OxyContin Abuse and Diversion and Efforts to Address the Problem. Report to Congressional Requesters. December 2003. Available at: http://www.gao.gov/new.items/ d04110.pdf. Accessed September 24, 2017.

Weiss A, Bailey M, O'Malley L, et al: Statistical brief #224. Patient characteristics of opioid-related inpatient stays and emergency department visits nationally and by state, 2014. June 2017a. Available at: https://www.hcup-us.ahrq.gov/ reports/statbriefs/sb224-Patient-Characteristics-Opioid-Hospital-Stays-ED-Visits-by-State.pdf. Accessed March 29, 2018.

Weiss A, Bailey M, O'Malley L, et al: Statistical brief #226. Patient residence characteristics of opioid-related inpatient stays and emergency department visits nationally and by state, 2014. July 2017b. Available at: https:// www.hcup-us.ahrq.gov/reports/statbriefs/sb226-Patient-Residence-Opioid-Hospital-Stays-ED-Visits-by-State.pdf. Accessed March 29, 2018.

Wood W, Neal DT: A new look at habits and the habit-goal interface. Psychol Rev 114(4):843–863, 2007 17907866

3

Heroin and Other Illicit Opioids

Abhishek Jain, M.D.
Carl E. Fisher, M.D.

Clinical Vignette: Liam's Escalating Heroin Problem

Liam is a 30-year-old man working in the financial services field, with no formal psychiatric or medical history, but with a long history of binge drinking of alcohol, intermittent use of various substances, and most recently heroin use. He reports consuming more than five drinks each evening and describes his alcohol use as unproblematic and without consequences. In his early 20s, he began taking opioid pills "recreationally" at parties when offered to him by acquaintances; his use gradually increased to almost every weekend, but the amounts still remained relatively low (usually 1–3 oxycodone-acetaminophen pills each Saturday and Sunday). He first used heroin intranasally 1 year ago when friends offered it to him at a party, after which he began obtaining his own heroin and using it regularly on weekend nights to "unwind and relax." He reports that he did not perceive difficulties with this practice at first and that his work (often 12-hour days from Monday to Saturday) never suffered, but in a short time, he became more socially withdrawn and stopped his usual recreational activities. Additionally, his then girlfriend left him due to his behavior changes. His life centered around work during the week and solitary heroin use on the weekends.

One month ago, his heroin dealer demonstrated to him how to prepare and inject heroin intravenously, after which point his use dramatically escalated. He began using on weekdays and often several times daily at work—a line he once thought he would never cross. He began having greater cognitive dissonance and intrapersonal struggles about his use. Despite making resolutions to cut down or stop entirely, he required larger and larger amounts to feel the same relief or "high." He began experiencing powerful physical symptoms of withdrawal between doses. His work, his last outlet for any personal fulfillment, began to suffer, and his supervisors openly criticized his performance and frequently reprimanded him in front of coworkers. Heroin became the organizing principle of his life. He continued to use and did not seek help.

One recent night, Liam's withdrawal symptoms were particularly troubling, and he asked his heroin dealer for antianxiety medications along with his usual supply of powder heroin. He was given an unknown pill "to take the edge off," but after he injected his heroin, he put the pills aside unused with the rest of his supply. He took his heroin and pills with him to work the next morning. He attempted as usual to administer small doses throughout the day to maintain a basic level of functioning, but he soon became preoccupied with anxious thoughts that he could not achieve the desired middle ground between withdrawal and sedation. For his next dose, he went to his usual low-traffic bathroom and took one of the purported antianxiety pills along with a small dose of heroin.

A coworker noticed Liam's feet sticking out from under the stall, and after he could not awaken Liam, he called 911. Emergency responders saw Liam's drug paraphernalia and found his pupils to be miotic (constricted) and his respiratory rate to be dangerously low. They administered emergency naloxone in the bathroom and took him to a local emergency department, where, after supportive measures, he recovered. After discussions with the medical providers there and a consultation with his Employee Assistance Program, he agreed to take a leave of absence from work, see an addiction psychiatrist for a consultation, and enter an intensive outpatient treatment program.

Liam's case raises a number of questions for mental health professionals to consider. When did humans first start using opium and related opioids such as heroin and how have the substances evolved over the years? Where and how are opioids produced today, and how do they ultimately reach those who use them? What are the physiological and psychological effects of opioids? What are the current trends pertaining to heroin use and addiction in the United States? What characterizes heroin overdose, what are its risk factors, and how can it be recognized, treated, and prevented?

Introduction

The alarming increase in the number of opioid-related overdose deaths since 1999 has been described as America's worst drug crisis in history. It has impacted all demographic groups. In 2016, more than 42,000 overdose deaths were attributed to opioids; of those, more than 15,000 were heroin related (National Vital Statistics System 2017). According to the White House Council of Economic Advisers (2017), in 2015, illicit opioid use cost the U.S. economy over $500 billion, or about 2.8% of the gross domestic product. Dr. Nora Volkow, Director of the National Institute on Drug Abuse, has called for an "all hands on deck" approach to end this concerning trend of opioid-related overdose deaths, including encouraging public-private partnerships and laying out a plan to accelerate research in overdose reversal, addiction treatment, and pain management (Volkow and Collins 2017). To better grasp this major current U.S. public health emergency, and the impact on individuals such as Liam, it is useful to gain a deeper understanding of the history, use, production, and pharmacology of these drugs.

From Poppies to Pain Relief: History, Production, and Classification of Opioids

Historical Overview

Evidence suggests that humans have used opium for at least 8,000 years (Brook et al. 2017). Ancient Sumerians cultivated the opium poppy to extract opium as far back as 3000 B.C.; the Greek poet Homer described its effects in the "Odyssey" around 800 B.C.; and Europeans used it in an alcoholic concoction (called laudanum) for medical purposes between the 1500s and 1800s (Blakemore and White 2002). Opium's profound impact on world history and global events is remarkable, as demonstrated, for example, by the Opium Wars in 1839–1842 and 1856–1860; the creation of the first multinational drug control treaty, the International Opium Convention, in 1912; and the estimated upward of 36 million people worldwide who used illicit opioids in 2012 (U.S. Department of Health and Human Services 2014).

In its most basic form, opium is produced from the opium poppy flower, or *Papaver somniferum*, by the laborious process of obtaining and drying the milky latex "poppy tears" from the plant's seedpods. The Latin word *somniferum* essentially translates to "sleep-inducing," referring to the sedative property of opium's naturally occurring alkaloid compounds called opiates (Brook et al. 2017). Opium contains 10%–15% of its most well-known analgesic opiate, *morphine* (Blakemore and White 2002), named for Morpheus, the Greek god of dreams (Brook et al. 2017). Morphine was chemically isolated around 1805 by German pharmacist Friedrich Sertürner; its chemical formula was deduced by the French chemist Auguste Laurent around 1847; and its chemical structure was identified by Sir Robert Robinson around 1925, for which he won the Nobel Prize in 1947 (Blakemore and White 2002; Brook et al. 2017; Williams 2008). Opium's other alkaloid compounds include analgesic (pain-relieving) *codeine*, the smooth muscle relaxant *papaverine*, and *thebaine*, which is used to produce various synthetic opioids (Williams 2008).

After morphine was isolated, it became more widely used following the invention of the hypodermic needle in 1853. Direct injection into the bloodstream, compared with oral administration, allowed for greater bioavailability and quicker onset of pain relief and euphoric effects. Morphine is the principal active ingredient of opium (even today the World Health Organization identifies it as the "gold standard opioid analgesic for cancer-related pain" [Brook et al. 2017]); thus, there has been great motivation to synthetically mass-produce it. Although Marshall Gates and Gilg Tschudi were eventually able to synthesize morphine in a laboratory from simple compounds in 1952, it required a 28-step process. An efficient and useful process to synthesize morphine on a large scale remains elusive, and growing and harvesting the poppy plant continues to be a more practical and cost-effective way to obtain morphine (Blakemore and White 2002; Brook et al. 2017).

Opioid importation, production, and distribution became more restricted in the United States with federal legislation such as the Food and Drug Act of 1906 and the Harrison Anti-Narcotic Tax Act of 1914. The Harrison Act was a response to the growing problem of addiction to various forms of opium, as well as coca products such as cocaine; however, historians have also described its racial and political undertones. This act was additionally used as a basis to prosecute physicians for prescribing to "addicts." Although the U.S. Supreme Court's

1925 decision in *Linder v. United States* loosened the Harrison Act's federal regulations, state medical boards continued to have their own regulations, and over the years *Linder* itself has largely been superseded by various laws. Nonetheless, this series of legislation serves as an example of how government control of physician prescribing practices has been, and remains, a complex issue (Herzberg 2017).

The Comprehensive Drug Abuse Prevention and Control Act of 1970 regulated the pharmaceutical industry and established the classification of controlled substances into five categories: Schedules I–V (Drug Enforcement Agency 2018). These categories are still used today and are grouped from most to least regulated. For example, Schedule I drugs are the most regulated, have no accepted medical purposes, and are considered unsafe with a high potential for abuse, and Schedule II drugs can be prescribed by physicians but have a high potential for abuse and dependence. Currently, various opioids and opium derivatives, such as heroin, are classified as Schedule I drugs, and most of the prescribed opioids, such as morphine, oxycodone, hydrocodone, and products containing more than 90 mg of codeine per dosage unit, are classified as Schedule II drugs (Drug Enforcement Agency 2008).

Production and Distribution: 1960s to Today

Individuals like Liam come into contact with illicit opium and its derivatives, such as heroin, through a variety of production and distribution channels. Under the United Nations (UN) Single Convention on Narcotic Drugs of 1961, only certain countries, such as India, Turkey, and Australia, were permitted to legally produce opium. In 1979, the UN adopted Resolution 471 to limit overproduction of opium, to support traditional suppliers, and to minimize illicit production. Responding to this UN resolution, the United States in 1981 passed the 80/20 rule, which states that at least 80% of opium imported legally into the United States must be from India and Turkey, and no more than 20% can be from France, Poland, Hungary, Australia, and Yugoslavia. In 2008, the U.S. Drug Enforcement Agency (DEA) continued the rule but amended it by removing Yugoslavia and adding Spain to the approved countries (Drug Enforcement Agency 2008).

Currently, most worldwide opium continues to be produced and distributed illicitly, especially from two major regions: the "Golden Crescent," which includes parts of Afghanistan, Iran, and Pakistan, and the

"Golden Triangle," which includes parts of Myanmar (Burma), Laos, and Thailand. Afghanistan alone accounted for about 80% of the world's illicit opium and heroin production in 2014, with the Golden Triangle producing about 10%, Mexico and Colombia combined producing about 5%, and another 40 or so countries combined producing about 5% (Miltenburg 2018). The $1.4 billion farm gate value (i.e., the net profit of the raw product sold by the farm, as opposed to the "retail" price paid by consumers farther down the production line, and not including profits from trafficking or opium's derivative by-products) of Afghanistan's opium alone was equivalent to roughly 7% of the country's estimated gross domestic product in 2017 (United Nations Office on Drugs and Crime 2017). According to the Afghan Ministry of Counter Narcotics and the UN Office on Drugs and Crime, 328,000 hectares (or more than 810,000 acres) of illicit opium poppy were cultivated and about 9,000 tons of illicit opium were produced in Afghanistan in 2017, representing increases of 63% and 87%, respectively, compared with the previous year (United Nations Office on Drugs and Crime 2017). Exploring potential solutions to minimize opium production and trafficking from this region has been of global interest, not just because of the harmful consequences of increased worldwide access to and consumption of opium and its derivatives such as heroin, but also because of the potential link to funding terrorism (Clark et al. 2010). For example, some have proposed allowing Afghan farmers to continue growing the opium poppy, under closely regulated licensing and monitoring, to provide cost-effective medications for third-world nations and to reduce the illicit drug trade (Clark et al. 2010). Others have suggested financial incentives and governmental efforts for farmers to cultivate alternative crops (Greenfield et al. 2017).

With such a worldwide demand for opium and concerns about illicit distribution, a great deal of energy and scientific effort has been expended over the years to develop more accessible, safer, and less addictive chemically manufactured alternatives (Table 3–1). Collectively, the naturally occurring opiates, along with the manufactured semisynthetic and synthetic compounds, are referred to as *opioids* (Williams 2008). One of the first semisynthetic opioids, diacetylmorphine—better known by its brand name Heroin—was developed in the late 1800s by researchers at the German pharmaceutical company Bayer (Huecker and Marraffa 2017; Sneader 1998). It was marketed in 1898 as a cough and pain remedy with the intention of its being a more favorable alternative to

TABLE 3–1. Various opioids and about when they were first isolated or synthesized

Morphine	1805
Codeine	1832
Diacetylmorphine (heroin)	1874
Oxymorphone	1914
Oxycodone	1916
Hydrocodone	1920
Hydromorphone	1921
Methadone	1937
Meperidine	1939
Fentanyl	1960
Tramadol	1962
Buprenorphine	1969
Carfentanil	1974

codeine and morphine, and many even thought of it as nonaddictive (Hosztafi 2001; Huecker and Marraffa 2017; Sneader 1998), which is obviously jarring in retrospect. Other semisynthetic opioids include oxycodone, synthesized from thebaine and first used in clinical practice around 1917, and hydrocodone, synthesized from codeine and first developed around 1920. Fully synthetic compounds, such as methadone, were developed in the 1930s. Methadone, with its slower onset and longer duration of action, is now a major treatment for pain and is a primary form of medication-assisted treatment for opioid use disorders (OUDs).

Fentanyl, another synthetic opioid (with 50–100 times the potency of morphine), was developed around 1960, and its even more potent analogues, including carfentanil, were developed in the 1970s (Duarte 2005). Although fentanyl is currently the most widely used synthetic opioid in medicine (National Institutes of Health, National Library of Medicine 2018)—its relatively rapid onset and offset are useful in anesthesia, and the 72-hour fentanyl patch is frequently used in palliative care—introduction of illicitly manufactured fentanyl into the drug market has resulted in a sharp increase in unintentional overdose deaths (Ciccarone 2017), as described in more detail in the subsection "'Cutting' With Fentanyl and Carfentanil."

Today, the United States is the largest consumer of legally prescribed opioids worldwide. In 2013, Americans consumed about 81% of the world's oxycodone and almost all of the world's hydrocodone, and the United States experienced a surge of opioid prescriptions from 76 million in 1991 to 207 million in 2013 (U.S. Department of Health and Human Services 2014). In 2015, about 98 million Americans, or 36% of the U.S. population age 12 and over, used a prescribed opioid (Hughes et al. 2016). Although the relationship between the availability of medications and their illicit use is certainly complex, the pervasiveness of prescribed opioids in the general public may explain how someone like Liam was able to readily obtain oxycodone-acetaminophen pills on a weekly basis without a prescription. For example, according to the National Survey on Drug Use and Health (NSDUH), among persons age 12 or older who in 2015 misused prescription opioids (defined as use of opioids "in any way that a doctor did not direct you to use them"), the majority (54%) most recently obtained them from a friend or relative, whereas only a minority (36%) obtained them through a prescription directly from a doctor (additionally, about 5% obtained them from a drug dealer or a stranger, and another 5% obtained them "some other way") (Hughes et al. 2016). Thus, addressing these ongoing questions, such as the relationship between prescribed medications, their misuse, and their illicit diversion, remains especially important with the increasing number of opioid overdose deaths over the past three decades—including a tripling between 1990 and 2010 (U.S. Department of Health and Human Services 2014).

Classification of Opioids

Besides being classified as naturally occurring, semisynthetic, or synthetic, opioids can also be categorized based on their action at the opioid receptor. Agonists (e.g., morphine, fentanyl) produce a full response at the receptor, partial agonists (e.g., buprenorphine) produce a limited response at the receptor, and antagonists (e.g., naloxone) block the receptor (Williams 2008). Opioids may also be categorized as long acting, short acting, or rapid onset, a designation that also depends on the compound's specific formulation and route of administration.

Furthermore, opioids can be differentiated based on their affinity for opioid receptors, as well as the specific type of opioid receptor on which they act. Traditionally, three types of opioid receptors, discovered in the

1970s, have been described: μ, δ, and κ opioid receptors. Although activation of each type of receptor can produce analgesic effects, other functional effects may also occur. For example, stimulation of the μ opioid receptor may cause sedation, euphoria, and respiratory depression; stimulation of the δ opioid receptor may cause reduced gastrointestinal motility; and stimulation of the κ opioid receptor may cause sedation and depressed mood. These effects correlate with the potential signs and symptoms of opioid intoxication and withdrawal. Additionally, humans and various animals naturally produce ligands (enkephalins, dynorphins, and endorphins) that bind to their opioid receptors to regulate various physiological responses, including pain (Blakemore and White 2002; Williams 2008). In fact, the term *endorphin* is shortened from *endogenous morphine*.

Heroin Use

As mentioned in the section on production and distribution, heroin (generic names diacetylmorphine or diamorphine) was originally marketed by the Bayer pharmaceutical company in 1898 as a cough and pain remedy. The company's researchers initially claimed it had a stimulant effect on the respiratory system; however, it was soon evident that it actually causes respiratory depression. It was even, for a time, surprisingly thought of as nonaddictive or at least less addictive than codeine or morphine. With its ready availability and increasing cases of heroin addiction, it became more closely regulated in the United States after the Harrison Act in 1914 and was officially banned in 1924 (Sneader 1998). By comparison, the United Kingdom continues to permit heroin to be prescribed in certain cases for the treatment of addiction or pain relief, for example, for postoperative analgesia or palliative care (Huecker and Marraffa 2017).

Although Afghanistan produces the majority of the world's opium, the majority of heroin in the United States has recently been produced and trafficked from Mexico or Colombia. In 2014, for example, 79% of the heroin in the United States was sourced from Mexico. The less pure "black tar" heroin, found mainly in western and southern parts of the United States, typically originates from Mexico; the more pure "white powder" heroin is more common in eastern parts of the United States and typically originates from Colombia (Ciccarone 2017). In general, farmers sell dried opium latex for about $1,400 per 10 kg (about 10 kg of opium is needed to produce 1 kg of heroin); however, after the various profit markups and "cutting" (mixing) and diluting along the supply chain by brokers, opium labs, heroin labs, wholesalers, local distributors, and local retailers, the final heroin product on the street is sold for roughly the equivalent of $200,000 per 1 kg (Miltenburg 2018). Thus, from the growers to the street dealers, heroin involves a major profitable business network. However, owing to the increased supply of heroin, along with the addition of various adulterants, it is available at historically low prices, with street prices reduced to almost half from 2010 to 2014 (Ciccarone 2017).

The unfortunate reality is that with the increasing availability and the decreased price of heroin, stories such as Liam's have become more common. The reported lifetime prevalence of heroin use in the United States has increased from 0.33% in 2001–2002 to 1.6% in 2012–2013 (Martins et al. 2017). According to the NSDUH, in 2013, an estimated 681,000 people used heroin, of whom 169,000 individuals (including 21,000 adolescents) used heroin for the first time. This represents about 460 people initiating heroin use daily, with the average age of first use being about 24 years (Lipari and Hughes 2015).

Pharmacology

Heroin is considered a semisynthetic opioid because it is derived from opium's naturally occurring morphine alkaloid, which is then chemically acetylated in heroin labs through a multistep chemical process involving various substances, including acetic anhydride, hydrochloric acid, and acetone (Miltenburg 2018). If taken orally, heroin undergoes a first-pass metabolism and is converted back to morphine through deacetylation. This process can delay the onset of its effects by about 30 minutes. When administered through more bioavailable methods, such as intravenously, it reaches peak serum levels in less than 1 minute, and its highly lipophilic property allows it to cross the blood-brain barrier in 15–20 seconds. Furthermore, intravenous heroin has more than 10 times the blood-brain permeability of intravenous morphine; about 68% of intravenous heroin, compared with about 5% of intravenous morphine, reaches the brain (Huecker and Marraffa 2017; Sporer 1999).

Although heroin itself has a weak affinity for the brain's opioid receptors, within 5–10 minutes it is deacetylated through a four-step enzymatic hydrolysis pathway in the central nervous system (CNS) into

6-monoacetylmorphine (6-MAM), which is then further metabolized to morphine via acetylcholinesterase over the next 20–30 minutes. Although heroin has some agonist properties at μ and δ receptors, 6-MAM has been described as heroin's most active metabolite, rapidly concentrating in the brain and having a higher μ receptor affinity than heroin or morphine (Qiao et al. 2014). Peripheral tissue can also hydrolyze heroin to 6-MAM and then to morphine. Morphine that is circulating in the serum is converted to morphine-3-glucuronide or morphine-6-glucuronide mainly by the liver and somewhat by the kidneys. Morphine-6-glucuronide also has significant analgesic properties. Although heroin has a short half-life of only a few minutes, its duration of action is 4–5 hours because of these various active metabolites. These compounds are then excreted in urine or bile (Sporer 1999).

Although other opioids and their metabolites may be detected in urine for 1–3 days, heroin—specifically through its metabolite 6-MAM—might only be detected for less than 8 hours. However, because 6-MAM is a unique metabolite of heroin, its presence in urine confirms heroin use and distinguishes heroin from other opioids (Staub et al. 2001). Additionally, although heroin generally has a very short half-life, various factors, such as impaired renal or hepatic function, genetics, and age, may play a role in its metabolism (Sporer 1999) and subsequently its detection by screening tests.

Physiological and Subjective Effects

Heroin's active metabolites stimulate various opioid receptors, as previously described. More specifically, by stimulating the $μ_1$ opioid receptor, they induce analgesia, respiratory depression, and euphoria, and by stimulating the $μ_2$ receptor, they cause pupillary constriction, reduced gastrointestinal motility, and physiological dependence. Stimulating κ and δ receptors also has the effect of analgesia (Huecker and Marraffa 2017). In addition, κ agonism plays a role in respiratory depression, pupillary constriction, and depressed mood. Although they are also found in the cortical regions, δ receptors specifically mediate spinal analgesia. In general, the respiratory depression through opioid agonism is caused by a direct effect on brain stem respiratory centers through a reduction in carbon dioxide responsiveness (Sporer 1999).

In an even closer look at the cellular level, the transmembrane opioid receptors (μ, κ, and δ) are coupled with G proteins that initiate intracellular signal transduction. Activation of these opioid receptors leads to effects on messenger-generating enzymes, such as adenyl cyclase and phospholipase C, along with a decrease in secondary messengers, such as cyclic adenosine monophosphate. Opioids, through this mechanism of action, can disrupt the body's complex neuromodulatory system, affecting neurotransmitters, including dopamine, γ-aminobutyric acid (GABA), and glutamate (Lutz and Kieffer 2013). The specific effect of modulating these neurotransmitter systems depends on the given receptor's location, such as in the central versus the peripheral nervous system. For example, the feeling of euphoria is driven by the release of high levels of dopamine in particular brain regions.

Subjectively, individuals who use heroin may characterize its euphoric feeling as both a "rush" and a "high." Some have described a rush as the intense orgasm-like sensation 1 or 2 minutes immediately after injecting the substance, which is then followed by a warm and pleasant high or even a profound feeling of satisfaction (Seecof and Tennant 1986). During a high, individuals may also experience a sedative, drowsy state, sometimes referred to as "going on the nod" or "nodding off"; excessive activity and talking, sometimes referred to as "drive"; or fluctuating states between nodding off and drive. To an observer, this may either be noticeable or the individual might simply appear to be functioning normally. The mental sluggishness and slurred speech can last for a few hours (Stimmel 1992). As described further in the section "Heroin Overdose," this is a particularly vulnerable state in which the individual may experience unintentional severe respiratory depression leading to hypoxia or even death.

Routes of Administration and Street Terminology

Thinking about heroin's pharmacology based on its various routes of administration may help elucidate how Liam's heroin use dramatically escalated after he started injecting it. Although injecting intravenously is common, heroin can also be administered by other means, such as subcutaneously as "skin-popping," intramuscularly as "muscling," inhaling as "chasing the dragon," intranasally as "snorting," or, less commonly, orally. Individuals might attempt using heroin via these alternative methods, perhaps due to fears of needles or of blood-borne infections spread through needle sharing; however, the drug's bioavailability is significantly lower and onset of action is slower through nonintravenous administration. For example, peak serum levels are reached in 5–10 minutes when heroin is administered subcutaneously and in 3–5 minutes when administered intramuscularly or intranasally but, as described previously, in less than 1 minute when administered intravenously (Sporer 1999). Anecdotally, patients have also described using heroin via anal or vaginal insertion in a process called "plugging," with a reportedly quicker high than with oral ingestion or snorting but not as rapid an effect as with intravenous use. Thus, not surprisingly, many individuals who may initially be averse to needles eventually turn to or "graduate" to intravenous use to achieve a sufficient rush or high. Furthermore, evidence suggests that administering heroin intravenously results in a quicker and more likely transition to daily heroin use compared with using heroin by inhaling or snorting. For example, according to a study in London involving 395 participants, individuals whose first use of heroin was intravenous had a 4.7-fold increased likelihood of progressing to daily heroin use within 1–3 weeks, compared with those whose first use was through inhalation or snorting (Hines et al. 2017).

Regarding additional terminology, although in clinical settings opioids are typically quantified by their weight in milligrams or as morphine equivalents, in street slang, heroin is frequently described as "bags" or "stamp bags," "bundles," and "bricks." Although exact measurements are often unclear, a bag is typically a small bag containing a quantity of heroin about the size of a person's smallest (pinkie) fingernail, or roughly 50–100 mg; a bundle is 10 bags; and a brick is 50 bags. Bags often have their "brand name" stamped on them, hence the reason they are sometimes referred to as stamp bags.

"Cutting" With Fentanyl and Carfentanil

As previously mentioned, heroin supply in the United States has been increasingly adulterated with synthetic opioids, such as fentanyl and carfentanil. These synthetic opioids, unlike heroin, can be manufactured without opium, and the removal of this agricultural restriction allows supplies of street drugs to keep up with the unfortunately growing demand. According to data from the DEA, law enforcement reports of finding heroin that tested positive for fentanyl increased by 1,400% from 2013 to 2015; also, according to preliminary data from the Office of National Drug Control Policy, fentanyl originating from China increased by 426% from 2015 to 2016 (Miltenburg 2018). Although producing or selling fentanyl or its analogues became illegal in China after March 2017 (Miltenburg 2018), these analogues continue to be widely manufactured and can still be found through illicit sources, such as the darknet (i.e., private or restricted computer networks). Cutting with the cheaper and more potent fentanyl allows for greater potency per volume of heroin product that is trafficked and sold; for example, 1 kg of fentanyl mixed into heroin can produce about 10 kg of "cut heroin," yielding about $2 million (instead of $200,000) per kilogram of heroin (Miltenburg 2018). The concentration of various synthesis by-products and adulterants can help identify the drug's country of origin.

Whereas fentanyl may be 50–100 times more potent than morphine, other analogues, such as carfentanil (intended for use in large nonhuman animals), may be up to 10,000 times as potent, thus making these particular adulterants extremely dangerous even with one-time use. A 2016 search found 118 darknet websites selling carfentanil, with mail shipments ranging from $800 to $2,500 per kilogram (Misailidi et al. 2018). Thus, with recently increased public access to fentanyl analogues such as carfentanil, researchers and clinicians have called for more toxicology screening and advanced analytic testing specific to these analogues, as well as adherence to guidelines regarding investigating deaths. Screening tests using gas chromatography and enzyme-linked immunosorbent assay (ELISA) that detect fentanyl analogues, including carfentanil and even ocfentanil—which has also recently been involved in lethal intoxication cases—have recently been developed (Misailidi et al. 2018).

Some proposed harm reduction strategies attempt to manage the consequences of dangerous, high-potency synthetic adulterants. One strategy focuses on detection through rapid testing at the point of use, such as drug-checking services (also known as pill testing or adulterant screening), which helps people who use opioids to avoid ingesting harmful adulterants. Supervised injection facilities have also been suggested as a way to reduce the risk of fatal overdose (Ciccarone 2017).

Heroin Addiction

Although heroin addiction is not a distinct diagnosis in the *Diagnostic and Statistical Manual of Mental Disorders*, Fifth Edition (DSM-5; American Psychiatric Association 2013), it is essentially subsumed under opioid use disorder, which is formally defined as "a problematic pattern of opioid use leading to clinically significant impairment or distress" as manifested by at least two of the criteria listed in Box 3–1 occurring within a 12-month period. The terms *opioid abuse* and *opioid dependence* were separately defined in DSM-IV (American Psychiatric Association 1994) but have now been combined into the single diagnosis of OUD. Nonetheless, terms such as *abuse, addiction, misuse, overuse,* and *dependence* are still used clinically and in scientific literature but may be vague and generally require further clarification depending on the context. In this section, we use the term *addiction* interchangeably with *OUD*.

BOX 3–1. Diagnostic Criteria, Opioid Use Disorder

A. A problematic pattern of opioid use leading to clinically significant impairment or distress, as manifested by at least two of the following, occurring within a 12-month period:

  1. Opioids are often taken in larger amounts or over a longer period than was intended.
  2. There is a persistent desire or unsuccessful efforts to cut down or control opioid use.
  3. A great deal of time is spent in activities necessary to obtain the opioid, use the opioid, or recover from its effects.
  4. Craving, or a strong desire or urge to use opioids.
  5. Recurrent opioid use resulting in a failure to fulfill major role obligations at work, school, or home.
  6. Continued opioid use despite having persistent or recurrent social or interpersonal problems caused or exacerbated by the effects of opioids.
  7. Important social, occupational, or recreational activities are given up or reduced because of opioid use.
  8. Recurrent opioid use in situations in which it is physically hazardous.
  9. Continued opioid use despite knowledge of having a persistent or recurrent physical or psychological problem that is likely to have been caused or exacerbated by the substance.
  10. Tolerance, as defined by either of the following:
     a. A need for markedly increased amounts of opioids to achieve intoxication or desired effect.

    b. A markedly diminished effect with continued use of the same amount of an opioid.

Note: This criterion is not considered to be met for those taking opioids solely under appropriate medical supervision.

11. Withdrawal, as manifested by either of the following:

    a. The characteristic opioid withdrawal syndrome (refer to Criteria A and B of the criteria set for opioid withdrawal).

    b. Opioids (or a closely related substance) are taken to relieve or avoid withdrawal symptoms.

Note: This criterion is not considered to be met for those individuals taking opioids solely under appropriate medical supervision.

Specify if:

In early remission: After full criteria for opioid use disorder were previously met, none of the criteria for opioid use disorder have been met for at least 3 months but for less than 12 months (with the exception that Criterion A4, "Craving, or a strong desire or urge to use opioids," may be met).

In sustained remission: After full criteria for opioid use disorder were previously met, none of the criteria for opioid use disorder have been met at any time during a period of 12 months or longer (with the exception that Criterion A4, "Craving, or a strong desire or urge to use opioids," may be met).

Specify if:

On maintenance therapy: This additional specifier is used if the individual is taking a prescribed agonist medication such as methadone or buprenorphine and none of the criteria for opioid use disorder have been met for that class of medication (except tolerance to, or withdrawal from, the agonist). This category also applies to those individuals being maintained on a partial agonist, an agonist/antagonist, or a full antagonist such as oral naltrexone or depot naltrexone.

In a controlled environment: This additional specifier is used if the individual is in an environment where access to opioids is restricted.

Note. For specific coding and coding notes for opioid withdrawal in DSM-5, visit www.PsychiatryOnline.org for the free DSM-5 Update.

Source. Adapted from American Psychiatric Association: *Diagnostic and Statistical Manual of Mental Disorders*, 5th Edition. Arlington, VA, American Psychiatric Association, 2013. Copyright © 2013 American Psychiatric Association. Used with permission.

Epidemiology and Current Trends

According to data from the NSDUH, about 517,000 people were *dependent on or abused heroin* (i.e., had an OUD related to heroin) in 2013, which was about 0.2% of the U.S. population age 12 or older and represents 8% of all individuals who had a substance use disorder. Of the 2.2 million Americans age 12 or older receiving treatment for a problem related to illicit drug use, about 526,000 people, or 24%, indicated they received treatment for heroin use in the past year. Overall, the number of individuals age 12 years and older who reported using heroin in the past year increased by 83% from 2007 to 2013 (Lipari and Hughes 2015). According to the Centers for Disease Control and Prevention, past-year heroin use rates in 2011–2013 were highest among males and persons ages 18–25 years and those having an annual household income of less than $20,000, living in urban settings, and having no health insurance. Although rates of use increased in almost all demographic groups, they notably doubled among females and among non-Hispanic whites (Jones et al. 2015). Particularly concerning are the perceptions about and availability of heroin among adolescents. Whereas 82% of people in the general population perceived great risk in trying heroin only once or twice, only 58% of individuals ages 12–17 perceived it as a great risk. Furthermore, 15% of all individuals age 12 and older reported it would be "very easy" or "fairly easy" to obtain heroin, and specifically 1 in 11 adolescents ages 12–17 thought it would be "very easy" or "fairly easy" to obtain it (Lipari and Hughes 2015).

The current prevalence of heroin use and addiction is likely due to a confluence of factors. For example, numerous commentaries have pointed toward the relationship between the increasing availability of prescription opioids and heroin use. According to pooled data from 2002 to 2011, fewer than 1 in 27 people who misused opioids (the study formally refers to this misuse as "nonmedical pain reliever use," which the NSDUH defines as "use of drugs that were not prescribed for the respondent or used only for the experience or feeling they caused") started using heroin within 5 years after initiating their misuse of opioids (Muhuri et al. 2013). Moreover, whereas past-year heroin use was 19 times higher among those who had ever misused opioids than among those who had not, and an overwhelming majority (almost 80%) of people who had previously used heroin had also misused opioids, only about 1% of people who misused opioids in the past year had previously used heroin. Thus, although there is a strong association between opioid misuse and initiation of heroin use, most who misuse prescription opioids do not progress to using heroin. Certainly, increased prescribing of and access to opioid pain medications are concerning, but these factors alone may not account for the increased rates of heroin use, and addressing heroin use and addiction will likely require a multipronged approach.

Tolerance and Withdrawal

As described in the section "Heroin Use," the use of heroin is strongly reinforced by its pharmacology, including its almost immediate effects on opioid receptors, especially when the drug is administered intravenously. This reinforcement may be due to a combination of behavioral and physiological factors. Opioid tolerance is more likely to develop as the effects of opioids have a decreased intensity and shortened duration on the person using the opioid, thus often requiring the person to use more of the substance to achieve the desired effect. Unfortunately, the body's tolerance to euphoria is generally quicker than its tolerance to respiratory depression; therefore, an individual may continue increasing the amount of his or her use to achieve the intended rush or high, without recognizing the increased risk of developing respiratory depression. On a cellular level, tolerance may be due to phosphorylation of the opioid receptors, which alters their normal function, or it may be due to a downregulation of the number of opioid receptors on the cell (Williams et al. 2013). Various biological factors, such as genetics, also play a role in an individual's pharmacokinetics.

Physiological dependence results after repeated administration of high doses of heroin and necessitates continued administration of the drug to prevent withdrawal, which often begins within a few hours of the last heroin dose. In addition to formal DSM-5 diagnostic criteria for opioid withdrawal (see criteria in Chapter 9, "Opioid Withdrawal Management and Transition to Treatment"), withdrawal symptoms seen clinically include restlessness, drug cravings, cold flashes, gooseflesh skin, and bone pain; symptoms peak about 48–72 hours after the last heroin use (Hosztafi 2011). The idiom "kicking the habit" originated from the muscle spasms and leg movements experienced during opioid withdrawal (Pierce and Vanderschuren 2010). Although opioid withdrawal symptoms typically are not life threatening and resolve after about 1 week, they are very uncomfortable and create a vulnerable period for relapse. Furthermore, people who use heroin chronically may experience protracted feelings of withdrawal, including nausea and depressed mood. Thus, treatment interventions (discussed in Chapters 8–11) become critical for individuals with heroin dependence, especially those who are experiencing withdrawal.

Comorbidity

Polysubstance use is very common among individuals who use heroin. In 2013, about 96% of those using heroin reported using at least one other drug during the past year, and 61% reported using at least three different drugs. The percentage of people who used heroin and also illicitly used prescribed opioid medications doubled from about 21% in 2002–2004 to about 45% in 2011–2013. About one in three people who used heroin had alcohol use disorder, one in four had cannabis use disorder, and one in four had cocaine use disorder (Jones et al. 2015). Significant other comorbidities among individuals who inject opioids include infections such as hepatitis A, B, and C; human immunodeficiency virus (HIV); and bacterial endocarditis. Additionally, psychiatric conditions, such as depressive disorders, posttraumatic stress disorder, and antisocial personality disorder, are more common among those with OUD. Conduct disorder in youth has particularly been identified as a significant risk factor for later opioid use and addiction. OUD is also often associated with criminal activity, such as possession and distribution of drugs, forgery, and robbery, and its detrimental impact on sociooccupational functioning, as in Liam's case, is unfortunately common (American Psychiatric Association 2013).

Heroin Overdose

Broadly, the concept of opioid overdose is straightforward: a dose in excess of an individual's physiological limits leads to acute opioid toxicity, resulting in possible symptoms and consequences that range from depressed mental status and mild respiratory depression to hypoxia and death. Moreover, it is important to note that the term *overdose* can refer to both fatal and nonfatal overdoses, and nonfatal overdoses can still carry with them significant consequences. However, *overdose* is an imprecise term and can also refer to complicated and multifactorial presentations, including polydrug use. For example, many deaths attributed to heroin overdose might actually be due to polypharmacy, because other CNS depressants are commonly detected in heroin overdose victims (Darke and Hall 2003). Thus, it should be kept in mind that the term *heroin overdose* may sometimes refer to these more complex presentations, such as Liam's coadministration of heroin and an unknown pill (likely a sedative-hypnotic).

Morbidity and Mortality

CNS control of breathing is localized in three main groups of neurons in the brain stem, and opioid drugs exert an effect at several sites within that system to depress neuronal activity, which leads to decreased tidal volume and respiratory frequency (White and Irvine 1999). At peripheral chemoreceptors, the inhibitory activity of opioids acts to diminish sensitivity to oxygen and carbon dioxide. The combined effect of these central and peripheral factors is depression of overall respiratory function and, when severe enough, hypoxia and death. These factors may be influenced by individual differences, such as variations in drug metabolism. Heroin in particular is subject to significant individual differences; it has several active metabolites, as described in the section "Heroin Use," so there is a significant potential for large variation in drug effect due to interindividual differences in metabolism.

Although the term *heroin overdose* often invokes the notion of fatal overdose, nonfatal overdoses are also clinically significant. Nonfatal overdose is extremely common among individuals who use heroin, with 50% or more of cross-sectional samples of heroin users reporting a history of overdose, usually on multiple occasions (Darke and Hall 2003). Overdose is a difficult phenomenon to study, and researchers have found wide variability in overdose prevalence. A worldwide systematic review found that the lifetime prevalence of personally experiencing a nonfatal overdose among people who use drugs ranged from 16.6% to 68.0%, with a mean of 45.4%, highlighting just how common overdose is in this population (Martins et al. 2015). Nonfatal overdoses can have major consequences; in one sample of people who experienced a nonfatal overdose, 33% required hospital treatment for overdose and 14% experienced overdose-related complications of sufficient severity that they had to be admitted to a hospital ward, rather than undergo the usual procedure of being treated in an emergency department and then discharged (Warner-Smith et al. 2002).

In terms of specific physiological consequences, nonfatal overdoses expose victims to high risk of morbidity in multiple physiological systems. Pulmonary conditions are the most common complications of overdose, of which the most widely reported is pulmonary edema, a buildup of fluid in the lungs (Warner-Smith et al. 2001). Pulmonary edema has a good prognosis when medical care is available—the condition usually resolves within a matter of days—but it may leave residual impairment, and it exposes individuals who use heroin to a higher risk of pneumonia (the risk of which can also be magnified by aspiration of vomit following an overdose). Furthermore, the residual pulmonary dysfunction increases the chances of dying from respiratory depression after any subsequent heroin overdoses.

Nonfatal overdose is also associated with rhabdomyolysis, which, although rarer than pulmonary edema, can also be very serious. Rhabdomyolysis is a breakdown of skeletal muscle, leading to the release of its products (such as the protein myoglobin) into the blood and urine, which can damage the kidneys and cause other systemic problems. This condition is usually associated with "crush injuries," but it is often described in people who use heroin, occurring as the result of limb compression by another part of their body while they were comatose. Rhabdomyolysis can lead to permanent muscular impairment and diminished renal function.

Heroin overdose is also associated with a wide range of cardiac complications, including potentially fatal arrhythmia and cardiomyopathy (Ghuran and Nolan 2000). Finally, hypoxia during an overdose has the potential to cause significant neurological damage. Nonfatal overdose is associated with cognitive impairment, and people who use heroin long term are likely to have a significant burden of cognitive morbidity proportional to their nonfatal overdose experience, leading to a potential vicious cycle in which older individuals suffer from neurologically based impaired decision making (Warner-Smith et al. 2001).

Risk Factors for Heroin Overdose

A long history of research into heroin overdose has identified a range of risk factors for fatal and nonfatal overdoses (Darke and Hall 2003). Route of administration is of chief importance: although there are documented fatal heroin overdoses by smoking, oral ingestion, and nasal ingestion, injection is associated with substantially increased risk of death. Purity level of heroin may be only moderately related to overdose deaths. Contrary to some popular assumptions, fatal heroin overdoses are more common in individuals with long-term dependence than in young and heroin-naïve individuals. Individuals who experience fatal overdose typically have a 10-year history of heroin use (Darke and Hall 2003).

As mentioned above, the term *overdose* is not necessarily limited to the use of heroin alone, even when heroin appears to be a person's primary substance. Perhaps the most significant finding regarding risk factors for fatal heroin overdose is that the overwhelming majority of overdoses involve the consumption of heroin with other drugs (Darke and Hall 2003). The major drugs associated with an increased risk of overdose are alcohol and benzodiazepines.

A key complication regarding heroin overdose is the recent trend of contamination or cutting of heroin with high-potency, nonpharmaceutical (i.e., illicitly manufactured) synthetic opioids such as fentanyl, carfentanil, and other fentanyl analogues (Butler et al. 2017). Although it has long been standard practice to cut illicit heroin with a wide variety of substitutes and adulterants, it is increasingly common for synthetic opioids to be used in this way. Synthetic opioids are generally more potent than heroin, and accordingly overdose deaths involving fentanyl and other synthetic analogues more than doubled from 2015 to 2016 (National Vital Statistics System 2017). As described in previous sections, many synthetic opioids are even more potent than fentanyl. For example, carfentanil can be 5,000 times as potent as heroin and 100 times as potent as fentanyl. Some synthetic opioids may even be absorbed through the skin, leading to concerns for first responders (e.g., emergency personnel and police), who may "overdose" after casual contact with powders or paraphernalia or through accidental inhalation.

Recognizing, Treating, and Preventing Overdose

Opioid intoxication is traditionally described as the triad of depressed level of consciousness, miotic (constricted) pupils, and decreased respiration (Sporer 1999). More recently, opioid intoxication has also been diagnosed by response to naloxone, a competitive opioid receptor antagonist. The attraction of using naloxone to confirm opioid intoxication comes from the sometimes challenging differential diagnosis of opioid intoxication, which may include intoxication on sedative-hypnotics, alcohol, and other CNS depressants. However, some clinical studies have suggested that using a naloxone challenge does not help diagnosis and may actually worsen the sensitivity for making a diagnosis of acute opioid intoxication. In one study, using clinical criteria alone to diagnose opioid overdose had a sensitivity of 92% and specificity of 76%, and adding a complete naloxone response to the clinical criteria resulted in a sensitivity of 86% and a specificity of 97%; in other words, naloxone may lead to more false negatives and missed diagnoses of overdose (Hoffman and Goldfrank 1995). A careful history, physical examination, and laboratory studies are paramount for diagnosing acute heroin overdose.

The assessment and treatment of possible acute heroin overdose begin with attention to the adequacy of ventilation. Many patients have inadequate respiration and need bag-valve-mask ventilation. Intubation is avoided except when patients are unable to ventilate adequately with bag-valve-mask ventilation or when they are oxygenating poorly despite adequate ventilation. All patients requiring ventilation support are treated with parenteral naloxone therapy. Naloxone can be administered through a variety of means, but in a clinical setting, the parenteral route is preferred because nasal, subcutaneous, and intramuscular routes of administration are associated with slower absorption. The proper dose of naloxone is a matter of some debate, with sources from different fields recommending a relatively wide range of doses. Some recent evidence suggests that a low initial dose (0.04 mg) followed by careful dose titration is sufficient and may help avoid complications from severe acute precipitated withdrawal, such as pulmonary edema and dangerous agitation (Kim and Nelson 2016). That said, in practice, apneic patients are often given a much higher starting dose. Regardless, naloxone is titrated with an end goal of adequate ventilation (i.e., not a normal level of consciousness). Although recommended observation periods can vary, patients with a complete naloxone response are typically observed for 4–6 hours for complications or for reemergence of sedation, and naloxone is repeated for clinically significant hypoventilation.

Of course, the preceding discussion assumes a certain level of access to medical supplies, as would be found in emergency departments or other hospital-based settings. There has also been significant recent attention to the community prevention and reversal of overdose, particularly through the distribution of home doses of naloxone. In recent years, several countries and U.S. jurisdictions have implemented plans to make take-home emergency doses of naloxone more available. In one survey of 140 U.S. organizations from 1996 through June 2014, naloxone kits were provided to 152,283 laypersons, and the organizations received reports of 26,463 overdose reversals (Wheeler et al. 2015). A meta-analysis also found that bystander administration of naloxone was associated with significantly increased odds of recovery compared with no naloxone administration (odds ratio = 8.58; 95% confidence interval, 3.90–13.25) (Giglio et al. 2015). Additionally, jurisdictions have enacted a variety of clarifications and other legal protections to attempt to enable resuscitation by members of the public (Strang et al. 2014). Nonetheless, community use and availability of naloxone continue to vary greatly depending on local public health and legislative efforts, and research on these efforts and outcomes is still developing.

Naloxone reversal is not the only prevention effort, however, and several other policy strategies have been attempted to reduce rates of lethal overdoses (Darke and Hall 2003). Because lack of engagement in treatment and other drug use are both strong risk factors for overdose deaths, one important prevention effort is to increase treatment enrollment, which, of course, aims not only to reduce lethal overdoses but also to detect and reduce the harm from OUD in general. Other harm reduction methods have also been attempted, such as supervised injection rooms and, outside the United States, medically supervised heroin maintenance (also known as heroin-assisted treatment, in which people with severe OUD receive regulated and controlled prescriptions of heroin). Additionally, more states are considering various legal strategies, such as court-ordered treatment, for these disorders. These methods are currently subject to ongoing debate.

Key Chapter Points

▶ Currently, worldwide, most opium is produced and distributed illicitly. The two major regions involved are the Golden Crescent (including parts of Afghanistan, Iran, and Pakistan) and the Golden Triangle (including parts of Myanmar [Burma], Laos, and Thailand). In 2014, Afghanistan produced about 80% of the world's illicit opium and heroin, the Golden Triangle produced about 10%, and Mexico and Colombia produced about 5%, and another 40 or so countries combined produced about 5%.

▶ Opium and its derivatives are classified as naturally occurring, semisynthetic, or synthetic and are collectively termed *opioids*. Their mechanism of action is generally via stimulating μ, δ, and κ opioid receptors, with a wide range of effects, including analgesia, euphoria, sedation, and respiratory depression. Many opioids have been discovered and synthesized over the past 200 years, and they have varying properties with regard to potency and duration of action.

▶ The reported lifetime prevalence of heroin use in the United States has increased from 0.33% in 2001–2002 to 1.6% in 2012–2013. The number of individuals age 12 years and older who reported using heroin in the past year has increased by 83% from 2007 to 2013. In 2013, an estimated 681,000 people used heroin, of whom 169,000 (including 21,000 adolescents) used heroin for the first time. This represents about 460 people initiating heroin use daily, with the average age of first use about 24 years old.

▶ Individuals who use heroin have significant comorbidities with regard to other substance use disorders. Individuals who inject opioids are at significant risk for infections such as hepatitis C virus, HIV, and bacterial endocarditis. Psychiatric conditions, such as depressive disorders, posttraumatic stress disorder, and antisocial personality disorder, are more common among those with OUD.

▶ Overdose is a complicated phenomenon, and often arises from the combined effects of polydrug use. Clinicians must take great care in the evaluation and treatment of suspected overdoses.

References

American Psychiatric Association: Diagnostic and Statistical Manual of Mental Disorders, 4th Edition. Washington, DC, American Psychiatric Association, 1994

American Psychiatric Association: Diagnostic and Statistical Manual of Mental Disorders, 5th Edition. Arlington, VA, American Psychiatric Association, 2013

Blakemore PR, White JD: Morphine, the Proteus of organic molecules. Chem Commun (Camb) (11):1159–1168, 2002 12109065

Brook K, Bennett J, Desai SP: The chemical history of morphine: an 8000-year journey, from resin to de-novo synthesis. J Anesth Hist 3(2):50–55, 2017 28641826

Butler DC, Shanks K, Behonick GS, et al: Three cases of fatal acrylfentanyl toxicity in the United States and a review of literature. J Anal Toxicol 42(1):e6–e11, 2017 29036502

Ciccarone D: Fentanyl in the U.S. heroin supply: a rapidly changing risk environment. Int J Drug Policy 46:107–111, 2017 28735776

Clark PA, Sillup GP, Capo JA: Afghanistan, poppies, and the global pain crisis. Med Sci Monit 16(3):RA49–RA57, 2010 20190697

Darke S, Hall W: Heroin overdose: research and evidence-based intervention. J Urban Health 80(2):189–200, 2003 12791795

Drug Enforcement Administration: Final rule: authorized sources of narcotic raw materials. February 6, 2008. Available at: https://www.deadiversion.usdoj.gov/fed_regs/rules/2008/fr0206.htm. Accessed March 29, 2018.

Drug Enforcement Administration: Controlled substance schedules. 2018. Available at: https://www.deadiversion.usdoj.gov/schedules/. Accessed January 9, 2018.

Duarte DF: Opium and opioids: a brief history [in Portuguese]. Rev Bras Anestesiol 55(1):135–146, 2005 19471817

Ghuran A, Nolan J: Recreational drug misuse: issues for the cardiologist. Heart 83(6):627–633, 2000 10814617

Giglio RE, Li G, DiMaggio CJ: Effectiveness of bystander naloxone administration and overdose education programs: a meta-analysis. Inj Epidemiol 2(1):10, 2015 27747742

Greenfield VA, Bond CA, Crane K: A household model of opium-poppy cultivation in Afghanistan. J Policy Model 39(5):741–761, 2017

Herzberg D: Entitled to addiction? Pharmaceuticals, race, and America's first drug war. Bull Hist Med 91(3):586–623, 2017 29081434

Hines LA, Lynskey M, Morley KI, et al: The relationship between initial route of heroin administration and speed of transition to daily heroin use. Drug Alcohol Rev 36(5):633–638, 2017 28470826

Hoffman RS, Goldfrank LR: The poisoned patient with altered consciousness: controversies in the use of a "coma cocktail." JAMA 274(7):562–569, 1995 7629986

Hosztafi S: The history of heroin [in Hungarian]. Acta Pharm Hung 71(2):233–242, 2001 11862675

Hosztafi S: Heroin addiction [in Hungarian]. Acta Pharm Hung 81(4):173–183, 2011 22329304

Huecker MR, Marraffa J: Heroin. Treasure Island, FL, StatPearls Publishing, 2017

Hughes A, Williams MR, Lipari RN, et al: Prescription drug use and misuse in the United States: results from the 2015 National Survey on Drug Use and Health. NSDUH Data Review. September 2016. Available at: www.sam-hsa.gov/data/sites/default/files/NSDUH-FFR2-2015/NSDUH-FFR2-2015.htm. Accessed January 11, 2018.

Jones CM, Logan J, Gladden RM, et al: Vital signs: demographic and substance use trends among heroin users—United States, 2002–2013. MMWR Morb Mortal Wkly Rep 64(26):719–725, 2015 26158353

Kim HK, Nelson LS: Reversal of opioid-induced ventilatory depression using low-dose naloxone (0.04 mg): a case series. J Med Toxicol 12(1):107–110, 2016 26289651

Lipari RN, Hughes A: Trends in heroin use in the United States: 2002 to 2013. The CBHSQ Report, April 23, 2015. Available at: https://www.samhsa.gov/data/sites/default/files/report_1943/ShortReport-1943.html. Accessed March 29, 2018.

Lutz PE, Kieffer BL: Opioid receptors: distinct roles in mood disorders. Trends Neurosci 36(3):195–206, 2013 23219016

Martins SS, Sampson L, Cerdá M, et al: Worldwide prevalence and trends in unintentional drug overdose: a systematic review of the literature. Am J Public Health 105(11):e29–e49, 2015 26451760

Martins SS, Sarvet A, Santaella-Tenorio J, et al: Changes in U.S. lifetime heroin use and heroin use disorder: prevalence from the 2001–2002 to 2012–2013 National Epidemiologic Survey on Alcohol and Related Conditions. JAMA Psychiatry 74(5):445–455, 2017 28355458

Miltenburg J: Supply chains for illicit products: case study of the global opiate production networks. Cogent Business & Management 5:1423871, 2018

Misailidi N, Papoutsis I, Nikolaou P, et al: Fentanyls continue to replace heroin in the drug arena: the cases of ocfentanil and carfentanil. Forensic Toxicol 36(1):12–32, 2018 29367860

Muhuri PK, Gfroerer JC, Davies MC; Substance Abuse and Mental Health Services Administration: Associations of nonmedical pain reliever use and initiation of heroin use in the United States. CBHSQ Data Review. Available at: https://www.samhsa.gov/data/sites/default/files/DR006/DR006/nonmedical-pain-reliever-use-2013.htm. August 2013. Accessed December 12, 2017.

National Institutes of Health, National Library of Medicine: Drug record. Fentanyl and analogues: alfentanil, remifentanil, sufentanil. 2018. Available at: https://livertox.nlm.nih.gov//FentanylAndAnalogues.htm. Accessed January 11, 2018.

National Vital Statistics System: Drug overdose deaths in the United States, 1999–2016, Data table for Figure 4: Age-adjusted drug overdose death rates, by opioid category: United States, 1999–2016. NCHS Data Brief No 294, December 2017. Available at: https://www.cdc.gov/nchs/data/databriefs/ db294_table.pdf. Accessed December 21, 2017.

Pierce RC, Vanderschuren LJ: Kicking the habit: the neural basis of ingrained behaviors in cocaine addiction. Neurosci Biobehav Rev 35(2):212–219, 2010 20097224

Qiao Y, Han K, Zhan CG: Reaction pathways and free energy profiles for cholinesterase-catalyzed hydrolysis of 6-monoacetylmorphine. Org Biomol Chem 12(14):2214–2227, 2014 24595354

Seecof R, Tennant FS Jr: Subjective perceptions to the intravenous "rush" of heroin and cocaine in opioid addicts. Am J Drug Alcohol Abuse 12(1–2):79–87, 1986 3788901

Sneader W: The discovery of heroin. Lancet 352(9141):1697–1699, 1998 9853457

Sporer KA: Acute heroin overdose. Ann Intern Med 130(7):584–590, 1999 10189329

Staub C, Marset M, Mino A, et al: Detection of acetylcodeine in urine as an indicator of illicit heroin use: method validation and results of a pilot study. Clin Chem 47(2):301–307, 2001 11159779

Stimmel B: The Facts About Drug Use: Coping With Drugs and Alcohol in Your Family, at Work, in Your Community. Binghamton, NY, Hawthorne Medical Press, 1992

Strang J, Bird SM, Dietze P, et al: Take-home emergency naloxone to prevent deaths from heroin overdose (editorial). BMJ 349:g6580, 2014 25378248

United Nations Office on Drugs and Crime: Afghanistan opium survey 2017: cultivation and production. November 2017. Available at: https:// www.unodc.org/documents/crop-monitoring/Afghanistan/Afghan _opium_survey_2017_cult_prod_web.pdf. Accessed December 12, 2017.

U.S. Department of Health and Human Services: Prescription opioid and heroin abuse, testimony by Nora Volkow, MD, Director, National Institute on Drug Abuse. National Institutes of Health, 2014. Available at: https:// www.drugabuse.gov/about-nida/legislative-activities/testimony-to-congress/2014/prescription-opioid-heroin-abuse. Accessed December 12, 2017.

Volkow ND, Collins FS: The role of science in addressing the opioid crisis. N Engl J Med 377(4):391–394, 2017 28564549

Warner-Smith M, Darke S, Lynskey M, et al: Heroin overdose: causes and consequences. Addiction 96(8):1113–1125, 2001 11487418

Warner-Smith M, Darke S, Day C: Morbidity associated with non-fatal heroin overdose. Addiction 97(8):963–967, 2002 12144598

Wheeler E, Jones TS, Gilbert MK, et al; Centers for Disease Control and Prevention: Opioid overdose prevention programs providing naloxone to laypersons—United States, 2014. MMWR Morb Mortal Wkly Rep 64(23):631–635, 2015 26086633

White JM, Irvine RJ: Mechanisms of fatal opioid overdose. Addiction 94(7):961–972, 1999 10707430

White House Council of Economic Advisers: The underestimated cost of the opioid crisis. November 2017. Available at: https://www.whitehouse.gov/sites/whitehouse.gov/files/images/The%20Underestimated%20Cost%20of%20the%20Opioid%20Crisis.pdf. Accessed January 8, 2018.

Williams J: Basic opioid pharmacology. Rev Pain 1(2):2–5, 2008 26524987

Williams JT, Ingram SL, Henderson G, et al: Regulation of μ-opioid receptors: desensitization, phosphorylation, internalization, and tolerance. Pharmacol Rev 65(1):223–254, 2013 23321159

4

Opioid Overdose, Toxicity, and Poisoning

Nathan M. Kunzler, M.D.
Katherine Devin, M.D.
Kavita Babu, M.D.
Edward W. Boyer, M.D., Ph.D.

Clinical Vignette: A Quick Emergency Department Visit

A 31-year-old woman walked into the emergency department (ED); at intake, she said to the triage nurse, "I don't feel so..." and, mid sentence, abruptly lost consciousness. The nurse immediately took the patient back to the treatment area. Her vital signs were notable for a temperature of 99°F, a pulse of 96 beats per minute, a blood pressure of 110/65 mm Hg, and a respiratory rate of 4 breaths per minute. On physical examination, the patient was comatose and unresponsive; she had miosis and crackles on lung auscultation. An intravenous catheter was placed and a dose of naloxone 0.04 mg was administered, resulting in moderate improvement in respiratory rate and consciousness. Upon awakening, the woman adamantly denied illicit drug use, particularly heroin, despite the presence of track marks and other signs of recent injection on her skin. She demanded to be discharged from the ED, but the supervising physician persuaded her to remain as a patient under care. In the midst of the discussion, she again lost consciousness and became apneic. Escalating doses of naloxone were administered intravenously until a total dose of 10 mg had been administered. When this amount of naloxone failed to reverse the presumed overdose, the attending physician decided to perform orotracheal intubation and admit the patient to the intensive care unit. Only when she was intubated were clinicians able to obtain blood and urine for laboratory analysis.

Initially, the patient required no sedation. Approximately 20 minutes following intubation, however, she became so agitated that she needed propofol for behavioral control. When propofol failed to provide control, the attending physician elected to extubate the patient. She again demanded to be discharged, but she finally agreed to remain for a brief period of observation. The woman, however, absconded, only to arrive again with opioid overdose 10 hours after leaving the ED.

A qualitative screen for drugs of abuse in urine (i.e., a toxicology screen) revealed the presence of monoacetylmorphine, but a dedicated opioid panel also identified codeine, morphine, and fentanyl. Liquid chromatography/mass spectroscopy, however, confirmed the presence of furanylfentanyl. Notably, during the patient's second presentation, she complained of a sore throat and demanded oxycodone for treatment.

The rising tide of deaths associated with opioid overdose impels us to understand several important questions, such as the following: Which individuals are most affected by the opioid epidemic? How does opioid overdose happen? What is the natural history of opioid overdose? Does the clinical presentation of overdose vary across the different opioids? How should opioid overdose be managed? Finally, what pitfalls or special considerations threaten patient outcomes?

Epidemiology of Opioid Overdose

Outbreaks of opioid overdose are not new; however, the breadth and scale of opioid overdose as of late are new. Opiates (and later opioids more generally) first gained popularity in the United States, mostly in California, in the 1890s with the use of opium. Although morphine was a popular choice among soldiers being mustered out of service, heroin use also began to emerge. The recognition of the addictive potential of opioids culminated in the criminalization of heroin in the Anti-Heroin Act of 1924 (P.L. 68-274).

Although misuse of opioids has been a problem for many decades, the past few decades have seen an astonishing increase in the levels of opioid analgesic prescribing, as well as in deaths associated with their use, misuse, and abuse. This increase in prescribing and use may have arisen from changing attitudes about pain management, aggressive (or illegal) marketing by pharmaceutical companies, shifting opinions about addiction, and increasingly sophisticated organic chemistry synthesis capacities of illicit drug manufacturers. Between 1999 and 2010, the amount of opioid analgesics prescribed by physicians tripled (Guy et al. 2017). In 2012, providers wrote 259 million prescriptions for opioid pain relievers, more than enough to give an opioid prescription to every American adult (Centers for Disease Control and Prevention 2014). As the availability of prescription opioids has increased, so too has the use of heroin. The observed increase in heroin use may be driven by a "gateway effect," as demonstrated by the fact that four out of five individuals who initiated heroin use self-reported using prescription drugs first (Jones 2013). For instance, a 2014 survey of patients seeking treatment for heroin use or dependence showed that 94% chose to use heroin because prescription opioids were more expensive and difficult to obtain (Cicero et al. 2014). Therefore, much of the increased use of heroin occurring in recent years may have arisen from new restrictions in opioid prescribing practices adopted by health care systems and clinicians, or as a paradoxical result of new "abuse-deterrent" opioid formulations. For example, in 2010, when an abuse-deterrent formulation of extended-release oxycodone (OxyContin) entered clinical practice, heroin use increased because the new composition of OxyContin could be injected or insufflated only with great difficulty (Cicero and Ellis 2015). Recent data from the Centers for Disease Control and Prevention (CDC) underscore the magnitude of the current opioid epidemic. In 2015 alone, an estimated 12.5 million people misused prescription opioids and 33,091 people died from opioid overdose (Centers for Disease Control and Prevention 2017a). A 2016 CDC report showed that the number of people who have died from opioid overdoses had tripled since 2000 (Rudd et al. 2016).

Another important change is the demographics of those using opioids. In the 1960s, opioid abuse among whites and nonwhites occurred in nearly equal proportions; by 2015, however, 90% of those seeking treatment for opioid use disorders (OUDs) were white. A substantial proportion (84%) of overdose deaths occurred in whites as well. Men were much more likely to abuse heroin in the past, but the prevalence of heroin use is now nearly equal between men and women in treatment-seeking samples (Cicero et al. 2014). Drug use, misuse, and abuse have long been considered problems of large urban centers; however, recent data demonstrate that mortality from overdose is now roughly equal across urban and nonurban settings (Paulozzi and Xi 2008).

Certain groups are at greatly increased risk for overdose. For example, individuals either discharged from inpatient drug treatment or released from prison are at substantially higher risk for lethal overdose (Binswanger et al. 2007). This association was first identified in recently released inmates. In that population, incarceration was associated not only with greater all-cause mortality following release, but also with overdose mortality that occurred at a rate far higher than that in the general population (Binswanger et al. 2007). Excess mortality in these two groups may be due in part to loss of *tolerance*, the condition in which escalating doses of drug are needed to produce the same psychological and physical effects. Individuals who enter drug treatment or become incarcerated frequently have decreased exposure to opioids; as opioid use lessens, tolerance to opioids is lost. Relapse to drug use in a person who has lost tolerance potentially leads to fatal overdose, particularly if the individual uses the same amount of drug as when tolerance was higher.

Pathophysiology of Opioid Overdose

Opioids agonize a group of G protein–coupled transmembrane receptor molecules known as the μ, δ, and κ opioid receptors. Additional genetic diversity is derived from splicing, posttranslational modification, and the formation of heterodimers and homodimers (Waldhoer et al. 2004). Each class of opioid receptor can be activated by both endogenous and exogenous ligands. Excessive administration of a μ opioid receptor agonist leads to overdose.

Opioid receptors distributed throughout the body are responsible for producing the classic constellation of findings observed in overdose: miosis, bradypnea or apnea, and coma. Receptors found in the anterior and ventrolateral thalamus, the amygdala, and the dorsal root ganglion, which mediate nociception and analgesia, are responsible for the diminished consciousness of overdose (Stein 1995). Brain stem μ opioid receptors modulate the respiratory response of the body to both hypercarbia and hypoxemia and are therefore responsible for the hypopnea seen with opioid overdose. Agonism of receptors in the Edinger-Westphal nucleus of the oculomotor nerve affects pupillary constriction and leads to the typical miosis seen in opioid intoxication and overdose (Lalley 2008). Although not considered a cardinal feature of overdose, agonism of opioid receptors in the gut leads to decreased motility, constipation, and hypoactive bowel sounds.

Knockout mouse studies have shown that the μ receptor mediates both the analgesic effects of opioids and the dependence seen in chronic opioid use (Matthes et al. 1996). The physiology of tolerance is an important consideration in overdose. Tolerance develops via desensitization of the μ opioid receptor, which results in a progressive inability of the receptor to propagate a signal after binding. This occurs through uncoupling of the receptors from their cell surface membrane–linked G proteins and incorporation into intracellular compartments (Whistler 2012). Once intracellular, these receptors can be returned to the cell surface and used again for signaling. The process of endocytosis and recycling to the cellular surface is thought to modulate the ability of the body to develop tolerance.

Endogenous ligands, which as short polypeptides undergo rapid hydrolysis and inactivation, also exhibit diurnal variation in their concentration; these two processes enhance receptor recycling and prevent significant tolerance from developing. In contrast, exogenous ligands persist—and are present at relatively stable concentrations—in the extracellular matrix, where they can stimulate μ receptor signaling for a prolonged period of time. The persistent binding of these ligands is thought to blunt receptor cycling and desensitize the receptor itself (Whistler 2012). Tolerance to exogenous opioids is therefore believed to arise from decreased receptor recycling and desensitization of the receptors themselves to ligands. Tolerance can be reversed following periods of abstinence, and this reversal of tolerance can cause a higher risk of overdose and death from opioid use following abstinence.

Recent data on the signaling pathways of the μ opioid receptor have further delineated the specific mechanisms behind analgesia as well as respiratory depression from exogenous ligands. Notably, a small protein known as β-arrestin appears to mediate the respiratory effects of opioids by modulating internalization of the μ opioid receptor. This is in contrast to the analgesic effects of the μ receptor, which are thought to be mediated through the G protein–coupled mechanism of the μ receptor

(Manglik et al. 2016). Despite the interest in developing opioid ligands that signal through the G protein–coupled pathway while avoiding the β-arrestin pathway, a viable medication has not yet been produced.

Toxicokinetics of Overdose

When discussing overdose, an important distinction must be made between the pharmacokinetics and the toxicokinetics of a drug. Although a robust body of literature describing the pharmacokinetics of many opioid ligands exists, the data are limited to therapeutic dosing and, consequently, therapeutic blood concentrations of the drug. In contrast, overdose arises from administration of excessive doses of drug, which, in turn, lead to supratherapeutic concentrations of drug in the bloodstream, which have important clinical implications.

Most drugs, including opioid agonists, undergo hepatic enzymatic metabolism by first-order kinetics. This condition, in which a constant proportion of the drug is eliminated via enzymatic degradation over a given unit of time, occurs in therapeutic dosing. In overdose, however, the enzymes responsible for degrading a xenobiotic can be overwhelmed by the high concentration of substrate in the blood, a process known as *saturation*. When saturation occurs, enzyme kinetics transition from first order to zero order. An enzyme operating under zero-order kinetics clears a constant *amount* of a substance rather than a constant *proportion*. In other words, drugs remain at higher concentrations for longer periods of time than observed in therapeutic dosing.

This change in enzyme kinetics has two important clinical implications. First, poisoning may be more severe and more protracted than the effects expected in therapeutic dosing. Second, when processes become saturated, small additional amounts of a substance can lead to disproportionate increases in the serum concentration, as well as a longer duration over which substances remain in the blood. This can lead to significant dangers for patients who are already intoxicated.

Drug use behaviors can also contribute to aberrant toxicokinetics. For example, ingestion of a large number of pills can lead to bezoar formation in the stomach and intestinal tract. Absorption from bezoars is erratic, culminating in unpredictable spikes of exacerbated toxicity that may persist for prolonged periods of time. Other common drug use behaviors among individuals with OUD—including *insufflation* (i.e., snorting), injection of powder obtained by grinding oral tablet formulations, heating of opioid analgesic patches, application of multiple patches, and ingesting opioid analgesic patches or their contents—can lead to an increased rate of absorption compared with traditional kinetic models for these drugs. In addition, this increased rate of absorption is often highly variable. For example, people who abuse prescription opioids may have difficulty controlling how finely they grind tablets, and they may insufflate the drug at an inconsistent dose or rate. They may apply whatever number of patches are available, apply them to different parts of the body, or inconsistently heat the patches to accelerate absorption across the skin. Each of these and other similar conditions can lead to intra-user and inter-user variability, which contributes to unpredictable rates of absorption.

Clinical Manifestations of Opioid Overdose

Evaluation of the Overdose Patient: General Principles

Evaluation of the overdose patient should always begin with the cardinal ABCs, a thorough but efficient assessment of the airway, breathing, and circulation. Assessment of the airway begins with ensuring that the airway is patent and that there is no obstruction or impedance to air traveling into the lungs. Evaluation of breathing focuses on the patient's respiratory drive and whether the rate itself is increased or decreased. Assessment of the body's circulation includes evaluation of heart rate, blood pressure, and peripheral pulses/tissue perfusion.

After the patient is stabilized, a more thorough evaluation should be completed. Clinicians should note signs of intravenous drug use, patches applied to the body (including the mouth, scrotum, vagina, rectum, perineum, and axillae), and trauma. Clinicians should search belongings for empty pill bottles or drug paraphernalia, interview friends and family for pertinent information, and review available medical information. Part of this assessment should include an evaluation of suicidality; although many overdoses are inadvertent, many others are intentional and arise from suicidal ideation coupled with the lethal means provided by opioids.

The Opioid Toxic Patient

The opioid toxidrome consists of the triad of respiratory depression, central nervous system (CNS) depression, and miosis. Exceptions to this rule do exist and are discussed below. Also, clinicians should recognize that polypharmacy overdose can present with a mixed picture that may not include each feature.

Respiratory depression is the sine qua non of opioid poisoning (Boyer 2012). Although opioids affect all parameters of respiratory activity, the respiratory rate is the easiest for clinicians to evaluate at the bedside. A respiratory rate under 12 breaths per minute occurs in severe overdose, can progress to apnea without intervention, and can occur after intentional or unintentional overdose of prescribed medications (Boyer 2012). In addition to evaluating respiratory rate, clinicians should assess for other physical examination findings associated with respiratory insufficiency, such as cyanosis and decreased oxygen saturations. Each of these is a late finding and is not a substitute for evaluating the depth and frequency of breathing. The type of opioid, its dose, and the route of administration affect the severity of the respiratory depression. Pulmonary edema can be a significant contributor to decreased oxygen saturation in an overdose; pulmonary edema can present as crackles or rales on lung auscultation, or as pink, frothy sputum emanating from the nose (referred to as a "nose cone"), within the oropharynx, or in the endotracheal tube (Boyer 2012).

Another cardinal feature of the opioid-poisoned patient is CNS depression, the severity of which may range from mild somnolence to complete unresponsiveness. Because somnolence relies on the drug crossing the blood-brain barrier to bind to μ receptors, it is more prominent as the lipophilicity of the causative agent increases. Some μ opioid agonists do not cross the blood-brain barrier; for example, the antidiarrheal loperamide, a congener of methadone, has negligible CNS penetrance unless the ingested dose significantly exceeds recommended dosing. The lack of CNS depression does not rule out ingestion of an opioid, because use of multiple substances can include sympathomimetic agents that produce CNS stimulation.

Although the typical opioid-poisoned patient will exhibit CNS depression, a subset of patients may experience seizures. Convulsant activity is typically associated with the atypical opioid analgesics meperidine, tramadol, propoxyphene, and tapentadol (Boyer 2012). Administration of elevated doses of meperidine to patients with renal insufficiency causes the proconvulsant metabolite normeperidine to accumulate. Tramadol is unique in its ability to produce seizures (that occur without prodrome) at any point in the therapeutic arc: seizures may occur after initiation of tramadol therapy, after long-term administration, following overdose, or in the setting of routine therapeutic use. Hypoxia is another frequent cause of opioid-related seizures, due to brain injury caused by prolonged oxygen deprivation.

Miosis from opioid intoxication is often described as "pinpoint pupils," although this finding is not universal, particularly in patients who have ingested multiple substances. Importantly, miosis can also be caused by ingestion of other classes of substances (e.g., sedative-hypnotics, alcohol, clonidine, nicotine, decongestants such as oxymetazoline) and by medical conditions (e.g., coma, pontine hemorrhage) (Boyer 2012). Furthermore, the absence of miosis does not exclude opioid toxicity, and in the case of polypharmacy ingestion (e.g., opioid and cocaine), the other drug(s) may produce pupillary dilation. Overdose with tramadol, meperidine, or propoxyphene is associated with normally reactive pupils or even mydriasis.

Other Considerations

Aside from the subset of atypical opioid analgesics described in the previous subsection, intoxication from one opioid brings about a clinical appearance that is nearly identical to that associated with any other opioid; the major difference in poisoning from individual opioids is the duration of action. Opioids have potent pharmacological activity following virtually all modes of administration (e.g., inhalational, rectal, oral, or parenteral administration), but inconsistencies in the time to onset as well as duration of action can occur from each route. Similarly, the existence of immediate- and extended-release formulations introduces additional complexity in anticipating how long a patient may be intoxicated or experience signs of poisoning or overdose.

A final consideration is that opioid abuse in different geographic areas carries unique local risks, of which the treating clinician should be aware. As an example, an outbreak of human immunodeficiency virus (HIV) in Indiana was related to the injection of oxymorphone from an abuse-deterrent formulation; in Tennessee, however, the injection of the same opioid but a different formulation was associated with the development of a syndrome similar to thrombotic thrombocytopenic purpura (Centers for Disease Control and Prevention 2013; Peters et al. 2016). Clinicians must make every effort to educate themselves not only on the risks of specific opioids but also about the unique risks of use in the area in which they practice.

Specific Opioids

According to CDC data, from 1999 to 2014, hydrocodone, oxycodone, and methadone were the most common prescription opioids associated with overdose deaths (Centers for Disease Control and Prevention 2017b). The relationship between each of these—as well as buprenorphine, fentanyl, and heroin—and overdose is described below.

Hydrocodone (Immediate and Extended Release)

Hydrocodone is a μ receptor agonist commonly used to treat pain in the outpatient setting. Prior to 2014, hydrocodone-acetaminophen was classified as a Schedule III drug; under this scheduling, hydrocodone prescriptions could be written and filled for a 6-month duration. This regulatory approach increased the convenience of prescribing hydrocodone and likely contributed to the high frequency with which it was misused in the U.S. population. Once the Drug Enforcement Administration (DEA) reclassified hydrocodone as a Schedule II drug, the numbers of prescriptions for hydrocodone-acetaminophen decreased nationally (Jones et al. 2016b). Hydrocodone is available in the United States in extended- and immediate-release formulations. The immediate-release form, also known by the brand name Norco, is coformulated with acetaminophen and most commonly used orally, but several reports describe its misuse by intranasal administration (Butler et al. 2011; Cassidy et al. 2017). Although death from hydrocodone overdose is not frequently encountered, the acetaminophen with which it is coformulated contributes to the overall incidence of acute hepatic injury observed in the United States.

The extended-release formulation of hydrocodone, known by the brand names Zohydro ER and Hysingla ER, does not contain acetaminophen and is intended to be administered every 12 or 24 hours, respectively. While the extended-release formulations are prepared using abuse deterrents (discussed later in section "Management of Opioid Overdose"), they are also available in much higher doses than their immediate-release counterparts; therefore, an overdose, whether intentional or unintentional, has the potential to expose the patient to a larger dose of opioid medication lasting for a longer period of time.

Oxycodone (Immediate and Extended Release)

Oxycodone is a commonly prescribed opioid with indications to treat both acute and chronic pain. CDC data show that oxycodone formulations are some of the most common prescriptions involved in death resulting from overdose (Centers for Disease Control and Prevention 2017b). Oxycodone is prescribed as either an immediate- or an extended-release formulation, under a variety of brand names. Whereas the immediate-release formulation has an onset of action and time to peak concentration of approximately 15 minutes and 1 hour, respectively, the extended-release formulations have a delayed onset of action of up to 1 hour, and peak concentrations are not achieved for nearly 2–3 hours (Lugo and Kern 2004). Perhaps the most crucial difference between immediate- and extended-release formulations is the duration of action: an immediate-release oxycodone dose will provide analgesia for approximately 3–4 hours, whereas the extended-release doses are intended to have lasting effects for up to 12 hours. These differences can lead not only to a delayed presentation of opioid overdose but also to a protracted intoxicated state, making it difficult for clinicians to manage an overdose. As with hydrocodone, the acetaminophen with which oxycodone is sometimes formulated can produce toxic hepatitis when taken in large amounts or repeatedly over an extended time period.

The abuse potential for extended-release oxycodone formulations arises from the relatively large quantity of opioid contained in a single pill. An attempt at preventing behaviors that increase the likelihood of abuse (e.g., crushing pills for injection or snorting) has led to the introduction of abuse-deterrent formulations. These include the use of matrices that form a gel upon exposure to an aqueous medium or that are resistant to crushing, chewing, or other physical destruction. Coformulation with an opioid antagonist such as naloxone is another deterrent method. In such a formulation, ingestion of the intact pill produces analgesia because naloxone has virtually no oral bioavailability; however, naloxone has opioid antagonist effects when administered via other routes, and therefore its inclusion in oxycodone formulations prevents misuse by injecting or snorting the crushed pill (Butler et al. 2011). Some epidemiological evidence indicates that modifying oxycodone to an abuse-deterrent formulation prevents misuse and potentially diversion (Schaeffer 2012).

Methadone

Methadone is a long-acting opioid agonist that is indicated for chronic pain control as well as medication-assisted treatment (MAT) of OUD. Following oral administration, methadone has an elimination half-life ranging between 8 and 59 hours (on average, roughly 24 hours), providing the patient with long-acting μ agonism. Methadone has been proven to be beneficial in decreasing the use of heroin, which in turn improves the overall health of individuals under treatment (Sordo et al. 2017). Current recommendations are that treating facilities require the recipient, at least initially, to present to a pharmacy or clinic daily to receive a supervised dose of methadone, which decreases the risk that the patient will divert the methadone for either recreational consumption or sale (Saulle et al. 2017). Patients with chronic pain, however, can receive prescriptions for methadone to take on an outpatient basis; the dose may exceed that normally used for treating OUD. When taken for chronic pain, methadone is dosed multiple times daily (in contrast to the once-daily use in MAT) because the analgesic effects of methadone wear off more rapidly than withdrawal and cravings begin.

Methadone for chronic pain, therefore, is a source of the drug that can be misused or diverted to illicit use. Methadone has been implicated in a substantial proportion of overdose deaths that arise from unintentional overdose during exploratory use, inappropriate dosing of the drug to self-treat pain, or rapid up-titration of dosing by physicians without considering the impact of the long half-life of methadone. After 2003, the U.S. Food and Drug Administration and DEA sought to educate prescribers and the public on the danger of methadone use for long-term chronic pain; this effort led to an overall decrease in the number of methadone-related deaths by the year 2014 (Jones et al. 2016a).

The elevated doses of methadone used to treat chronic pain relative to OUD revealed an idiosyncratic effect of the drug: QT interval prolongation. Typically occurring at oral doses of more than 300 mg of methadone per day, prolongation of the QT interval places patients at higher risk for polymorphic ventricular tachycardia, also known as torsades de pointes. The risk of torsades de pointes is higher early in the course of methadone therapy and is exacerbated by polypharmacy with other QT interval–prolonging medications, such as azoles, macrolides, some antipsychotic agents, and several common antiemetics.

Buprenorphine

Buprenorphine is a long-acting partial opioid agonist used in the treatment of OUD, as another form of MAT. Despite potent binding at μ receptors, buprenorphine does not exert the same degree of agonism as opioids that are full agonists (Orman and Keating 2009). The form of buprenorphine most commonly encountered in clinical practice is coformulated with naloxone. However, it is also dispensed as buprenorphine alone, intended to be used mainly for chronic pain (or for MAT in special populations, such as pregnant women). Buprenorphine-naloxone combinations are formulated for buccal mucosal absorption. The addition of the naloxone is intended to prevent misuse by injection because parenteral administration of naloxone will precipitate withdrawal.

The dosing of buprenorphine-naloxone is determined largely by subjective criteria, which may lead to the prescribing of greater daily doses of the medication than necessary for some patients. At the same time, buprenorphine-naloxone is dispensed by outpatient pharmacies for home use by recipients (without the daily supervision required by methadone clinics). These two circumstances have converged to increase the potential for diversion of buprenorphine-naloxone, which has contributed to pediatric exposures culminating in toxicity, overdose, and death (Monte et al. 2009). Clinicians prescribing buprenorphine-containing products should therefore have safeguards to check for and prevent diversion (e.g., random urine toxicology, pill counts, careful patient psychoeducation) and should take care to prescribe the minimum effective dose for an individual patient's current stage of treatment.

Fentanyl

Fentanyl is a synthetic, short-acting opioid used for both acute and chronic pain that is 50–100 times more potent than morphine. Of the numerous formulations that are available, the ones responsible for the majority of overdoses among prescription fentanyl products are transdermal delivery systems (i.e., fentanyl patches). Fentanyl poisoning from patches typically occurs in the setting of misuse, excessive application, miscalculation of patch size, or aggressive titration of dose (Fox et al. 2017). Recently, fentanyl and its congeners—other high-potency opioids with a chemical structure based on the fentanyl nucleus—have become a significant source of mortality among individuals who inject heroin. In some studies, up to 94% of people who overdosed on heroin had received a fentanyl analogue despite the fact that none of them intended to use fentanyl. Although the adulteration of heroin with fentanyl is not new, what is new is the breadth and scale of the current crisis (Peterson et al. 2016). Commonly identified fentanyl analogues in these deaths include furanylfentanyl, acrylfentanyl, and carfentanil, although numerous others have been found in circulation (Daniulaityte et al. 2017). What makes these fentanyl analogues lethal, in addition to their potency, is their unregulated manufacture without rigorous quality control. Inconsistencies in mixing micrograms of fentanyl into grams of heroin can lead to a lack of homogeneity in the drug mixture. This variability means that one dose of heroin can contain no fentanyl, whereas another can contain a lethal amount of the adulterant. Persons using heroin, therefore, cannot know the exact amount of fentanyl they are receiving, even if they purchase heroin from a trusted source.

Fentanyl patches are a common intentionally abused formulation of the drug. Patches contain literally milligrams of fentanyl; the enormous amount of fentanyl is needed to create a concentration gradient that drives the drug across the skin, into the body. Patches remain in place for a 72-hour period, but even at the end of this time period (when the patch is supposedly "consumed"), milligram amounts of fentanyl remain (Marquardt et al. 1995). Some people misuse patches by ingesting them, placing them in body orifices, or extracting the remaining drug for the purpose of recreational use (Mrvos et al. 2012). Because the rate of absorption of fentanyl is temperature dependent, placing patches in the axillae or perineum can lead to elevated blood concentrations of fentanyl. Fatalities resulting from ingestion of patch contents, intentional misapplication, and placement of patches within the oropharynx are well described in the literature (Arvanitis and Satonik 2002). Importantly, poisoning from fentanyl patches can be severe and long lasting; even though the duration of action in therapeutic doses is approximately 20–45 minutes, fentanyl poisoning from patches may persist for up to 24 hours following exposure, because fentanyl leaches from the pharmacological compartments in the skin.

Heroin

Heroin, an illicit opioid with no medically accepted uses in the United States, has nonetheless been approved for medical use in Canada and some European countries as a harm reduction measure to decrease deaths from adulterated heroin. A highly trafficked drug that has been associated with considerable morbidity and mortality, heroin is active following administration via parenteral, mucosal, and pulmonary routes and has a duration of action of 4–6 hours. Intravenous use is associated with significant risks, including contracting blood-borne illnesses such as HIV and hepatitis C virus infections, development of abscesses at injection sites, endocarditis, septic emboli, epidural abscesses, osteomyelitis, and talc emboli, as well as bacteremia and septicemia. Heroin use is associated with a significant economic cost, not only from the purchase costs for individuals using it but also from hospitalizations and long-term care associated with addiction and overdoses.

Heroin is administered via several routes, and some of these pose unique risks. The most common modes of administration are injection and intranasal use, but pulmonary administration by smoking is also possible. "Chasing the dragon"—a method of heating heroin on aluminum foil to produce fumes that are inhaled—has been associated with irreversible spongiform leukoencephalopathy, characterized by altered mental status, dysarthria, ataxia, coma, paralysis, cerebellar dysfunction, and death (Kass-Hout et al. 2011). Pathognomonic findings from magnetic resonance imaging include bilateral hyperintense lesions in the cerebellum, occipital lobe, internal capsule, and brain stem, while the frontal lobe is spared (Bartlett and Mikulis 2005; Long et al. 2003).

Management of Opioid Overdose

The management of opioid overdose centers on reversing respiratory depression. Patients with apnea require a pharmacological or mechanical stimulus to breathe. For patients with depressed mental status and a respiratory rate of 12 or fewer breaths per minute, ventilation should be assisted using a bag-valve mask in concert with chin-lift and jaw-thrust maneuvers. These airway manipulation techniques ensure anatomical optimization of the naso-oropharyngeal structures and, along with assistive ventilation, help to reduce hypercarbia. Although the exact relationship between hypercarbia and acute lung injury is not well defined, simple assistive ventilation with a bag-valve mask is relatively low risk and provides the benefit of oxygenation.

Naloxone is the antidote for opioid overdose. It is a competitive μ opioid receptor antagonist that reverses all elements of opioid intoxication.

Naloxone is highly active when administered via parenteral, intranasal, or pulmonary routes. When administered orally, it has minimal bioavailability because it undergoes extensive first-pass metabolism (a feature that is exploited in many abuse-deterrent formulations, as discussed in a previous section of this chapter) (Pond and Tozer 1984). The kinetics of naloxone are altered in patients with opioid dependence, potentially leading to lower plasma levels, larger volumes of distribution, and longer elimination half-lives (Fishman et al. 1973). When naloxone is given intravenously, onset of action can be less than 2 minutes; however, the clinical duration of naloxone activity is only 20–90 minutes. This is much shorter than the duration of action of many opioids, which may therefore create the need for redosing of naloxone in intervals based on clinical need (Berkowitz 1976; Evans et al. 1974).

If opioid overdose is suspected, naloxone should be administered. Naloxone has few if any side effects. Precipitating withdrawal in patients with opioid dependence is of secondary concern when compared with reversing the life-threatening apnea of overdose. The symptoms of opioid abstinence and withdrawal (e.g., yawning, lacrimation, piloerection, diaphoresis, myalgia, vomiting, diarrhea) can be extremely uncomfortable but are not fatal by themselves (Berkowitz 1976).

Naloxone dosing is based on clinical presentation and response and should be titrated to reversal of respiratory depression. The dose of naloxone needed to reverse overdose is affected by many factors, including the causative opioid and its affinity for the μ opioid receptor, the affinity of naloxone for the receptor, the patient's weight, the amount of opioid used, and the extent of the opioid's penetration across the blood-brain barrier into the CNS (Berkowitz 1976; Tenenbein 1984). The initial dose of naloxone should be 0.04 mg; if this dose fails, the clinician can increase the naloxone dose every 15 minutes. Failure of 15 mg of intravenous naloxone to produce any effect should compel reconsideration of the therapeutic approach. New, potent analogues of fentanyl—such as carfentanil and furanylfentanyl—may require higher doses of naloxone than have been commonly required in the past.

Because the dosing of naloxone is empirical, the clinician should attempt to find the lowest effective dose that restores adequate ventilation for the patient. In patients with opioid dependence, the dose that will restore a normal breathing pattern is often low enough that frank withdrawal will not be provoked. This is the ideal circumstance and makes the treatment interaction more tolerable for the patient and clinician. As mentioned earlier, the duration of action of naloxone is markedly shorter than that of many opioids; consequently, patients treated with naloxone should be observed, typically for 4–6 hours, following naloxone administration.

An alternative to pharmacological reversal is the use of extrinsic ventilation. Orotracheal intubation with mechanical ventilation provides ventilatory support as well as adequate oxygenation and can protect against aspiration (Prosser et al. 2010). The use of activated charcoal in opioid overdose is typically discouraged; it is only effective if given within 1 hour of ingestion, can complicate the view of the airway if orotracheal intubation is required, and can increase the risk of aspiration in opioid toxic patients who have depressed mental status (Chyka and Seger 1997). The ingestion of extended-release preparations of opioids can necessitate the use of multiple doses of intravenous naloxone, often at intervals that are difficult to predict. When this medical situation is suspected, admission to an intensive care unit and the use of a continuous infusion of naloxone are warranted (Nelsen et al. 2010).

A thorough physical examination should be performed to search for fentanyl patches, even when fentanyl is not considered the primary intoxicant. Fentanyl patches have caused delayed toxicity in cases where only a cursory physical examination was performed (Moon and Chun 2011). Areas where patches may be missed include the axillae, perineum, scrotum, and oropharynx. Any patch that is found should be removed, and the area(s) should be rinsed with clean, cool water (Nelson and Schwaner 2009). Ingestion of fentanyl patches can also cause systemic toxicity; patients who have done so may benefit from whole bowel irrigation (Prosser et al. 2010).

Persistent hypoxia after the administration of naloxone and the return of adequate ventilation effort may indicate the presence of negative-pressure pulmonary edema. This complication exists on a spectrum from mild cases resolving within 24 hours with supportive care only, to more severe cases that may require orotracheal intubation and positive-pressure ventilation. Naloxone has been implicated erroneously as the cause of pulmonary edema in opioid overdose (Boyer 2012). Pulmonary edema, however, is present in almost all cases of opioid overdose, including those that occurred before the advent of naloxone. In clinical studies in which patients received large doses of naloxone via continuous infusion, the patients did not develop pulmonary edema (Peters et al. 1981). Because pulmonary edema is caused by negative pressure, not fluid overload, the use of diuretic agents is ineffective and should be avoided.

Rhabdomyolysis can develop in the opioid toxic patient who remains immobile while intoxicated. Rhabdomyolysis should be treated with volume resuscitation to prevent the crystallization of myoglobin in the renal tubules, and urine output should be closely monitored. The use of bicarbonate infusions for rhabdomyolysis does not improve outcomes and should be avoided (Gabow et al. 1982). The presence of rhabdomyolysis can also herald the development of compartment syndrome. Clinicians should scrupulously search for the development of compartment syndrome, which warrants emergent surgical consultation and fasciotomy.

Hypoxic brain injury is a feared complication of opioid overdose. Because no treatments improve neurological function after hypoxic injury, the most important goal is prevention. This can be facilitated by clinicians maintaining a high index of suspicion for opioid overdose, having a low threshold to initiate treatment for acute opioid overdose (i.e., administration of naloxone), and taking aggressive measures to maintain adequate oxygenation (i.e., simple assistive ventilation with a bag-valve mask or mechanical ventilation when clinically indicated). Prevention of hypoxic injury can also be enhanced by education and training for prehospital providers such as police, fire, and emergency medical services; public access and training programs for bystander naloxone use; and harm reduction strategies such as supervised injection sites.

Several pitfalls threaten successful outcomes in treating an opioid-poisoned patient. The first is failure to realize that naloxone will not truncate the course of toxicity. The use of naloxone will not prevent the recurrence of toxicity in a patient who has overdosed; observation even after reversal of an overdose is warranted. The second pitfall is that clinicians may erroneously believe that the dose of naloxone is related to the severity of the overdose. As mentioned earlier in this section, the dose of naloxone is empiric in nature, and many opioid-dependent patients will not require a large dose of naloxone for reversal of their respiratory depression, particularly if opioid tolerant. Third is the assumption that the timing of respiratory depression and peak plasma opioid concentrations coincide. The respiratory depression associated with opioid intoxication is unrelated to the peak concentration of opioid, and the timing of the respiratory depression cannot be reliably determined in overdose (Rigg 1978). Fourth is the failure to remember that many opioids are coformulated with acetaminophen, and toxicity from acetaminophen may thus go unnoticed during the period in which treatment is most effective. The final pitfall is failure to recognize that the pharmacokinetics and toxicokinetics of opioids in children and elderly patients differ from those in young, healthy adults and therefore necessitate longer observation periods.

Key Chapter Points

▶ Opioid use and abuse have increased dramatically in recent years, with a concomitant increase in overdose and fatalities. Fentanyl and its analogues, which are added to heroin as adulterants, have contributed substantially to recent increases in opioid overdose mortality.

▶ Clinicians should recognize the signs of opioid toxicity, as well as the unique threats posed by various opioids. Respiratory depression remains the cardinal sign of opioid overdose, along with coma and pinpoint pupils.

▶ Opioids, when used in overdose, have a consistent presentation; a clinician at the bedside cannot discriminate between an opioid that is short acting, long acting, or contained in an extended-release formulation. The duration of observation should be determined solely by clinical improvement.

▶ Naloxone, the antidote for opioid overdose, has almost no adverse effects but has a duration of action that is shorter than that of most opioids encountered in clinical practice. Repeated naloxone dosing will be necessary for treatment of overdose on long-acting opioid analgesics.

References

Arvanitis ML, Satonik RC: Transdermal fentanyl abuse and misuse. Am J Emerg Med 20(1):58–59, 2002 11781919

Bartlett E, Mikulis DJ: Chasing "chasing the dragon" with MRI: leukoencephalopathy in drug abuse. Br J Radiol 78(935):997–1004, 2005 16249600

Berkowitz BA: The relationship of pharmacokinetics to pharmacological activity: morphine, methadone and naloxone. Clin Pharmacokinet 1(3):219–230, 1976 13957

Binswanger IA, Stern MF, Deyo RA, et al: Release from prison—a high risk of death for former inmates. N Engl J Med 356(2):157–165, 2007 17215533

Boyer EW: Management of opioid analgesic overdose. N Engl J Med 367(2):146–155, 2012 22784117

Butler SF, Black RA, Cassidy TA, et al: Abuse risks and routes of administration of different prescription opioid compounds and formulations. Harm Reduct J 8:29, 2011 22011626

Cassidy TA, Oyedele N, Mickle TC, et al: Patterns of abuse and routes of administration for immediate-release hydrocodone combination products. Pharmacoepidemiol Drug Saf 26(9):1071–1082, 2017 28771942

Centers for Disease Control and Prevention: Thrombotic thrombocytopenic purpura (TTP)–like illness associated with intravenous Opana ER abuse—Tennessee, 2012. January 11, 2013. Available at: https://www.cdc.gov/mmwr/preview/mmwrhtml/mm6201a1.htm. Accessed January 25, 2018.

Centers for Disease Control and Prevention: Opioid Painkiller Prescribing. July 2014. Available at: https://www.cdc.gov/vitalsigns/opioid-prescribing/index.html. Accessed January 25, 2018.

Centers for Disease Control and Prevention: Drug Overdose Death Data. December 2017a. Available at: www.cdc.gov/drugoverdose/data/statedeaths.html. Accessed August 24, 2018.

Centers for Disease Control and Prevention: Prescription Opioid Overdose Data. August 1, 2017b. Available at: https://www.cdc.gov/drugoverdose/data/overdose.html. Accessed January 24, 2018.

Chyka PA, Seger D: Position statement: single-dose activated charcoal. American Academy of Clinical Toxicology; European Association of Poisons Centres and Clinical Toxicologists. J Toxicol Clin Toxicol 35(7):721–741, 1997 9482427

Cicero TJ, Ellis MS: Abuse-deterrent formulations and the prescription opioid abuse epidemic in the United States: lessons learned from OxyContin. JAMA Psychiatry 72(5):424–430, 2015 25760692

Cicero TJ, Ellis MS, Surratt HL, et al: The changing face of heroin use in the United States: a retrospective analysis of the past 50 years. JAMA Psychiatry 71(7):821–826, 2014 24871348

Daniulaityte R, Juhascik MP, Strayer KE, et al: Overdose deaths related to fentanyl and its analogs—Ohio, January–February 2017. MMWR Morb Mortal Wkly Rep 66(34):904–908, 2017 28859050

Evans JM, Hogg MI, Lunn JN, et al: Degree and duration of reversal by naloxone of effects of morphine in conscious subjects. BMJ 2(5919):589–591, 1974 4833964

Fishman J, Roffwarg H, Hellman L: Disposition of naloxone-7,8,3H in normal and narcotic-dependent men. J Pharmacol Exp Ther 187(3):575–580, 1973 4588968

Fox LM, Hoffman RS, Vlahov D, et al: Risk factors for severe respiratory depression from prescription opioid overdose. Addiction 113(1):59–66, 2017 28646524

Gabow PA, Kaehny WD, Kelleher SP: The spectrum of rhabdomyolysis. Medicine (Baltimore) 61(3):141–152, 1982 7078398

Guy GP Jr, Zhang K, Bohm MK, et al: Vital signs: changes in opioid prescribing in the United States, 2006–2015. MMWR Morb Mortal Wkly Rep 66(26):697–704, 2017 28683056

Jones CM: Heroin use and heroin use risk behaviors among nonmedical users of prescription opioid pain relievers—United States, 2002–2004 and 2008–2010. Drug Alcohol Depend 132(1–2):95–100, 2013 23410617

Jones CM, Baldwin GT, Manocchio T, et al: Trends in methadone distribution for pain treatment, methadone diversion, and overdose deaths—United States, 2002–2014. MMWR Morb Mortal Wkly Rep 65(26):667–671, 2016a 27387857

Jones CM, Lurie PG, Throckmorton DC: Effect of U.S. Drug Enforcement Administration's rescheduling of hydrocodone combination analgesic products on opioid analgesic prescribing. JAMA Intern Med 176(3):399–402, 2016b 26809459

Kass-Hout T, Kass-Hout O, Darkhabani MZ, et al: "Chasing the dragon"—heroin-associated spongiform leukoencephalopathy. J Med Toxicol 7(3):240–242, 2011 21336801

Lalley PM: Opioidergic and dopaminergic modulation of respiration. Respir Physiol Neurobiol 164(1–2):160–167, 2008 18394974

Long H, Deore K, Hoffman RS, et al: A fatal case of spongiform leukoencephalopathy linked to "chasing the dragon." J Toxicol Clin Toxicol 41(6):887–891, 2003 14677803

Lugo RA, Kern SE: The pharmacokinetics of oxycodone. J Pain Palliat Care Pharmacother 18(4):17–30, 2004 15760805

Manglik A, Lin H, Aryal DK, et al: Structure-based discovery of opioid analgesics with reduced side effects. Nature 537(7619):185–190, 2016 27533032

Marquardt KA, Tharratt RS, Musallam NA: Fentanyl remaining in a transdermal system following three days of continuous use. Ann Pharmacother 29(10):969–971, 1995 8845555

Matthes HW, Maldonado R, Simonin F, et al: Loss of morphine-induced analgesia, reward effect and withdrawal symptoms in mice lacking the mu-opioid-receptor gene. Nature 383(6603):819–823, 1996 8893006

Monte AA, Mandell T, Wilford BB, et al: Diversion of buprenorphine/naloxone coformulated tablets in a region with high prescribing prevalence. J Addict Dis 28(3):226–231, 2009 20155591

Moon JM, Chun BJ: Fentanyl intoxication caused by abuse of transdermal fentanyl. J Emerg Med 40(1):37–40, 2011 18455903

Mrvos R, Feuchter AC, Katz KD, et al: Whole fentanyl patch ingestion: a multicenter case series. J Emerg Med 42(5):549–552, 2012 21683542

Nelsen JL, Marraffa JM, Jones L, et al: Management considerations following overdoses of modified-release morphine preparations. World J Emerg Med 1(1):75–76, 2010 25214946

Nelson L, Schwaner R: Transdermal fentanyl: pharmacology and toxicology. J Med Toxicol 5(4):230–241, 2009 19876859

Orman JS, Keating GM: Buprenorphine/naloxone: a review of its use in the treatment of opioid dependence. Drugs 69(5):577–607, 2009 19368419

Paulozzi LJ, Xi Y: Recent changes in drug poisoning mortality in the United States by urban-rural status and by drug type. Pharmacoepidemiol Drug Saf 17(10):997–1005, 2008 18512264

Peters PJ, Pontones P, Hoover KW, et al; Indiana HIV Outbreak Investigation Team: HIV infection linked to injection use of oxymorphone in Indiana, 2014–2015. N Engl J Med 375(3):229–239, 2016 27468059

Peters WP, Johnson MW, Friedman PA, et al: Pressor effect of naloxone in septic shock. Lancet 1(8219):529–532, 1981 6111636

Peterson AB, Gladden RM, Delcher C, et al: Increases in fentanyl-related overdose deaths—Florida and Ohio, 2013–2015. MMWR Morb Mortal Wkly Rep 65(33):844–849, 2016 27560948

Pond SM, Tozer TN: First-pass elimination: basic concepts and clinical consequences. Clin Pharmacokinet 9(1):1–25, 1984 6362950

Prosser JM, Jones BE, Nelson L: Complications of oral exposure to fentanyl transdermal delivery system patches. J Med Toxicol 6(4):443–447, 2010 20532845

Rigg JR: Ventilatory effects and plasma concentration of morphine in man. Br J Anaesth 50(8):759–765, 1978 678362

Rudd RA, Aleshire N, Zibbell JE, et al: Increases in drug and opioid overdose deaths—United States, 2000–2014. Centers for Disease Control and Prevention, January 1, 2016. Available at https://www.cdc.gov/mmwr/preview/mmwrhtml/mm6450a3.htm. Accessed January 25, 2018.

Saulle R, Vecchi S, Gowing L: Supervised dosing with a long-acting opioid medication in the management of opioid dependence. Cochrane Database Syst Rev 4:CD011983, 2017 28447766

Schaeffer T: Abuse-deterrent formulations, an evolving technology against the abuse and misuse of opioid analgesics. J Med Toxicol 8(4):400–407, 2012 23073726

Sordo L, Barrio G, Bravo MJ, et al: Mortality risk during and after opioid substitution treatment: systematic review and meta-analysis of cohort studies. BMJ 357:j1550, 2017 28446428

Stein C: The control of pain in peripheral tissue by opioids. N Engl J Med 332(25):1685–1690, 1995 7760870

Tenenbein M: Continuous naloxone infusion for opiate poisoning in infancy. J Pediatr 105(4):645–648, 1984 6481543

Waldhoer M, Bartlett SE, Whistler JL: Opioid receptors. Annu Rev Biochem 73:953–990, 2004 15189164

Whistler JL: Examining the role of mu opioid receptor endocytosis in the beneficial and side-effects of prolonged opioid use: from a symposium on new concepts in mu-opioid pharmacology. Drug Alcohol Depend 121(3):189–204, 2012 22226706

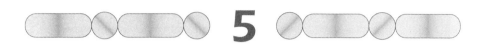

5

The Opioid Epidemic

Social Determinants and Health Inequities

Leila M. Vaezazizi, M.D.
Julie Netherland, Ph.D.
Helena Hansen, M.D., Ph.D.

Clinical Vignettes: Gabriel and Sara

Vignette 1: Gabriel

Gabriel is a 54-year-old Puerto Rican man with a medical history of hepatitis C virus (HCV) infection. He was born in Puerto Rico and came to the continental United States with his parents and siblings when he was 7 years old. He grew up in housing projects of an urban northeastern city. His neighborhood school was low performing, and he dropped out of high school in the eleventh grade, feeling that school was not relevant to his life. He was first arrested at age 19 for carrying a small amount of marijuana. While in his early 20s, he was exposed to heroin by friends who lived in his building, and he began injecting. He then started selling heroin as a way to financially support himself because he had few other employment opportunities given his legal history.

Gabriel was married when in his late 20s and had three children. His relationship with his wife was marked by domestic violence and multiple separations and reconciliations. Over the course of two decades, he served multiple sentences in jail for a mix of drug possession and domestic violence charges. During this time, he was in and out of drug treatment programs and was able to maintain his longest period of abstinence of 4 years after completing court-mandated, long-term residential treatment. He and his now ex-wife divorced several years ago. Most recently, he had been doing well in a methadone maintenance treatment program and working in construction with a family friend, although he continued to smoke marijuana.

When Gabriel was arrested 1 year ago for marijuana possession, he was in a methadone maintenance program, taking methadone 140 mg/day. There was no methadone program in his jail, and after going through a distressing involuntary detoxification while in jail awaiting his trial, he was charged and sentenced to 1 year in prison.

When he was released, he had nowhere to stay and therefore went to a local shelter near his old neighborhood. He tried to return to his old methadone program but was unable to start treatment because he did not have insurance or an identification card. Two weeks later, Gabriel encountered an old acquaintance with whom he used to use drugs, and he relapsed; he did five bags of heroin intravenously and overdosed. His acquaintance, however, had received naloxone training recently, and was able to rescue him with a naloxone nasal spray and by calling 911. While Gabriel was in the emergency department, the social worker helped him complete paperwork for emergency Medicaid and medical services, and made an appointment for him at an outpatient substance abuse program for the following week.

Vignette 2: Sara

Sara is a 33-year-old white woman living in a suburban area of a midsize midwestern city. She works as an accountant. She has had no serious medical problems, but was introduced to heroin by her partner, with whom she has been living for the past 3 years. She has an 8-year-old daughter from a previous relationship. Sara started using only occasionally with her partner, but then slowly began escalating her use, and for a year she used three bags of intranasal heroin daily. She experienced intolerable withdrawal symptoms when she tried to stop using. When she discovered that she was pregnant, she wanted to continue the pregnancy but was mortified that she was using heroin and was unable to stop without experiencing withdrawal symptoms.

She drove 45 minutes from her home to see a private addiction psychiatrist, Dr. Lee, to whom she was referred by a relative's friend. Dr. Lee charged her $200 per session, which Sara paid in full. She did not want to get reimbursed by her out-of-network insurance benefits because she did not want the diagnosis or treatment on her medical records. She reported to Dr. Lee that she was pregnant and had no idea what to do. She described feeling extremely guilty about using heroin while being pregnant and was very concerned that child protective services would get involved and take away her other child if she tried to get help. She stated that she really wanted help to stop using heroin and would do anything possible. Sara had already started seeing an obstetrician, who confirmed her 10-week pregnancy and said that her preliminary tests were all normal, although she chose not to tell the doctor about her substance use.

Dr. Lee reassured her, and together they decided that Sara would start taking buprenorphine, with the agreement that Sara would continue seeing her obstetrician regularly and would allow the two providers to be in contact. She began taking buprenorphine and was stabilized on 8 mg/day.

Sara was maintained on this dose, and at 39 weeks went into labor and was hospitalized. She gave birth to a healthy baby boy who was born with neonatal abstinence syndrome. Because Sara was not using any illicit substances and there were no concerns for the child's welfare, there were no state requirements for the clinical team to contact child protective services. The baby had an uncomplicated treatment course for neonatal abstinence syndrome and spent 7 days in the hospital before being discharged. Sara continued taking buprenorphine for 6 months after that and then made the decision to taper off, with ongoing, periodic follow-up care with Dr. Lee.

These two vignettes raise a number of questions, each of which will be addressed in this chapter. First, what are the populations most affected by the current opioid epidemic, and how do they compare with affected populations in previous opioid epidemics in American history? Second, what explains the shift in demographic groups most affected by today's opioid epidemic? Third, how do sociodemographic factors such as race/ethnicity, gender, and income influence the treatment and legal systems with which an individual with opioid use disorder (OUD) is likely to interact? Fourth, does treatment—such as the likelihood of being offered or prescribed buprenorphine, methadone, or long-acting injectable extended-release naltrexone (XR-naltrexone)—vary for individuals with OUD based on sociodemographic characteristics? Fifth, how have the U.S. federal government's "War on Drugs" and the American criminal justice approach to drug use impacted treatment access and outcomes for individuals with OUD? Sixth, how have pharmaceutical marketing and regulatory factors influenced the opioid epidemic and contributed to health inequities for individuals with OUD? Seventh, what are examples of local, state, and national policies currently in place that may have influenced the trajectory of both Gabriel and Sara, described in the clinical vignettes? Eighth, what kinds of clinical and policy research are most needed to understand the causes and consequences of the health care inequities illustrated by these cases?

Introduction

This chapter focuses on the social determinants and resulting demographic patterns of the current opioid epidemic. The phrase *social determinants of health* refers to the broad social and environmental contextual factors that influence individual health. These factors include neighborhood and institutional conditions, as well as political and economic forces that have shaped who is affected by the current opioid epidemic, which treatments are offered to what types of patients, and how communities and organizations respond to individuals struggling with OUD. Two individuals from different racial groups, or from a rural versus an urban area, may share the same condition of having an OUD but have a different structural relationship to it that may impact treatment engagement and outcomes over time. For instance, one individual may experience racial bias in the criminal justice system or be unable to obtain addiction treatment in his or her rural area. The importance of social determinants has been demonstrated for an array of health conditions; in a recent meta-analysis, one-third of deaths from all causes in the United States were estimated to be attributable to social factors such as racial segregation, poverty, and income inequality (Galea et al. 2011). The opioid epidemic is characterized by marked group differences in terms of race, ethnicity, socioeconomic status, gender, sexual orientation, age, and geography.

The current epidemic, beginning in the late 1990s, has expanded into regions and demographic groups that previously were not as severely affected by opioid dependence in the United States. This is due to a number of social and economic forces that have dramatically increased exposure and access to opioids over the past two decades, predominantly among white individuals. Some causal factors include aggressive pharmaceutical marketing and deregulation of prescription opioids, leading to rapid increases in prescribing for pain conditions in white suburban and rural areas, and declining economic and job opportunities in many of those areas, leading to psychological distress, chronic health conditions, and vulnerability to substance use. At the same time, the War on Drugs and unequal application of law enforcement and clinical care in nonwhite communities have driven inequalities in opioid-related health outcomes in the United States for decades. Ironically, lack of access to health care and opioid prescriptions among black and Latino populations had an unintended protective effect by reducing their exposure to prescription opioids in the first decade of the epidemic. However, ongoing racial discrimination in incarceration for heroin possession has led to disparities in the prison population, with rippling effects on the social and economic well-being of black, Latino, and American Indian individuals and families. In this chapter, we provide highlights from what is known regarding the interplay of these and other factors and the broader context that has sown the seeds for today's opioid epidemic. We trace the ways in which these forces have had an impact on treatment and outcomes for OUD, particularly with regard to race, gender, and rural versus urban differences.

Providers who understand the impact of social determinants on health, and resultant health inequities, are able to address them in clinical practice; for instance, providers can counteract possible racial bias in recommending buprenorphine, methadone, or XR-naltrexone for treatment of a patient with an OUD, or they can reduce institutional barriers to treatment, such as concerns regarding involvement of child protective services or child care needs for a pregnant woman seeking treatment. Such advocacy is necessary for health-promoting institutional and policy change. In addition, research is needed to develop effective interventions on the social determinants that drive opioid and heroin use, overdose, and related health and social outcomes.

Race and Gender in America's Opioid Epidemics: Past and Present

Historical Perspective: Opioids, Race, and Gender in Nineteenth- and Twentieth-Century America

Today's opioid epidemic began in the late 1990s, with the introduction of newly patented prescription opioids that were initially marketed as "minimally addictive," followed by a vast expansion of opioid prescribing in the United States. The expansion of opioid prescribing, reaching its peak in 2010 when there were 81.2 opioid prescriptions per 100 people in the United States, parallels the rapid rise in people newly initiated to opioid use, increased prevalence of OUD and drug overdose deaths, and the geographical shifting of the opioid addiction burden to predominantly white rural and suburban areas (Guy et al. 2017).

Pervasive opioid use is not a new phenomenon in the history of the United States. The current epidemic is at least the fourth opioid epidemic of its kind, with the first dating back to the turn of the nineteenth century. Each epidemic has had a specific demographic and geographic distribution, and the race, ethnicity, and socioeconomic status of those affected have strongly shaped the corresponding social and health interventions and outcomes. Examining historical patterns of previous opioid epidemics illustrates an important principle: that avenues of access largely determine who is most at risk for developing an opioid addiction, and the cultural beliefs about who is at risk for addiction influence policy and public health interventions for addiction.

Between 1840 and 1890, the use of opiates (opium and morphine) increased by an estimated 538%, in parallel with the development of the hypodermic needle, affecting diverse sociodemographic groups including Civil War soldiers, mothers treating themselves and their children, Chinese immigrants, and alcoholic individuals self-treating hangovers. Opiate-containing "patent medicines" were heavily marketed to women and children for a number of pain conditions, including dysmenorrhea. According to one estimate, there were enough opiates to support an addiction for 4.6/100,000 individuals, the majority of whom were women. Subsequent morphine prescribing declined after its peak in 1890, in part due to the development of new treatments for pain, such as aspirin, and increased caution about narcotic prescribing in the medical literature. By 1898, heroin (diacetylmorphine) was marketed by the pharmaceutical company Bayer as a "nonaddictive" treatment for morphine addiction. By the late 1910s, physicians had become more circumspect in opiate prescribing, including heroin prescribing (Kolodny et al. 2015; Terplan 2017). In addition, early twentieth-century developments in international drug policy, such as international pressure on the U.S. Congress to pass prohibitionist domestic policy in the wake of the Opium Wars in China, led policy makers and the popular media to associate opiates with urban poverty and ethnic minorities in newspaper articles. Such media reports invoked stereotypes of cocaine-crazed Negroes in the South and Chinese opium dens in coastal cities. This imagery built public support for narcotic prohibition. Physicians were banned from prescribing opiates to opiate-addicted patients with passage of the 1914 Harrison Act (P.L. 63-223), which also made illegal all medical uses of heroin by 1924 (Courtwright 1982; Musto 1999).

Despite prohibitionist policies, narcotic use and overdose among whites in the United States grew to record levels from World War II through the 1960s, largely due to legally prescribed nonopioid medications such as barbiturates and, later, meprobamate (Miltown) and the benzodiazepines, such as diazepam (Valium) (colloquially known as "Mother's Little Helper"), as well as stimulants that were heavily marketed to white, largely middle-class and predominantly female patients with private doctors. This marked a racialized, two-tiered system of drug policy that sharply distinguished between prescribed and illegal narcotics, a distinction that protected white drug consumers from law enforcement while enabling their high levels of prescription narcotic use and overdose (Herzberg 2009). This pattern presaged the 1990s to 2000s, when newly patented opioid pain relievers were heavily marketed to primary care physicians, who subsequently prescribed opioids in large volume to white patients in rural and suburban areas.

As noted above, after the initial opioid epidemic of the late nineteenth and early twentieth centuries, two subsequent opioid epidemics dotted the twentieth century—the first following World War II and the second beginning in the 1960s, with effects reverberating into the 1980s and 1990s. After World War II, heroin use increased among blacks and Puerto Ricans but was largely confined to a "hipster" subculture in major U.S. port cities and to Mexicans in the Southwest (Broz and Ouellet 2008).

Public officials and popular media coverage amplified racial stereotypes about the identity and moral irresponsibility of heroin users. Harry Anslinger, who ran the Federal Bureau of Narcotics from 1930 to 1962, stated that the majority of drug users were "Negroes, Hispanics, Filipinos, and entertainers." Few public health or educational measures were taken to curb the epidemic, and no evidence-based treatments were available at the time. The few hospital units for managing opioid withdrawal and counseling clinics that were started were eventually abandoned because of poor results (Hughes et al. 1972).

Federal crackdowns on organized crime in the 1950s and 1960s, with heightened sentencing for drug trafficking, led organized crime leaders to hand over lower-level heroin trade to blacks and Latinos in an era of rising unemployment in their neighborhoods and civil rights–related social unrest, fostering widespread increases in heroin use among blacks and Latinos through the 1960s (Agar and Reisinger 2002). These waves of heroin use were met with vigorous law enforcement and scant investment in public health or addiction treatment services (Frederique 2016). By 1971, on the heels of race riots in several major U.S. cities that had been linked to heroin and urban crime in the minds of middle-class white voters and fears about heroin-addicted veterans returning from Vietnam, President Richard Nixon launched the War on Drugs, aimed at combating addiction with a law enforcement approach. Two decades later, Nixon's former domestic policy chief John Ehrlichman went public with the explicit racial and political motivations for the War on Drugs when he stated:

> The Nixon White House had two enemies: the antiwar left and black people. We knew we couldn't make it illegal to be either against the war or black, but by getting the public to associate the hippies with marijuana and blacks with heroin, and then criminalizing both heavily, we could disrupt those communities. We could arrest their leaders, raid their homes, break up their meetings, and vilify them night after night on the evening news. Did we know we were lying about the drugs? Of course we did. (Baum 2016, p. 1)

Nixon's War on Drugs focused on supply-side law enforcement in the form of drug interdiction, searches, and arrests in low-income black and Latino urban neighborhoods, a strategy that was reinvigorated under President Ronald Reagan a decade later. The War on Drugs has cost over $1 trillion since its inception, has not reduced drug use (Dai 2012), and has led the United States to have the highest rate of incarceration in the world, with pronounced racial inequalities. In 2016, for example, black men were more than 5 times as likely as white men to be in prison (Nellis 2016).

Although heroin use prevalence remained fairly stable during the 1980s and 1990s, emergency room visits for heroin use quadrupled, reflecting increased morbidity and mortality primarily concentrated in urban minority communities (Hughes and Rieche 1995). The population of intravenous heroin users helped fuel the rapid spread of human immunodeficiency virus (HIV) in the 1980s, which contributed to grave consequences particularly in black and Latino communities (Broz and Ouellet 2008), where blacks are 7 times and Latinos 3 times more likely to become HIV positive than whites (Brooks et al. 2013).

The Current Opioid Epidemic: Late 1990s Onward

Today's opioid epidemic has largely been portrayed as demographically distinct from previous epidemics in that individuals new to heroin use in the past decade are 90% white and a dramatic increase in heroin and nonmedical prescription opioid use has been observed in suburban and rural areas (Cicero et al. 2014). Today's opioid epidemic also could be conceptualized as the interweaving of prescription opioid, heroin, and, more recently, fentanyl epidemics.

Social Determinants and Health Inequities in Opioid Use

Racial/Ethnic Differences

OUD has expanded to white rural and suburban areas, whereas previously it was concentrated in urban black and Latino communities (Cicero et al. 2014). Prevalence trends in heroin and nonmedical prescription opioid use as well as opioid overdose death rates have been reviewed in other chapters (see Chapters 2, "Prescription Opioids," and 3, "Heroin and Other Illicit Opioids"); however, here we report on select prevalence rates to highlight key differences by race/ethnicity. Lifetime heroin use has increased overall in the population between 2001–2002 and 2012–2013, with the greatest increase among non-Hispanic whites, from 0.34% to 1.90% (compared with 0.32% to 1.05% for nonwhites). Past-year nonmedical prescription opioid use has similarly increased significantly over the same time period (from 1.8% to 4.1%), with the highest 2010–2014 prevalence rates of nonmedical prescription opioid use among non-Hispanic whites and American Indians (4.6% and 7.1%, respectively, compared with 4.1% in non-Hispanic blacks). The proportion of whites reporting nonmedical prescription opioid use prior to initiating heroin use significantly increased between 2001–2002 and 2012–2013 (from 35.8% to 52.8%), and a significant trend in the opposite direction was observed for nonwhites (decreasing from 44.1% to 26.2%) (Martins et al. 2017).

Hypotheses for this racial patterning of opioid misuse are manifold. In parallel with the increase in opioid prescribing for noncancer pain, there has been a rapid rise in the uptake of prescription opioid medications, particularly in white communities. Findings from the Centers for Disease Control and Prevention (CDC) show that county-level factors associated with increased opioid prescribing include having a greater proportion of non-Hispanic whites, a higher prevalence of chronic and painful conditions (e.g., diabetes, arthritis), greater unemployment, and higher Medicaid enrollment (Guy et al. 2017). Extensive research has shown that physicians are more likely to prescribe opioids to whites compared with other racial/ethnic groups for the same conditions, disproportionately increasing both the number of whites newly exposed to prescription opioids and the amount of medication available for misuse and diversion in white communities (Pletcher et al. 2008; Singhal et al. 2016). Among patients entering substance abuse treatment programs for heroin dependence who had abused prescription opioids, heroin use is increasing due to cheaper prices and easier access (Cicero et al. 2014). Blacks and Latinos are less likely to be insured or to have access to health care, which may have had the unintended effect of protecting those populations from exposure to opioids.

A number of researchers attempting to explain the disproportionate increase in opioid and heroin use among whites over the past two decades have also pointed to the concentration of overdose in Rust Belt cities and towns experiencing high unemployment and downward mobility of their residents following the closure of manufacturing plants (Case and Deaton 2015), accompanied by declining social networks and increased isolation of people in these economically depressed areas (Zoorob and Salemi 2017). These theories do not explain the racial/ethnic distribution of increased heroin use and overdose, however, given that many black and Latino communities have experienced even more severe economic decline. Additional factors, including racialized drug development, deregulation, and marketing, as well as the media, likely have had a prominent role in channeling newly patented opioids, and, later, as those opioids became more restricted, new heroin distribution networks, toward white rural and suburban consumers (as detailed further in later sections of this chapter).

Although the current opioid epidemic has been largely defined and described in the mainstream media as a "white" epidemic, other racial/

ethnic groups are affected. Opioid overdose deaths remained relatively stable between 1999 and 2010 among blacks and Hispanics; however, since 2010 there has been an uptick in opioid overdose deaths in these groups, primarily driven by heroin and fentanyl. Despite the lower overall rates of opioid use and overdose deaths among blacks and Hispanics, morbidity and mortality from conditions related to intravenous opioid use, such as from HIV and HCV infections, are disproportionately high. For example, 2014 mortality rates among those diagnosed with HIV were sevenfold higher among blacks than among whites; these high rates are partially driven by viral transmission from intravenous drug use, which is more prevalent among blacks (Centers for Disease Control and Prevention 2016).

American Indians, who have the highest rate of opioid overdose deaths of any racial/ethnic group, have been largely overlooked in the public discourse on the opioid epidemic. There are currently 567 federally recognized tribes and nearly 3 million American Indians in the United States, a large portion of whom live in rural or small-town areas. The high rate of opioid use and drug overdoses occurs in the context of persistent inequities in rates of depression, posttraumatic stress disorder, violence, and suicide, along with limited treatment resources in tribal and Indian Health Service facilities (Gone and Trimble 2012). The incidence and mortality from HCV infection has been highest among American Indians compared with other racial/ethnic groups over the past 10 years (Centers for Disease Control and Prevention 2017a). Although data are limited regarding whether a disproportionate amount of opioid prescribing has occurred among American Indians, some tribes are suing companies that are alleged to have flooded their communities with opioid medications or turned a blind eye to suspicious opioid prescribing and dispensing practices (Heygi 2017).

There are many limitations in fully describing racial/ethnic differences in opioid use and their causes. National surveys used to estimate drug and alcohol use prevalence, such as the National Survey on Drug Use and Health (NSDUH) and the National Epidemiologic Survey on Alcohol and Related Conditions (NESARC), frequently do not have sample sizes large enough to obtain accurate prevalence estimates for smaller racial/ethnic groups like American Indians. These surveys also do not sample individuals in institutionalized settings such as jails and prisons, which may lead to underestimation of substance use prevalence among blacks and Latinos, who are incarcerated for drug offenses at higher rates than whites. Last, the majority of studies that examine racial/ethnic differences do not take an intersectional approach in which the interplay of more than one sociodemographic characteristic or social risk factor (e.g., race and gender) is examined more closely. Not doing so can lead to incomplete or misleading findings. For example, a reanalysis of data from a widely cited report identifying white men as the group most affected by drug-related reductions in life expectancy, and largely covered in the media as an affliction primarily of disenfranchised white men, found that when the data were disaggregated by gender and state, increasing mortality rates among whites were driven by deaths among women (Case and Deaton 2017; Gelman and Auerbach 2016).

Gender Differences

As described above (see subsection "Historical Perspective"), the current opioid epidemic is notable in that people newly using heroin in the past 10 years include a higher proportion of women; currently, heroin-using treatment seekers are about equally men and women, whereas close to 90% of heroin-using treatment seekers in the 1960s were men (Cicero et al. 2014). Regarding past-year nonmedical prescription opioid use, men have significantly greater prevalence rates compared with women (4.4% vs. 3.8%), according to results from the 2012–2013 NESARC-III; with respect to heroin use, men were estimated, according to 2011–2013 NSDUH data, to have more than twice the odds compared with women of having heroin abuse or dependence after controlling for other demographic characteristics and other substance use disorders (SUDs) (Jones et al. 2015). Despite this, between 1999 and 2010, the increase in death rate from prescription opioid overdoses was greater among women (400%) than among men (265%), although men are still more likely to die from a prescription opioid overdose. Hospitalizations for prescription opioid overdoses, however, were higher for women than men in every year studied from 1993 to 2009, whereas hospitalizations for heroin overdose were consistently higher in men (Centers for Disease Control and Prevention 2013; Unick et al. 2013). The proportion of infants born with neonatal abstinence syndrome increased by nearly 300% between 2000 and 2009 (Patrick et al. 2012). These demographic shifts in the burden of the opioid epidemic are significant and highlight the changing landscape of risk.

In terms of differences in patterns and riskiness of use, women frequently report initiating opioid use to relieve pain, whereas men often report euphoria as the motivation for first use. Women are prescribed opioids more frequently than men (21.8 prescriptions/100 people among women vs. 16.4/100 among men) and receive higher doses of opioid medications for a longer period of time (Centers for Disease Control and Prevention 2017b; Hemsing et al. 2016). In addition, women report chronic conditions more often and make more frequent health care visits. The prevalence of posttraumatic stress disorder and depression is higher among women; trauma, chronic pain, and the misuse of prescription opioids are closely intertwined (Hemsing et al. 2016). Women have a higher rate of being prescribed opioids and other controlled medications, such as benzodiazepines, that increase overdose risk (Kolodny et al. 2015). Whereas the discourse on the opioid epidemic has largely focused on the impact on white men, it is important to realize that the burden of morbidity and mortality is increasingly shifting to women.

Rural Versus Urban Differences

The first reports of extended-release oxycodone (OxyContin) abuse arose in rural areas, particularly in Appalachia. Opioid analgesic prescribing varies widely nationwide by county, and geographic rurality is a risk factor for higher rates of opioid prescribing (Guy et al. 2017), making available more opioids for diversion and misuse in these areas. Although the overall rate of drug overdose deaths was still highest in metropolitan areas as of 2015, the drug overdose rate increase from 1999 to 2015 was greater in nonmetropolitan areas (325%) than in metropolitan areas (198%), particularly among women (Mack et al. 2017). Nonmedical prescription opioid use is more prevalent in rural than in urban areas, and several hypotheses have been suggested to explain this. Higher opioid prescription sales, a higher concentration of heavy labor occupations in which narcotic use is common, and worsening unemployment and economic deprivation, as well as older average age and worse overall health, may together contribute to increased rural nonmedical prescription opioid use (Keyes et al. 2014; Monnat and Rigg 2016).

There was a significant increase in past-year heroin use in both urban and nonurban areas between 2002–2004 and 2011–2013, but over a similar time period, there was a shift in heroin overdose deaths to increasingly nonurban areas (Jones et al. 2015; Stewart et al. 2017). In a treatment-based sample, the demographics of patients seeking treatment for heroin use were shown to have shifted from predominantly racial/ethnic minority men living in urban areas in the 1960s and 1970s to white men and women living outside large urban areas by 2010, who had largely used prescription opioids before initiating heroin. Some suggested mechanisms for the expansion of heroin use in nonmetropolitan areas include the increase in opioid prescribing leading to increased numbers of individuals newly exposed to opioids, and increased experimentation with heroin among individuals misusing prescription opioids. Lower cost and easier accessibility to heroin further fueled a transition from prescription opioid misuse to heroin use (Cicero et al. 2014; Monnat and Rigg 2016).

Social Determinants and Health Inequities in Treatment and Outcomes

In this section, we review what is currently known regarding treatment variability for OUD. Overall, rates of treatment for any SUD are low, and figures from the Substance Abuse and Mental Health Services Administration (SAMHSA) show that in 2012, less than 11% of individuals with a drug or alcohol problem sought specialty treatment (Substance Abuse and Mental Health Services Administration 2014). For those who do interact with the treatment system, there are major population-level disparities in rates of treatment referral, treatment entry, and use of medication for OUD.

Evidence-based pharmacological treatments for OUD are referred to collectively as *medication-assisted treatment* (MAT) and include two opioid agonists (buprenorphine and methadone) and one antagonist (XR-naltrexone [Vivitrol]). Each of these medications carries a different burden of stigma and varying levels of federal prescribing oversight, with methadone being the most restrictive and stigmatized, requiring daily dispensation at federally licensed methadone clinics that are frequently located in poor, urban neighborhoods. Buprenorphine, on the other hand, can be prescribed in an office-based setting but requires a physician who has received a special waiver. XR-naltrexone is not a scheduled medication and thus is not subject to any federal restrictions. Later in this chapter, we discuss the different federal requirements for prescribing MAT and the political context for these differences.

Expansion of buprenorphine prescribing is a national priority in the current opioid epidemic. Buprenorphine has many advantages over methadone: it can be prescribed in an office-based setting, and when combined with naloxone, it has lower overdose and abuse liability than methadone. Buprenorphine and methadone have comparable levels of efficacy for treatment of OUD.

Racial/Ethnic Differences

Despite the advantages of buprenorphine treatment, there has been limited uptake in buprenorphine prescribing, particularly for racial/ethnic minorities with OUD. According to a 2006 national study that compared the demographics of buprenorphine and methadone users, buprenorphine users were disproportionately more likely than methadone users to be white (91% vs. 53%), to be employed (58% vs. 29%), and to have some secondary education (56% vs. 19%) (Stanton et al. 2006). In a more recent U.S. Department of Veterans Affairs study, Manhapra and colleagues (2016) examined patient factors associated with receiving buprenorphine or methadone for OUD and concluded that demographic factors, rather than clinical indicators, largely predicted buprenorphine utilization; being black, urban residence, and older age were most associated with receiving methadone over buprenorphine. In a retrospective study examining the extent to which buprenorphine and XR-naltrexone were prescribed for OUD in a privately insured sample of youth ages 13–25 from 2001 to 2014, non-Hispanic blacks and Hispanics were less likely than whites to be prescribed any medication (14.8%, 20.0%, and 23.1%, respectively); females were also less likely than males to receive any medication (20.3% vs. 24.4%). With respect to XR-naltrexone, this same study found that factors associated with a greater likelihood of receiving XR-naltrexone over buprenorphine included younger age, being female, and residing in a metropolitan neighborhood with higher education levels and lower poverty; no differences between whites and nonwhites were identified, although sample sizes were too small to stratify further by race/ethnicity (Hadland et al. 2017). Additional information regarding the demographics of XR-naltrexone users is limited given that it was FDA approved in late 2010.

The reasons for the racial/ethnic inequities in MAT are unclear. Analogous to the disproportionate dispensation of prescription opioids for white patients with pain conditions, there may be inherent physician bias for who is considered an ideal candidate for buprenorphine treatment, which is less restrictive than methadone treatment. Another possibility is that there may be less demand for buprenorphine among blacks and Latinos with OUD, although there is no published evidence for this; rather, one study found that black patients reported a preference for buprenorphine given that methadone treatment carried substantial stigma (Gryczynski et al. 2013). Also, there is evidence that the racial distribution of MAT is in part due to the geographic location of substance abuse programs, methadone clinics, and buprenorphine providers. Substance abuse programs accepting Medicaid (these programs may not offer MAT) exist in 60% of all U.S. counties but are less likely to be found in counties with a higher proportion of black and/or uninsured residents (Cummings et al. 2014). Methadone clinics, on the other hand, are frequently located in poor, urban, racial/ethnic minority communities and are highly stigmatized. Between 2002 and 2011, buprenorphine provider availability expanded, particularly in nonmetropolitan areas; otherwise, little is known about the location of buprenorphine providers with respect to neighborhood demographics (Dick et al. 2015). Racial and ethnic disparities in pharmaceutical marketing and regulation of buprenorphine likely contributed to disparities in MAT use, as discussed further below. Acceptability and availability of treatment choices regarding type of medication used to treat OUD are important considerations; black and Latino patients are significantly less likely to complete treatment for OUD than whites, and limited treatment options may contribute to this disparity (Mennis and Stahler 2016).

Gender Differences

Screening and referral from the emergency department for detoxification are overall lower for women (3.2%) than for men (5.9%) presenting with any drug use, and men have higher odds of being referred for opioid detoxification (Ryoo and Choo 2016). In addition, women are less likely than men to be screened for substance use when presenting for trauma (Beasley et al. 2014). However, national samples show that men and women are equally likely to be treated for past-year or lifetime nonmedical opioid use (Kerridge et al. 2015) and that about equal numbers of men and women are in treatment for heroin use (Cicero et al. 2014).

For pregnant women, addiction treatment carries additional stigma and legal ramifications. Many states criminalize substance use during pregnancy. As a result, treatment seeking is lower among pregnant women than in other populations (Brown et al. 2017). Those who seek treatment face additional barriers: only 12 states provide priority access to substance abuse treatment for pregnant women, and only 4 states prohibit discrimination against pregnant women seeking treatment. Twenty-four states and the District of Columbia consider substance use during pregnancy to be child abuse under civil child-welfare statutes, and 3 consider it grounds for civil commitment. Twenty-three states and the District of Columbia require health care professionals to report suspected prenatal drug use, and 7 states require them to test for prenatal drug exposure if they suspect drug use. Only 19 states have either created or funded drug treatment programs specifically targeted to pregnant women, and 17 states and the District of Columbia provide pregnant women with priority access to state-funded drug treatment programs (Back et al. 2010; Terplan and Minkoff 2017).

Rural Versus Urban Differences

There is a severe shortage of MAT providers in rural areas, where demand outpaces supply and there are often long waiting lists for treatment programs. There are few buprenorphine prescribers in rural areas: 90.4% of buprenorphine-certified physicians practice in urban counties, leaving the majority of U.S. counties—53.4%, most of them rural—with no certified prescribers (Rosenblatt et al. 2015). In addition, fewer treatment facilities in rural areas accept Medicaid. Sixty percent of U.S. counties have at least one Medicaid-accepting facility for the treatment of SUDs; these facilities are less likely to be in rural areas, particularly in southern and midwestern states. These gaps are further compounded for areas with a higher proportion of racial and ethnic minorities. As of 2017, a total of 18 states opted out of Medicaid expansion, and 5 of the 10 states with the highest proportion of counties without an SUD treatment facility opted out, which places these already hard-hit states in an even more vulnerable position if there were to be federal funding cuts for SUD treatment (Cummings et al. 2014). With respect to federally qualified health centers, rural facilities are about half as likely to offer MAT as urban health centers (Jones et al. 2017). Rural residents face additional barriers to care: they travel greater distances to get treatment, and they often lack access to public transportation. These issues commonly result in missed visits and missed medication doses (Sigmon 2014).

Race, Addiction, and the Criminal Justice System

Racialized imagery surrounding illegal drug use has bolstered public support for a punitive War on Drugs approach to drug policy in the United States during the past five decades, which has led to racially disparate health and social outcomes. In the 1980s, thinly concealed references to the supposed threat that black and Latino crack cocaine–addicted people posed to white communities were pervasive in political debates and media coverage leading up to the passage of the 1986 Anti-Drug Abuse Act (P.L. 99-570). This law mandated a minimum 5-year prison sentence for possession of 1/100th the weight of crack cocaine that would lead to the same sentence for powder cocaine, at a time when powder cocaine was perceived as a drug of the white middle and upper classes. The legislation appropriated an additional $1.7 billion for the War on Drugs and established 29 new mandatory minimum sentences for offenses that also involved heroin. After passage of the act, narcotics searches and arrests were geographically targeted to communities of color and led to sharp increases in mass incarceration (Alexander 2010), with disproportionate public spending on incarceration among residents of low-income black and Latino neighborhoods, made visible in maps of "million-dollar blocks" (defined as blocks where more than $1 million per year was spent on sending residents to jails and prisons). In urban areas such as Chicago, New York City, and New Orleans, these blocks are concentrated in poor, minority communities (Badger 2015).

A history of arrest in itself further marginalizes low-income people of color from employment in the formal economy and increases the likelihood of future involvement in drug trade. Employers discriminate against applicants with an arrest record, and a drug conviction disqualifies convicted people from many benefits, including public housing. In addition, welfare reform, including the 1996 Temporary Assistance for Needy Families bill limiting welfare payments to 5 years and the 1996 discontinuation of Social Security disability benefits for people with a disabling substance dependence diagnosis, has left many low-income people who have a history of drug dependence and arrest with few sources of income (Hansen et al. 2014). The resulting vicious cycle of concentrated drug trade, violence, joblessness, homelessness, and re-lated chronic diseases including HIV infection and psychiatric disorders in low-income communities has been termed a "syndemic," and is associated with increased inequities in life expectancy by race, ethnicity, and neighborhood (Drucker 2013; Singer 2009).

Increasing opioid use among suburban and rural whites starting in the late 1990s was met with a less punitive response. This difference was first apparent in the distinction that law enforcement made between manufactured opioids and heroin. Although by 2004 prescription opioids had overtaken heroin as the primary opioid of abuse in the United States, the arrest rate for their illegal possession was one-fourth that for possession of heroin. The arrest rate for illegal sale of prescription drugs was less than one-fifth that for selling heroin (U.S. Census Bureau 2009). Not coincidentally, at the time, the nonmedical use of prescription opioids was twice as high among whites as blacks (Substance Abuse and Mental Health Services Administration 2010), while rates of heroin use among blacks, Latinos, and whites were almost identical (Office of National Drug Control Policy 2011). The more recent shift from nonmedical use of prescription opioids to heroin use in white communities has been followed by bipartisan calls for less punitive law enforcement and an emphasis on diversion from jail or prison to treatment and supportive services (Seelye 2015).

Amid these changes in drug policy, the Drug Enforcement Administration (DEA) and other regulators shifted their surveillance and enforcement to prescription opioid prescribers and suppliers through prescription drug monitoring programs (PDMPs), which have been enacted in 49 states, half of which mandate prescriber participation with threats of loss of license and prosecution (Finklea et al. 2014). Other recent shifts away from incarceration include court-sponsored diversion from sentencing to treatment; public support for training and engagement of police officers as first responders who administer naloxone during overdose, and accompanying Good Samaritan laws protecting overdose bystanders from drug charges; use of MAT, such as buprenorphine maintenance; and harm reduction measures, such as widespread naloxone distribution and training, naloxone availability in pharmacies, and syringe exchange programs.

Pharmaceutical Marketing and Regulatory Considerations

Pharmaceutical Development and Regulation

The shifting demographics of prescription opioid use and related increases in heroin use are best understood in the context of late twentieth-century opioid pharmaceutical development, regulation, and marketing. These changes unfolded on the backdrop of the Decade of the Brain (1990–2000), an era in which President George H.W. Bush directed the National Institute on Drug Abuse (NIDA) to study the neuromolecular bases for addiction, in anticipation of breakthroughs from the Human Genome Project.

Alan Leshner, director of NIDA at the time, lobbied to rebrand addiction as a "chronic relapsing brain disease." In 1997, Leshner published a landmark article titled "Addiction Is a Brain Disease, and It Matters." Pharmaceutical manufacturers built on this ethos of molecular bases for addiction and corresponding biotechnological solutions in ways that made the social contexts of addiction less visible to regulators. In 1996, Purdue Pharma received approval from the U.S. Food and Drug Administration (FDA) to market OxyContin as a "minimally addictive opioid pain reliever" suitable for chronic management of moderate pain.

This approval was based on OxyContin's patented sustained-release capsule technology, which in theory lowered the reward for those using the medication by preventing the euphoria that immediate-release, high-dose oxycodone would otherwise cause (Seppala 2010). What the model of addiction-proof biotechnology left out was the social context of drug use: because oxycodone is more potent than morphine, OxyContin users interested in a rush quickly learned to crush and snort or inject the oxycodone in each capsule. Also in the mid-1990s, the Joint Commission on hospital accreditation called for pain to be aggressively monitored and treated as the "fifth vital sign," leading to widespread prescription of OxyContin and other opioids for moderate pain, such as that due to lower back injury (Van Zee 2009).

Office-based buprenorphine maintenance treatment was developed specifically in response to this largely white, suburban and rural prescription opioid epidemic. In the 1990s, NIDA subsidized the manufacture of Suboxone (buprenorphine and naloxone) to test it for use in addiction treatment. Also, in an effort to sharply distinguish buprenorphine from methadone, NIDA lobbied Congress and the DEA to lower the abuse potential rating of buprenorphine from Schedule II, where oxycodone and methadone fall, to Schedule III, along with other widely prescribed medications such as codeine cough syrup. This then made it possible to prescribe buprenorphine in doctors' offices. For buprenorphine maintenance prescribing in office-based settings to be legalized, however, the federal law restricting physicians from prescribing opioids to opioid-dependent patients—the 1914 Harrison Act—had to be reversed. Buprenorphine's manufacturer collaborated with sympathetic members of Congress and addiction scientists to design a suitable bill (Jaffe and O'Keeffe 2003). In 2000, Congress passed the Drug Addiction Treatment Act (DATA 2000), which enabled certified physicians to prescribe buprenorphine in the privacy of their own offices.

The congressional testimony in support of DATA 2000 asserted that 1) buprenorphine was uniquely appropriate for a new kind of opioid user, as opposed to methadone, "which tends to concentrate in urban areas, is a poor fit for the suburban spread of narcotic addiction" (Congressional Record 1999, p. S1092) and 2) buprenorphine, as an alternative to methadone, would serve a new kind of addict, "including many citizens who would not ordinarily be associated with the term addiction" (Congressional Record 2000, p. S9113). The implication was that these new users are white.

To give additional assurance to the DEA that buprenorphine would not spill over into illicit markets, buprenorphine's manufacturer, along with SAMHSA, developed an 8-hour certification course that was required for doctors to prescribe buprenorphine, the first and only prescription drug in the United States to come with such a requirement. Physicians working in the public sector, often with heavy caseloads, may not have the same incentives to obtain an additional certification as do private-sector physicians, who can charge high fees for buprenorphine prescribing. As a result, uptake of buprenorphine maintenance has been most rapid among white, educated, and employed consumers with access to certified prescribers (Stanton et al. 2006), as well as in higher-income areas with higher percentages of white residents (Hansen et al. 2016). In public clinics and in low-income regions, a lack of physicians who are certified to prescribe buprenorphine has been a significant barrier to equity in access to treatment (Jones et al. 2017; Urada et al. 2014).

Ethnic Marketing and Media

When OxyContin was under review at the FDA, Purdue estimated the addictive potential of OxyContin to be "less than 1%" based on testing among terminally ill cancer patients for a 3-month period. Purdue referred to this minimized risk to sell OxyContin to a new, larger, and therefore lucrative market of patients with moderate chronic pain, hiring a cadre of 671 drug representatives who canvassed a call list of up to 94,000 physicians, mostly generalists in (predominantly white) suburban and rural areas nationwide. This led to a 10-fold increase in prescription opioids nationally (Van Zee 2009).

Major media outlets have contributed to the white racial image of the population newly using opioids and heroin. A content analysis of 100 randomly selected major national newspaper articles about opioids and heroin in 2001 and 2011 found two types of stories: one about urban black and Latino people using opioids and heroin that consistently mentioned crime and another about white suburban and rural people using opioids and heroin, who were portrayed sympathetically as victims of overprescription or as people struggling with real or existential pain (Netherland and Hansen 2016).

Suboxone, the targeted intervention for the population new to heroin and opioid use, was marketed to middle-class, insured patients over the Internet. The manufacturer's website prominently displayed public service announcements featuring white professionals and business owners taking Suboxone for maintenance. This same website featured a link to a Suboxone prescriber locator service created by SAMHSA; browsers could enter a zip code to generate a list of Suboxone prescribers, most of whom were in private practice rather than public clinics. These strategies created an exclusive yet lucrative segment of the market for Suboxone, making it a blockbuster drug at over $1.5 billion a year in sales in the United States by the end of its first decade (CESAR FAX 2012), second only to OxyContin, which by 2010 had reported annual sales of $3 billion, while prescription opioids as a drug class had generated $11 billion per year (Eban 2011).

Local, State, and National Policies and Their Impact on Health Inequities

As the opioid epidemic has grown and become perceived to be a problem affecting primarily white communities, less punitive approaches to drug use have emerged. In particular, harm reduction–oriented solutions, such as syringe exchange programs, naloxone, and Good Samaritan laws (protecting those who call for emergency assistance during an overdose from drug charges), have proliferated, and there is increased funding for MAT. Even supply-side interventions, which have typically been focused on arrest and incarceration, now include "softer" approaches, such as PDMP databases and law enforcement diversion programs. It is important to examine the ways that deployment of these seemingly race-neutral drug policies may reinforce, rather than mitigate, racial disparities, by monitoring whether and how these less punitive approaches are reaching communities of color. Unfortunately, data that indicate where and to whom these new policy approaches are being deployed are limited. However, the contrast between the ramping up of the drug war during the crack epidemic, which was perceived as a problem of the nonwhite community, and these gentler policy responses during an epidemic considered to be a problem for the white community is striking.

Harm Reduction

Harm reduction refers to a set of practical strategies aimed at reducing the harms associated with drug use. Although harm reduction programs have operated for decades in the United States, until recently they have received relatively little support and have been seen as controversial, despite a robust evidence base documenting their effectiveness in reducing drug-related harms, such as the transmission of blood-borne diseases. Among the most well-known and common harm reduction programs in the United States are needle and syringe exchange programs, which offer clean syringes to people who inject drugs, typically alongside an array of other services. Like methadone clinics, these highly stigmatized programs have typically been situated in low-income communities of color.

In recent years, however, support for syringe exchange programs has steadily grown, and they have been implemented in places that used to vociferously oppose them. In 2016, the federal ban on funding syringe exchange programs was lifted, although federal funds still cannot be used to pay for syringes themselves. These kinds of legislative changes, even in Republican-dominated states, were driven in part by outbreaks of HIV caused by the use of injection opioids, especially in white rural and suburban communities (Rich and Adashi 2015).

Similarly, programs to expand the use of naloxone have increased exponentially. Naloxone is a medication that when administered during an opioid overdose can reverse its effects. As the opioid crisis grew and spread to white suburban communities, efforts to expand access to naloxone increased. As of 2016, laws to increase access to naloxone were passed in 47 states and the District of Columbia. One study looking at naloxone administration in 42 states found that the odds of naloxone administration were highest in suburban and rural areas (Faul et al. 2015). Additionally, hundreds of law enforcement agencies, in states ranging from Washington to New York to North Carolina, now ask their police officers to carry and use naloxone. Police officers, whose previous purview had been to arrest those using drugs, are now responsible for saving their lives. It remains an open question whether communities of color that have been historically over-policed are benefiting from police-based naloxone programs to the same extent as white communities.

Another harm reduction policy that has proliferated in recent years is that 911 Good Samaritan laws protect those who call for emergency assistance during an overdose, as well as the overdosed person, from drug charges. Forty states and the District of Colombia have enacted some form of 911 Good Samaritan laws.

The opioid crisis in white America has even led several jurisdictions to consider drug consumption rooms, where people who use drugs can legally inject or consume drugs under medical supervision. Although the effectiveness of drug consumption rooms at reducing illness and public disorder is well documented in Canada and Europe, until very recently such programs were considered too controversial for public debate in the United States. For instance, a Google News search on "supervised injection facilities" between 2000 and 2010 yielded no news stories and only two opinion pieces, both authored by drug policy reform advocate Ethan Nadelmann. The situation began to change when the mayor of the small, predominantly white city of Ithaca, New York, which had experienced a number of overdose deaths, advocated publicly for a supervised injection facility. In 2017 alone, the same Google News search yielded almost 300 stories, and a number of national newspapers have portrayed drug consumption rooms as a reasonable response to the growing problem of drug overdoses (see, e.g., USA Today Editorial Board 2016).

Supply-Side and Law Enforcement Interventions

Prior to the white opioid crisis, drug policy focused on law enforcement, mandatory minimums, and mass incarceration—framed as the need to reduce supply. More recently, "softer" supply-side interventions, such as PDMPs, have become more common; 49 states had operational PDMPs by 2016 (National Alliance for Model State Drug Laws 2016). State PDMPs are highly varied. Some states have "proactive" PDMPs, which issue reports on clients without provider initiation, whereas others require a provider to request previous prescription data.

The research suggests that PDMPs are effective at decreasing the level of opioids prescribed, as well as doctor-shopping and pharmacy-shopping behaviors, but the research is divided on PDMPs' impacts on overall opioid use, including the degree to which they contribute to increased heroin use (Dasgupta et al. 2014). Also under-studied is the extent to which PDMPs might exacerbate the well-documented racial disparities in the prescription of pain medications. Numerous studies have shown that black Americans in particular are denied access to pain medication even when it is compellingly warranted. If physicians are already reluctant to prescribe opioids to people of color, having to check a PDMP prior to doing so may create an additional barrier. Moreover, pharmacies in poor, white neighborhoods are 54 times as likely as pharmacies in poor neighborhoods of color to have "adequate supplies" of opioids (Goodnough 2016).

Another supply-side innovation to curb the abuse of prescription opioids has been the DEA's National Prescription Drug Take Back Day (www.deadiversion.usdoj.gov/drug_disposal/takeback/), a yearly event that allows individuals to dispose of unused prescription medications. This strategy is notable for its focus on upstream causes of use and its refusal to penalize individual users. That the DEA is now involved in protecting people who use drugs and trying to assist them is a radical departure for an agency that has previously spent many millions of dollars pursuing punitive drug war tactics.

A significant change in law enforcement practices is the use of diversion programs, which divert people involved in low-level drug offenses directly to services or treatment. Perhaps the best known of these programs is Law Enforcement Assisted Diversion (LEAD), which originated in Seattle (Collins et al. 2017). Under LEAD, police officers have discretion to divert low-level drug and prostitution offenders into community-based treatment and support services—including housing, health care, job training, treatment, and mental health support—instead of processing them through traditional criminal justice system avenues. Similar programs, called Angel Programs, encourage people struggling with addiction to turn themselves in at local police stations, not to be arrested but to be directed to treatment. Launched in 2015 by the Police Department of Gloucester, Massachusetts, Angel Programs have reportedly been replicated by 128 police departments in 28 states. These programs represent a notable change from the role of the police during the prior drug crises such as the crack cocaine epidemic, which was seen as affecting primarily black and Latino communities, and during which police did not divert users to treatment. The following remain unknown: whether these kinds of diversion programs are being deployed equally in white communities and communities of color, and whether white people and people of color are diverted at proportional rates.

Policies on Treatment

Treatment admissions for OUD are increasing, especially for whites, who currently represent a larger proportion of those receiving publicly funded treatment slots. According to a survey of publicly funded treatment programs, in 2014, whites accounted for 84% of treatment admissions for nonheroin opioids and 69% of admissions for heroin. Between 2004 and 2014, the proportion of whites ages 20–34 among heroin admissions increased by 27% (Substance Abuse and Mental Health Services Administration, Center for Behavioral Health Statistics and Quality 2015). Among private insurers, spending on substance use treatment per enrollee increased from $9.81 in 2001 to $17.86 in 2009, a faster rate of growth than general price inflation and faster also than general medical prices. Moreover, the percentage of the population using any substance abuse medications (including methadone and buprenorphine) grew from 0.05% to 0.18% (Mark and Vandivort-Warren 2012).

At the federal level over the past few years, there has also been a steady increase in funding for prevention and treatment, while funding for law enforcement and interdiction has remained level. President Obama's fiscal year 2017 budget included $1 billion in new mandatory funding over 2 years to expand access to treatment and recovery support services specifically for those with OUD, including $50 million for MAT such as buprenorphine maintenance. These investments may not benefit all communities equally, however. One study found that the number of publicly owned drug treatment facilities declined between 2002 and 2010 by 17.2%, whereas the number of private, for-profit facilities grew by 19.1%. Counties with high percentages of black residents were disproportionately affected by the decline in public facilities (Cummings et al. 2016).

How treatment access plays out in the future will depend largely on the fate of the Patient Protection and Affordable Care Act of 2010 (ACA; P.L. 111-148). The ACA recognizes addiction as a health problem, and under the ACA, public and private insurance plans must provide health care services for addiction just as they would for diabetes or cancer. The ACA expanded Medicaid to millions of people who lacked health insurance, providing access to health care, opioid-related care, and mental health services. Having access to health care helps people who struggle with addiction address underlying health needs, reduce drug-related harm, reduce overdose risk, and get access to evidence-based MAT and other care. However, some research suggests that counties with a higher percentage of black, rural, and/or uninsured residents are less likely to have Medicaid-funded treatment facilities, meaning those communities not only are less helped by the ACA expansion but also are likely the first to suffer from cuts in terms of access to needed treatment (Cummings et al. 2014). Federal block grants, the other primary source of treatment funding, are also vulnerable to cuts by the federal government, which could be especially problematic for those states that have opted out of Medicaid expansion.

Pursuing Equity

The increased attention to opioid use in white communities has coincided with a sea change in drug policy. There is an unprecedented focus on treatment and harm reduction strategies heretofore unseen in the United States, as well as a transformation in the role of law enforcement in responding to drug use. These changes may be due in part to the growing recognition that the War on Drugs has been costly and detrimental to families and communities in terms of missed opportunities to promote public health, spending on ineffective law enforcement approaches, and mass incarceration. The shift in the public perception of who uses drugs and the corresponding increase in sympathetic media portrayals that foster a growing understanding of addiction as a health problem, rather than a moral failing, also contribute to this change (Netherland and Hansen 2016). Although this turn to more therapeutic approaches in policy is encouraging, in order to reduce inequities in the health and social outcomes of addiction, the geographic and demographic distribution of resources for addiction treatment and of changes to law enforcement practices must be made more equitable in our racially bifurcated system. It is also important to note that the racial divisiveness of past policy responses to drugs has undermined opportunities to respond more effectively to the current crisis. Low levels of investment in a public health infrastructure have left many of the communities now facing OUD problems without the treatment and harm reduction services they need. The failure to invest adequately in prevention, treatment, and public health when drug use was viewed as primarily a problem for communities of color means that all communities are now scrambling to address the problem. As the nation works to improve population health for all through comprehensive addiction treatment, harm reduction, and health care, it must be ensured that all communities are equitably served.

Future Directions for Clinical Training and Research

The available evidence on differences in opioid use and treatment by race, ethnicity, gender, and socioeconomic status indicates that the differences are driven by institutional and policy-level forces, including pharmaceutical marketing strategies, regulations with a geographically disparate impact, state- and federal-level decision making about distribution of funding for health care coverage and treatment services, and law enforcement practices such as diversion from drug possession sentencing to treatment or criminalization of substance use while pregnant. These systems-level drivers are compounded by provider-level biases in practice, such as differences in the likelihood of screening and referral for treatment of opioid dependence and differences in the likelihood of offering buprenorphine in primary care offices. However, individual-level biases in themselves do not explain the majority of population-level patterns regarding who is exposed to opioids and heroin, who receives treatment for dependence, and what the outcomes of treatment are. Such population-level patterns are best described by social determinants that require systemic, institutional levels of intervention.

To date, however, clinicians have not been sufficiently trained to intervene on the social determinants of health. The opioid epidemic calls for new approaches to clinical training that empower clinicians to see and act upon institutional barriers to their patients' health. An example is *structural competency*, which involves helping trainees to identify the structural and social factors impinging on patient care and outcomes and to observe and practice working with neighborhood organizations and local agencies as well as policy makers to address those factors (Hansen and Metzl 2017). Other key competencies include *cultural humility*, which involves recognition of unequal power relations between providers and patients and a posture of collaboration with patients as well as community representatives to rectify inequities in health (Tervalon and Murray-García 1998), as well as *critical thinking skills*, which involve training practitioners to reflect critically about the ways that clinical institutions are structured and how they may be harming patients (Bromley and Braslow 2008). These competencies call for innovative tools to prepare a clinical workforce for the challenges of socially determined health inequities such as those related to opioid use.

Researchers can help identify ways to intervene on social determinants to improve health outcomes. Research may involve stratifying population-level data by race/ethnicity and gender, as well as examining interactions between demographic and clinical variables while incorporating the concept of intersectionality—the additive effects of multiple marginalized identities (e.g., race, gender, sexual orientation). Mixed-method approaches drawing on both quantitative and qualitative data may better characterize the "social ecology" of addiction, including the ways that the costs and consequences of substance use are unequally distributed across populations (Wallace et al. 1999).

Key Chapter Points

▶ A social determinants approach to the opioid epidemic requires examination of the economic, social, and political structures that have shaped the disease burden of OUD, as well as treatment access and outcomes across race/ethnicity, gender, and geography.

▶ The United States has experienced multiple opioid epidemics, beginning in the mid-1800s, and the national response to each epidemic has ranged from punitive to more treatment focused, depending on the sociopolitical climate and the ethnicity, race, and socioeconomic status of the groups perceived to be affected.

▶ Opioid use—which in the 1970s and 1980s was portrayed as involving predominantly young, urban, minority males—was shown beginning in the 1990s to involve an increasingly white, older, suburban and rural, male and female population.

▶ Utilization of the three FDA-approved medications for OUD (methadone, buprenorphine, and extended-release naltrexone [XR-naltrexone]) varies significantly by race and ethnicity; for example, white patients are more likely than black patients to receive the newer, less restricted medications buprenorphine and XR-naltrexone.

▶ Emerging evidence indicates that without interventions to promote racial, ethnic, and socioeconomic equity in prevention and treatment of OUD, systemic, unequal application of public health versus law enforcement approaches to opioid dependence will persist.

▶ As the opioid epidemic has grown along with the perception that the problem primarily affects white communities, less punitive approaches to drug use have emerged. Ensuring that these approaches reach all communities equally requires deliberate attention to ameliorating existing racial inequities.

References

Agar M, Reisinger HS: A heroin epidemic at the intersection of histories: the 1960s epidemic among African Americans in Baltimore. Med Anthropol 21(2):115–156, 2002 12126273

Alexander M: The New Jim Crow: Mass Incarceration in the Age of Colorblindness. New York, New Press, 2010

Back SE, Payne RL, Simpson AN, et al: Gender and prescription opioids: findings from the National Survey on Drug Use and Health. Addict Behav 35(11):1001–1007, 2010 20598809

Badger E: How mass incarceration creates "million dollar blocks" in poor neighborhoods. Washington Post, July 30, 2015. Available at: https://

www.washingtonpost.com/news/wonk/wp/2015/07/30/how-mass-incarceration-creates-million-dollar-blocks-in-poor-neighborhoods/?utm_term=.327b286fa20. Accessed March 30, 2018.

Baum D: Legalize it all: how to win the war on drugs. Harper's Magazine, April 2016. Available at: https://harpers.org/archive/2016/04/legalize-it-all/. Accessed March 30, 2018.

Beasley GM, Ostbye T, Muhlbaier LH, et al: Age and gender differences in substance screening may underestimate injury severity: a study of 9793 patients at level 1 trauma center from 2006 to 2010. J Surg Res 188(1):190–197, 2014 24370454

Bromley E, Braslow JT: Teaching critical thinking in psychiatric training: a role for the social sciences. Am J Psychiatry 165(11):1396–1401, 2008 18981073

Brooks AJ, Lokhnygina Y, Meade CS, et al: Racial/ethnic differences in the rates and correlates of HIV risk behaviors among drug abusers. Am J Addict 22(2):136–147, 2013 23414499

Brown JD, Goodin AJ, Talbert JC: Rural and Appalachian disparities in neonatal abstinence syndrome incidence and access to opioid abuse treatment. J Rural Health 34(1):6–13, 2017 28685864

Broz D, Ouellet LJ: Racial and ethnic changes in heroin injection in the United States: implications for the HIV/AIDS epidemic. Drug Alcohol Depend 94(1–3):221–233, 2008 18242879

Case A, Deaton A: Rising morbidity and mortality in midlife among white non-Hispanic Americans in the 21st century. Proc Natl Acad Sci USA 112(49):15078–15083, 2015 26575631

Case A, Deaton A: Mortality and morbidity in the 21st century. Paper presented at the Brookings Panel on Economic Activity conference, March 23, 2017. Available at: https://www.brookings.edu/bpea-articles/mortality-and-morbidity-in-the-21st-century/. Accessed March 30, 2018.

Centers for Disease Control and Prevention: Vital signs: overdoses of prescription opioid pain relievers and other drugs among women—United States, 1999–2010. Morbidity and Mortality Weekly Report, July 5, 2013. Available at: https://www.cdc.gov/mmwr/preview/mmwrhtml/mm6226a3.htm. Accessed March 30, 2018.

Centers for Disease Control and Prevention: HIV surveillance report, 2015. 2016. Available at: http://www.cdc.gov/hiv/library/reports/hiv-surveillance.html. Accessed March 30, 2018.

Centers for Disease Control and Prevention: Annual surveillance report of drug-related risks and outcomes—United States, 2017. Surveillance Special Report 1. 2017a. Available at: https://www.cdc.gov/drugoverdose/pdf/pubs/2017-cdc-drug-surveillance-report.pdf. Accessed March 30, 2018.

Centers for Disease Control and Prevention: Surveillance for viral hepatitis—United States, 2015, 2017b. Available at: https://www.cdc.gov/hepatitis/statistics/2015surveillance/index.htm. Accessed March 30, 2018.

CESAR FAX: Suboxone® sales estimated to reach $1.4 billion in 2012—more than Viagra® or Adderall®. December 10, 2012. Available at: http://www.cesar.umd.edu/cesar/cesarfax/vol21/21-49.pdf. Accessed March 30, 2018.

Cicero TJ, Ellis MS, Surratt HL, et al: The changing face of heroin use in the United States: a retrospective analysis of the past 50 years. JAMA Psychiatry 71(7):821–826, 2014 24871348

Collins SE, Lonczak HS, Clifasefi SL: Seattle's Law Enforcement Assisted Diversion (LEAD): program effects on recidivism outcomes. Eval Program Plann 64:49–56, 2017 28531654

Congressional Record: Drug Addiction Treatment Act of 1999. Senate 106th Congress, 1999, pp S1089–S1093

Congressional Record: Drug Addiction Treatment Act of 2000. Congressional Record—Senate. 106th Congress, 2000, p S9113

Courtwright D: Dark Paradise: A History of Opiate Use in America. Cambridge, MA, Harvard University Press, 1982

Cummings JR, Wen H, Ko M, et al: Race/ethnicity and geographic access to Medicaid substance use disorder treatment facilities in the United States. JAMA Psychiatry 71(2):190–196, 2014 24369387

Cummings J, Wen H, Ko M: Decline in public substance use disorder treatment centers most serious in counties with high shares of black residents. Health Aff (Millwood) 35(6):1036–1044, 2016 27269020

Dai S: A chart that says the war on drugs isn't working. The Atlantic. October 12, 2012. Available at: https://www.theatlantic.com/national/archive/2012/10/chart-says-war-drugs-isnt-working/322592/. Accessed March 30, 2018.

Dasgupta N, Creppage K, Austin A, et al: Observed transition from opioid analgesic deaths toward heroin. Drug Alcohol Depend 145:238–241, 2014 25456574

Dick AW, Pacula RL, Gordon AJ, et al: Growth in buprenorphine waivers for physicians increased potential access to opioid agonist treatment, 2002–11. Health Aff (Millwood) 34(6):1028–1034, 2015 26056209

Drucker E: A Plague of Prisons: The Epidemiology of Mass Incarceration in America. New York, New Press, 2013

Eban K: OxyContin: Purdue Pharma's painful medicine. Fortune, November 9, 2011. Available at http://fortune.com/2011/11/09/oxycontin-purdue-pharmas-painful-medicine/. Accessed March 30, 2018.

Faul M, Dailey MW, Sugerman DE, et al: Disparity in naloxone administration by emergency medical service providers and the burden of drug overdose in U.S. rural communities. Am J Public Health 105 (suppl 3):e26–e32, 2015 25905856

Finklea K, Sacco LN, Bagalman E: Prescription drug monitoring programs. Congressional Research Service, March 24, 2014. Available at: https://fas.org/sgp/crs/misc/R42593.pdf. Accessed March 30, 2018.

Frederique K: The role race plays in the war on drugs. February 8, 2016. Available at: http://www.ebony.com/news-views/race-war-on-drugs. Accessed March 30, 2018.

Galea S, Tracy M, Hoggatt KJ, et al: Estimated deaths attributable to social factors in the United States. Am J Public Health 101(8):1456–1465, 2011 21680937

Gelman A, Auerbach J: Age-aggregation bias in mortality trends. Proc Natl Acad Sci USA 113(7):E816–E817, 2016 26858421

Gone JP, Trimble JE: American Indian and Alaska Native mental health: diverse perspectives on enduring disparities. Annu Rev Clin Psychol 8:131–160, 2012 22149479

Goodnough A: Finding good pain treatment is hard. If you're not white, it's harder. New York Times, August 9, 2016. Available at: https://www.nytimes.com/2016/08/10/us/how-race-plays-a-role-in-patients-pain-treatment.html?_r=0. Accessed March 30, 2018.

Gryczynski J, Jaffe JH, Schwartz RP, et al: Patient perspectives on choosing buprenorphine over methadone in an urban, equal-access system. Am J Addict 22(3):285–291, 2013 23617873

Guy GP Jr, Zhang K, Bohm MK, et al: Vital signs: changes in opioid prescribing in the United States, 2006–2015. MMWR Morb Mortal Wkly Rep 66(26):697–704, 2017 28683056

Hadland SE, Wharam JF, Schuster MA, et al: Trends in receipt of buprenorphine and naltrexone for opioid use disorder among adolescents and young adults, 2001–2014. JAMA Pediatr 171(8):747–755, 2017 28628701

Hansen H, Metzl JM: New medicine for the U.S. health care system: training physicians for structural interventions. Acad Med 92(3):279–281, 2017 28079725

Hansen H, Bourgois P, Drucker E: Pathologizing poverty: new forms of diagnosis, disability, and structural stigma under welfare reform. Soc Sci Med 103:126–133, 2014 24507913

Hansen H, Siegel C, Wanderling J, et al: Buprenorphine and methadone treatment for opioid dependence by income, ethnicity and race of neighborhoods in New York City. Drug Alcohol Depend 164:14–21, 2016 27179822

Hemsing N, Greaves L, Poole N, et al: Misuse of prescription opioid medication among women: a scoping review. Pain Res Manag 2016:1754195, 2016 27445597

Herzberg D: Happy Pills in America: From Miltown to Prozac. Baltimore, MD, Johns Hopkins University Press, 2009

Heygi N: Cherokee Nation sues Wal-Mart, CVS, Walgreens over tribal opioid crisis. April 25, 2017. Available at: https://www.npr.org/sections/codeswitch/2017/04/25/485887058/cherokee-nation-sues-wal-mart-cvs-walgreens-over-tribal-opioid-crisis. Accessed March 30, 2018.

Hughes PH, Rieche O: Heroin epidemics revisited. Epidemiol Rev 17(1):66–73, 1995 8521947

Hughes PH, Barker NW, Crawford GA, et al: The natural history of a heroin epidemic. Am J Public Health 62(7):995–1001, 1972 5039507

Jaffe JH, O'Keeffe C: From morphine clinics to buprenorphine: regulating opioid agonist treatment of addiction in the United States. Drug Alcohol Depend 70(2)(suppl):S3–S11, 2003 12738346

Jones CM, Logan J, Gladden RM, et al: Vital signs: demographic and substance use trends among heroin users—United States, 2002–2013. MMWR Morb Mortal Wkly Rep 64(26):719–725, 2015 26158353

Jones CM, Christensen A, Gladden RM: Increases in prescription opioid injection abuse among treatment admissions in the United States, 2004–2013. Drug Alcohol Depend 176:89–95, 2017 28531769

Kerridge BT, Saha TD, Chou SP, et al: Gender and nonmedical prescription opioid use and DSM-5 nonmedical prescription opioid use disorder: results from the National Epidemiologic Survey on Alcohol and Related Conditions—III. Drug Alcohol Depend 156:47–56, 2015 26374990

Keyes KM, Cerdá M, Brady JE, et al: Understanding the rural-urban differences in nonmedical prescription opioid use and abuse in the United States. Am J Public Health 104(2):e52–e59, 2014 24328642

Kolodny A, Courtwright DT, Hwang CS, et al: The prescription opioid and heroin crisis: a public health approach to an epidemic of addiction. Annu Rev Public Health 36:559–574, 2015 25581144

Leshner AI: Addiction is a brain disease, and it matters. Science 278(5335):45–47, 1997 9311924

Mack KA, Jones CM, Ballesteros MF: Illicit drug use, illicit drug use disorders, and drug overdose deaths in metropolitan and nonmetropolitan areas—United States. MMWR Surveill Summ 66(19):1–12, 2017 29049278

Manhapra A, Quinones L, Rosenheck R: Characteristics of veterans receiving buprenorphine vs. methadone for opioid use disorder nationally in the Veterans Health Administration. Drug Alcohol Depend 160:82–89, 2016 26804898

Mark TL, Vandivort-Warren R: Spending trends on substance abuse treatment under private employer-sponsored insurance, 2001–2009. Drug Alcohol Depend 125(3):203–207, 2012 22436972

Martins SS, Sarvet A, Santaella-Tenorio J, et al: Changes in U.S. lifetime heroin use and heroin use disorder: prevalence from the 2001–2002 to 2012–2013 National Epidemiologic Survey on Alcohol and Related Conditions. JAMA Psychiatry 74(5):445–455, 2017 28355458

Mennis J, Stahler GJ: Racial and ethnic disparities in outpatient substance use disorder treatment episode completion for different substances. J Subst Abuse Treat 63:25–33, 2016 26818489

Monnat SM, Rigg KK: Examining rural/urban differences in prescription opioid misuse among U.S. adolescents. J Rural Health 32(2):204–218, 2016 26344571

Musto DF: The American Disease: Origins of Narcotic Control. New York, Oxford University Press, 1999

National Alliance for Model State Drug Laws: Compilation of prescription monitoring program maps. May 2016. Available at: http://www.namsdl.org/library/CAE654BF-BBEA-211E-694C755E16C2DD21/. Accessed March 30, 2018.

Nellis A: The color of justice: racial and ethnic disparity in state prisons. The Sentencing Project, 2016. Available at: http://www.sentencingproject.org/publications/color-of-justice-racial-and-ethnic-disparity-in-state-prisons/. Accessed March 30, 2018.

Netherland J, Hansen HB: The war on drugs that wasn't: wasted whiteness, "dirty doctors," and race in media coverage of prescription opioid misuse. Cult Med Psychiatry 40(4):664–686, 2016 27272904

Office of National Drug Control Policy: Minorities and drugs: facts and figures. 2011. Available at: http://www.whitehousedrugpolicy.gov/drugfact/minorities/minorities_ff.html. Accessed December 15, 2015.

Patrick SW, Schumacher RE, Benneyworth BD, et al: Neonatal abstinence syndrome and associated health care expenditures: United States, 2000–2009. JAMA 307(18):1934–1940, 2012 22546608

Pletcher MJ, Kertesz SG, Kohn MA, et al: Trends in opioid prescribing by race/ethnicity for patients seeking care in U.S. emergency departments. JAMA 299(1):70–78, 2008 18167408

Rich JD, Adashi EY: Ideological anachronism involving needle and syringe exchange programs: lessons from the Indiana HIV outbreak. JAMA 314(1):23–24, 2015 26000661

Rosenblatt RA, Andrilla CH, Catlin M, et al: Geographic and specialty distribution of U.S. physicians trained to treat opioid use disorder. Ann Fam Med 13(1):23–26, 2015 25583888

Ryoo HJ, Choo EK: Gender differences in emergency department visits and detox referrals for illicit and nonmedical use of opioids. West J Emerg Med 17(3):295–301, 2016 27330662

Seelye K: In heroin crisis, white families seek gentler war on drugs. New York Times, October 30, 2015. Available at: https://www.nytimes.com/2015/10/31/us/heroin-war-on-drugs-parents.html. Accessed March 30, 2018.

Seppala M: Prescription Painkillers: History, Pharmacology, and Treatment. Center City, MN, Hazelden Publishing and Educational Services, 2010

Sigmon SC: Access to treatment for opioid dependence in rural America: challenges and future directions. JAMA Psychiatry 71(4):359–360, 2014 24500040

Singer M: Introduction to Syndemics: A Critical Systems Approach to Public and Community Health. San Francisco, CA, Jossey-Bass, 2009

Singhal A, Tien YY, Hsia RY: Racial-ethnic disparities in opioid prescriptions at emergency department visits for conditions commonly associated with prescription drug abuse. PLoS One 11(8):e0159224, 2016 27501459

Stanton A, McLeod C, Luckey B, et al: SAMHSA/CSAT evaluation of the buprenorphine waiver program: expanding treatment of opioid dependence: initial physician and patient experiences with the adoption of buprenorphine. Substance Abuse and Mental Health Services Administration, 2006. Available at: https://www.samhsa.gov/sites/default/files/programs_campaigns/medication_assisted/evaluation-buprenorphine-waiver-program-study-overview.pdf. Accessed August 29, 2018.

Stewart K, Cao Y, Hsu MH, et al: Geospatial analysis of drug poisoning deaths involving heroin in the USA, 2000–2014. J Urban Health 94(4):572–586, 2017 28639058

Substance Abuse and Mental Health Services Administration: Results From the 2009 National Survey on Drug Use and Health, Vol 1: Summary of National Findings (NSDUH Series H-38A, HHS Publ No SMA-10-4586). Rockville, MD, Substance Abuse and Mental Health Services Administration, 2010. Available at: http://www.gmhc.org/files/editor/file/a_pa_nat_drug_use_survey.pdf. Accessed March 30, 2018.

Substance Abuse and Mental Health Services Administration: Results From the 2013 National Survey on Drug Use and Health: Summary of National Findings (NSDUH Series H-48, HHS Publ No SMA-14-4863). Rockville, MD, Substance Abuse and Mental Health Services Administration, 2014. Available at: https://www.samhsa.gov/data/sites/default/files/NSDUHresultsPDFWHTML2013/Web/NSDUHresults2013.pdf. Accessed March 30, 2018.

Substance Abuse and Mental Health Services Administration, Center for Behavioral Health Statistics and Quality: Treatment Episode Data Set (TEDS): 2004–2014. State Admissions to Substance Abuse Treatment Services (BHSIS Series S-85, HHS Publ No SMA-16-4987). Rockville, MD,

Substance Abuse and Mental Health Services Administration, 2015. Available at: https://wwwdasis.samhsa.gov/dasis2/teds_pubs/ 2014_teds_rpt_st.pdf. Accessed March 30, 2018.

Terplan M: Women and the opioid crisis: historical context and public health solutions. Fertil Steril 108(2):195–199, 2017 28697909

Terplan M, Minkoff H: Neonatal abstinence syndrome and ethical approaches to the identification of pregnant women who use drugs. Obstet Gynecol 129(1):164–167, 2017 27926654

Tervalon M, Murray-García J: Cultural humility versus cultural competence: a critical distinction in defining physician training outcomes in multicultural education. J Health Care Poor Underserved 9(2):117–125, 1998 10073197

Unick GJ, Rosenblum D, Mars S, et al: Intertwined epidemics: national demographic trends in hospitalizations for heroin- and opioid-related overdoses, 1993–2009. PLoS One 8(2):e54496, 2013 23405084

Urada D, Teruya C, Gelberg L, et al: Integration of substance use disorder services with primary care: health center surveys and qualitative interviews. Subst Abuse Treat Prev Policy 9:15, 2014 24679108

USA Today Editorial Board: War on drugs requires new tactics: our view [editorial]. May 16, 2016. Available at: http://www.usatoday.com/story/opinion/ 2016/05/16/heroin-safe-injections-vancouver-opioids-overdose-editorials-debates/84421772/. Accessed March 30, 2018.

U.S. Census Bureau: Law enforcement, courts, and prisons: arrests. 2009. Available at: http://www.census.gov/compendia/ statab/cats/law _enforcement_courts_prisons/arrests.html. Accessed February 18, 2013.

Van Zee A: The promotion and marketing of OxyContin: commercial triumph, public health tragedy. Am J Public Health 99(2):221–227, 2009 18799767

Wallace R, Wallace D, Ullmann JE, et al: Deindustrialization, inner-city decay, and the hierarchical diffusion of AIDS in the USA: how neoliberal and cold war policies magnified the ecological niche for emerging infections and created a national security crisis. Environ Plan A 31(1):113–139, 1999

Zoorob MJ, Salemi JL: Bowling alone, dying together: the role of social capital in mitigating the drug overdose epidemic in the United States. Drug Alcohol Depend 173:1–9, 2017 28182980

Opioid Use Disorder and Medical Comorbidity

Aaron Fox, M.D., M.S.
Benjamin Hayes, M.D., M.P.H., M.S.W.

Clinical Vignette: Jason's Intravenous Drug Use Leads to Hepatitis C Virus Infection

Jason is a 24-year-old man with a history of major depressive disorder who started experimenting with opioid pain relievers as a teenager. His childhood in New Hampshire was filled with hiking, camping, and team sports. However, during high school, Jason developed dysphoria with sleeping problems and early morning awakening. He slowly lost interest in sports and withdrew from the friends with whom he had grown up. He began seeing Dr. Sanchez, a psychologist in private practice, who made the diagnosis of major depressive disorder and provided cognitive-behavioral therapy. As an eleventh grader, Jason disclosed to Dr. Sanchez that he sometimes would drink alcohol or take "oxys" at parties, because these substances helped him relax and fit in. He occasionally would steal oxycodone tablets from his parents' medicine cabinet and take them to fall asleep, but he never developed physical dependence on opioids. Despite some struggles socially, Jason excelled academically and graduated from high school with a 3.74 grade point average. He went away to college with the goal of becoming a fiction writer.

After several years, Jason has returned to see Dr. Sanchez, accompanied by his mother. The appointment was arranged by Jason's mother, who had urged Dr. Sanchez to fit him into her schedule because "his life is falling apart." Jason is thin, 6 feet tall and 140 pounds, but otherwise appears healthy. His affect is flat, and he seems embarrassed to be in the office. It is summertime, but Jason has on a long-sleeve shirt that completely covers his arms. Dr. Sanchez welcomes Jason, directs his mother to wait outside the office, and then asks him about the reason for the urgent appointment. He replies, "I'm on Suboxone [buprenorphine-naloxone], and the doctor needs me to bring proof that I'm getting counseling."

In this initial visit, Dr. Sanchez asks Jason about any updates to his medical history and current medications. Jason states that he was told that he has hepatitis C virus (HCV) infection, but he is not taking medication for it. They move on to talk about how his intermittent oxycodone use escalated during college, and how he was introduced to heroin. Jason explains that as his tolerance for opioids grew, he switched from oxycodone tablets to intranasal heroin because it became too expensive to buy oxycodone. He remembered telling himself that he would never use needles, but after about a year of sniffing heroin, he started to inject so that he could get a better high while spending less money. Jason bought sterile syringes from pharmacies when he could, and one of his friends would pick up supplies at a syringe exchange program weekly; however, frequently he was forced to reuse syringes and share drug paraphernalia (e.g., "cookers" used to dissolve heroin in water) with his friends. The conversation leads back to a discussion of HCV infection. Jason explains, "All of my friends have it—it's no big deal." Dr. Sanchez knows that new direct-acting antivirals for HCV are more effective than older medication, such as interferon, and have fewer side effects, and she reinforces that Jason should follow up with his medical doctor. Dr. Sanchez notes that Jason's lack of concern regarding HCV will be an important topic to explore in the future, and she seeks to learn more about HCV prognosis and treatment.

Jason's case highlights one of the major medical comorbidities of opioid use disorder (OUD), HCV infection, which is rapidly increasing among young people who inject drugs. The case raises several questions: What other medical conditions are common among individuals with OUD? Are there unique medical comorbidities due to Jason's injection drug use (IDU)? Is Jason also at risk for human immunodeficiency virus (HIV) infection? Should mental health providers wait to refer patients for medical treatment until they are no longer using drugs? If Jason continues opioid agonist treatment (OAT), are there harms that come from chronic exposure to opioids? How do medical comorbidities change the approach to treating OUD? Are there models of medical care in which Jason could receive treatment for both OUD and co-occurring medical conditions? What routine screening tests and preventive medical care should Jason be receiving?

Introduction

A common story line describing the "opioid epidemic" in the United States has focused on changes in physicians' attitudes toward chronic pain treatment, increases in opioid prescribing, and concomitant increases in OUD, opioid overdoses, and other harms of opioid misuse. The image of a middle-aged person, possibly a factory worker, having shoulder surgery, receiving prescription opioids for postsurgical pain, and becoming addicted to opioids, and then eventually moving on to heroin, informs the public's understanding of the crisis and has shifted attention to efforts to reduce opioid prescribing. Although chronic pain is an important factor in opioid overdose deaths, the pain narrative fails to include some of the most high-risk behaviors and medical conditions associated with OUD. According to the 2014 National Survey on Drug Use and Health, the age group most likely to have misused prescription opioids in the past year continues to be those ages 18–25 years (8.1%, compared with 2.0% among those over age 50 years), and a new generation of young adults from mostly suburban or rural areas is increasingly using heroin and injecting opioids (Cicero et al. 2014; Jones et al. 2017; Substance Abuse and Mental Health Services Administration 2017). The 2015 outbreak of HIV infection in Scott County, Indiana (Peters et al. 2016), and increases in HCV infection among young adults living in rural and suburban areas (Zibbell et al. 2015) are reminders that some of the most devastating consequences of OUD come from drug use behaviors (i.e., risky injection practices) rather than from direct opioid effects.

There is much variability among the individuals with OUD—at least 2.5 million of them—in the United States, and data representing the entire population of people with OUD are limited. Thus, determining which comorbidities are most commonly associated with OUD is difficult. However, age is an important factor to consider when gauging a patient's risk for specific comorbidities. As people with OUD age, mortality risk shifts from acute events, such as overdose, unintentional injuries, or suicide, to chronic medical conditions, such as cardiovascular disease, liver disease, pulmonary disease, and cancer (Degenhardt et al. 2014). Bahorik and colleagues (2017) found that chronic medical conditions, including asthma, coronary artery disease, chronic obstructive pulmonary disease, chronic pain, and others, were 2–20 times more common among individuals with OUD than among an age- and sex-matched comparison group within a large integrated U.S. health care system. Thus, although some health-promoting interventions, such as prevention of overdose and HCV or HIV infection, could be delivered outside medical settings, engagement in medical care is also critical, especially as people age.

In this chapter, we review medical comorbidities commonly seen in individuals seeking treatment for OUD, including medical conditions that are directly attributable to the effects of opioids, and introduce important considerations for providing OUD treatment to patients with chronic medical conditions. We also present necessary preventive care recommendations (e.g., vaccinations, screenings) for people with OUD and propose ideal models of integrated care that can engage this hard-to-reach population in both addiction treatment and medical care.

Comorbidities That Are Complications of Behaviors Associated With Opioid Use Disorder

Beyond the pharmacological effects of opioids, behaviors associated with OUD increase risk for a spectrum of medical complications. In this section, we differentiate the comorbidities associated with behaviors into those relating to the mode of opioid administration (injecting, sniffing, or smoking) and those relating to other behaviors, such as comorbid substance use disorders (SUDs) or sexual risk behaviors, that co-occur with OUD. Harms from oral opioid ingestion mostly stem from the direct effects of opioids and are discussed in the section "Comorbidities Due to Direct Opioid Effects." Behaviors associated with OUD can also have social consequences, such as incarceration or homelessness, which affect medical comorbidities and medical care access; however, in-depth discussion of these problems is beyond the scope of this chapter (see Chapters 5, "The Opioid Epidemic: Social Determinants and Health Inequities," and 12, "Harm Reduction: Caring for People Who Misuse Opioids").

Route of Opioid Administration

Percutaneous Injection

IDU is a conduit for common and serious complications of OUD. Injecting can be a private or communal behavior, and the process of preparing and injecting drugs presents several distinct risks. Commonly injected opioids include heroin, which comes as a white powder, darker brown powder, or sticky "black tar" variety; illicit synthetic opioids, such as fentanyl or similar analogues; and crushed or dissolved prescription opioids, such as oxycodone or oxymorphone. Powdered opioids may be "cut" with adulterants, such as lactose or quinine, which can have health consequences when injected. When preparing opioids for injection, people typically use a spoon or a small metal receptacle (i.e., "cooker") to mix and dissolve the drug. White powdered forms of heroin tend to dissolve in water alone, whereas some brown base forms need to be heated and combined with a mild acid (e.g., vitamin C) to dissolve. Typically, the dissolved drug is drawn into a syringe through a cotton filter, which may be saved and reused to extract any drug remnant within the filter. Therefore, syringes, cookers, water, and filters may each be involved in infectious disease transmission (Harm Reduction Coalition 2001).

People who inject drugs may have a particular preference for injecting into a vein ("mainlining"), muscle ("muscling"), or subcutaneous or intradermal tissue ("skin-popping"). Each site of injection carries risks: intravenous injection increases the risk of overdose, whereas intramuscular or subcutaneous injection increases the risk of soft tissue infection. Percutaneous injection may introduce bacteria beneath the skin and into the bloodstream, especially if needles or syringes are reused, drugs are dissolved in nonsterile water (e.g., water from sinks in public restrooms), cookers or filters are shared or reused, or the skin is not thoroughly cleaned (Harm Reduction Coalition 2001). For this reason, public injection in parks, alleyways, or homeless encampments is particularly risky, because people who inject drugs may be rushed, have inadequate lighting, and be unable to maintain a hygienic environment.

The most important medical complications of IDU of which health care providers should be aware are HCV, HIV, and skin and soft tissue infections (SSTIs). Additional comorbidities related to IDU are listed in Table 6–1. Despite increased awareness regarding HIV transmission, greater access to sterile syringes and injection supplies in some areas, and other prevention efforts, rates of HCV and HIV infection remain higher among people who inject drugs than in the general population. Infections of the skin, soft tissue, and heart valves are also increasingly frequent causes of hospitalizations. These serious complications are preventable.

In the United States, there are likely more than 5 million people living with HCV infection (Chak et al. 2011). Highly effective medications are available, yet deaths attributable to HCV continue to rise, making HCV infection the most fatal infectious disease in the United States (Ly et al. 2016). HCV infection is the primary cause of liver-related deaths, liver transplantation, cirrhosis, and hepatic cancer. HCV is highly infectious through blood exposure, and within 5 years of IDU initiation, more than one in five people who inject drugs becomes infected with HCV (Amon et al. 2008). Recently, the largest increases in HCV incidence have been in nonurban populations among people age 30 years or younger (Zibbell et al. 2015). This trend parallels increasing OUD and IDU in young, nonurban populations. These areas may have limited public health and preventive services, and over time, HCV-related morbidity and mortality are likely to increase further.

Acute HCV infection is generally asymptomatic, and approximately one-third of infected individuals will spontaneously clear the virus without developing chronic infection. Two-thirds of infected individuals develop chronic HCV infection, which can cause symptoms such as fatigue, muscle aches, and skin changes. Liver fibrosis and cirrhosis occurs slowly over several decades but may be accelerated by alcohol use disorder or concomitant HIV infection. Over a 20-year period, 15%–20% of those with chronic HCV infection will develop cirrhosis (Kim 2016). Outward signs of advanced liver disease include scleral icterus (yellowing of the eyes), swelling due to fluid retention in the legs and abdomen, and spider angiomas on the back and chest. Hepatocellular carcinoma, a primary malignancy of the liver occurring in approximately 3% of patients with HCV cirrhosis, causes significant mortality. HCV is also an important cause of chronic kidney disease, arthritis, diabetes, and non-Hodgkin's lymphoma (Kim 2016). Therefore, HCV treatment, ongoing preventive care, and medical surveillance are also indicated.

TABLE 6–1. Select medical comorbidities by route of opioid administration

Organ system or disease category	Conditions associated with injection drug use	Conditions associated with intranasal insufflation	Conditions associated with smoking or inhalation
Cardiovascular	Endocarditis	—	—
Cancer	Hepatocellular carcinoma (due to HCV)	—	—
Infectious diseases	Hepatitis A, B, C; HIV; soft tissue infections (abscess, cellulitis, necrotizing fasciitis); infective endocarditis; septic arthritis; osteomyelitis; brain abscess; pulmonary infections; TB; tetanus	Hepatitis A, B, C; pulmonary infections; TB	Hepatitis A, B, C; pulmonary infections; TB
Neurological	—	—	Progressive spongiform leukoencephalopathy
Respiratory	Pneumonia; septic pulmonary embolism, talc granulomatosis, emphysema, pulmonary hypertension, pulmonary edema, pneumothorax	Asthma exacerbation, sinus problems, hypersensitivity pneumonitis, nasal septum necrosis or perforation	Asthma exacerbation, emphysema, pulmonary edema, pneumothorax
Renal	Focal glomerular sclerosis, glomerulonephritis, nephrotic syndrome, chronic kidney disease	—	—

Note.   Dash indicates no known major comorbidities. HCV=hepatitis C virus; HIV=human immunodeficiency virus; TB=tuberculosis.
Source.   Adapted from Ries et al. 2014.

New directly acting antiviral therapies for HCV have exceptionally high cure rates (>90% in many populations) and are far better tolerated than older treatment regimens, such as interferon. Referral to medical care should happen at the time of diagnosis. Antiviral therapy is safe and effective even among people with active substance use. People who inject drugs should not be excluded from HCV treatment (Kim 2016). Ongoing IDU increases the risk of reinfection in the future, but offering HCV treatment to people who are at high risk of transmitting HCV infection to others—or "treatment as prevention"—can reduce new HCV infections (Martin et al. 2015). Patients enrolled in OAT programs (e.g., methadone maintenance) with good adherence are ideal candidates for HCV treatment. Guideline-recommended treatments vary based on the HCV genotype, presence of cirrhosis, and prior treatment history: however, common regimens are one pill daily for as few as 8–12 weeks. More detailed information about HCV care and treatment is available at www.hcvguidelines.org.

HCV complications may not be detected for decades, underscoring the importance of HCV awareness, prevention, and screening. Rapid screening tests can be performed using an oral swab, and results are available at the point of care. HCV testing recommendations are based on demographics, high-risk behaviors, and medical conditions, but all people who inject drugs should be offered HCV testing annually. People using intranasal drugs should also be offered periodic HCV testing because HCV transmission may occur by sharing contaminated implements for nasal inhalation (American Association for the Study of Liver Diseases and Infectious Diseases Society of America 2017). HCV is not transmitted through coughing, sneezing, or sharing of eating utensils or drinking glasses, but patients should be counseled about not sharing razors or toothbrushes because contact with blood may occur. Access to sterile injection equipment (syringes, needles, water, filters, cookers, spoons, or other devices for preparing and injecting drugs) and OAT reduce transmission of HCV (Turner et al. 2011). Mental health providers have many opportunities to participate in HCV prevention, screening, and referral to primary care or liver specialists.

HIV infection is also a common comorbidity among people who inject drugs in the United States. At the end of 2013, there were 1.1 million people living with HIV/acquired immune deficiency syndrome (AIDS), and IDU was the mode of transmission for 103,000 men and

68,000 women. From 2010 to 2014, IDU accounted for 11% of new infections among men and 23% among women (Centers for Disease Control and Prevention 2016b). HIV incidence among people who inject drugs is far below its peak in the early 1980s, but increasing IDU in the current opioid crisis puts at least 220 counties across the United States at high risk for HIV outbreaks (Van Handel et al. 2016). Young people who inject drugs (age < 30) are at highest risk for HIV infection because they are more likely than older people who inject drugs to share injection equipment and to participate in high-risk sexual behavior (Centers for Disease Control and Prevention 2016a). All people who inject drugs should be tested for HIV annually, and other people with OUD and reasons for elevated HIV risk (e.g., multiple sexual partners, exchanging sex for money or drugs, receptive anal intercourse) should also receive HIV testing regularly (Feinberg and Keeshin 2017). People who inject drugs should be linked to medical care at the time of diagnosis. HIV screening and prevention among people who inject drugs and improved linkage to and retention in HIV care are high-priority areas.

According to the classification scheme of the Centers for Disease Control and Prevention (1992), HIV infection can be categorized as asymptomatic HIV, symptomatic HIV, or AIDS, based on symptoms and the concentration of CD4$^+$ T-lymphocytes (i.e., called the "CD4 count"). After acute infection, most individuals will have symptoms, which include fever, sore throat, rash, muscle aches, and other flu-like symptoms. Symptoms of acute infection typically occur 2–4 weeks following exposure and may last up to 4 weeks. Standard HIV diagnostic testing relies on detection of antibodies that target HIV, which may not be detectable for up to 12 weeks following infection. During this initial "window period," diagnosis can still be made by directly testing for the presence of viral RNA (Feinberg and Keeshin 2017). After the acute infection, there is an asymptomatic phase that can last for years. As the CD4 count gradually decreases, the immune system weakens, and people with HIV/AIDS are at risk for atypical infections, such as oral thrush or shingles, and generalized symptoms, such as persistent diarrhea or fever. An AIDS diagnosis is made when the CD4 count decreases to below 200 cells/µL or when an AIDS-defining illness (e.g., *Pneumocystis jiroveci* pneumonia, esophageal candidiasis, Kaposi sarcoma) is present. Antiretroviral treatment initiation is recommended as soon as possible after diagnosis regardless of CD4 count because this can also prevent transmission of HIV to others (Feinberg and Keeshin 2017).

Over the past two decades, there have been remarkable improvements in HIV diagnostic tests, antiretroviral therapy, and overall longevity. Life expectancy for those who start antiretroviral therapy early is nearly equal to that of the general population. However, despite improvements in HIV care, people who inject drugs, nonwhites, and other marginalized groups who are HIV positive have experienced smaller reductions in HIV-related mortality (Antiretroviral Therapy Cohort Collaboration 2017). HIV health care providers may withhold antiretroviral therapy from people who inject drugs due to concerns about incomplete medication adherence; however, one-pill, once-daily antiretroviral therapy regimens or supportive interventions, such as pillboxes, daily reminders, or directly observed therapy, can improve adherence (Malta et al. 2008). Robust care delivery models that provide extra supports for people with OUD could reduce disparities in HIV-related mortality.

A full discussion of HIV prevention is beyond the scope of this chapter, but there are several preventive measures that are relevant for people who inject drugs. Syringe exchange programs are effective in reducing HIV transmission rates, and services should be expanded to cover all communities at risk for outbreaks (Fernandes et al. 2017). Where available, supervised injection facilities provide a space where people who inject drugs can bring drugs to inject more safely. Typically, these spaces have well-lit stalls, sterile injection equipment, and medical supervision, in order to reduce the risk of HIV transmission, soft tissue infections, or overdose. Pharmacological HIV prevention is possible with pre-exposure prophylaxis (PrEP). A tablet combining two HIV medications, emtricitabine and tenofovir disoproxil fumarate (Truvada), can be taken daily to prevent HIV infection. PrEP has been shown to prevent HIV infection among people who inject drugs (Choopanya et al. 2013). These services, along with condoms and counseling on safer sexual practices, should be available to all people who inject drugs.

SSTIs are among the most serious complications of IDU and are the most common reason for hospital admission among people who inject drugs, having doubled between 1993 and 2010 (Ciccarone et al. 2016). OUD treatment providers should maintain heightened suspicion for acute infections because patients may present with nonspecific symptoms, such as fatigue, sweating, or impaired mental status, which could be attributed to opioid intoxication or withdrawal (Center for Substance Abuse Treatment 2005). Female gender, injecting intramuscularly, more frequent injection, using mixtures of heroin and cocaine (i.e., "speed balls"), and using black tar heroin are associated with increased infection risk (Smith et al. 2015). Injecting crushed prescription opioids can also lead to adverse skin reactions due to inactive ingredients in tablets. Harm reduction practices, such as sterile syringe distribution or counseling on safer injection techniques, could reduce SSTI risk.

SSTIs are part of a larger spectrum of bacterial infections that includes abscesses, cellulitis, systemic sepsis, necrotizing fasciitis, infective endocarditis, pyomyositis (abscesses of skeletal muscle), abscesses of visceral organs, and bone and joint infections. Abscesses are the most frequent SSTIs among people who inject drugs and present as red, tender fluctuant areas in the skin (Larney et al. 2017). The most important aspects of abscess care are cleaning the infected area and incision and drainage.

Necrotizing fasciitis, which also has a high incidence among people who inject drugs, is a more serious SSTI, involving deeper layers of subcutaneous tissue. Severe pain out of proportion to the skin appearance, rapid spread of skin findings, or unstable vital signs can be a clue to a more serious infection. Necrotizing fasciitis is a medical emergency and often requires advanced imaging, surgical exploration, debridement of infected skin and muscle, and intravenous antibiotics.

Infective endocarditis refers to infection of the heart valves and cardiac tissue; lifetime prevalence among people who inject drugs is 0.5%–12% (Larney et al. 2017). Signs and symptoms of this life-threatening infection can be subtle, including fever, night sweats, joint and muscle pain, and weight loss, or more severe, including heart failure, cardiac arrhythmias, abscesses of visceral organs, distinctive skin findings, and other immune-mediated phenomena. When people who inject drugs present with fever and a new heart murmur, additional investigation with blood cultures and echocardiography is necessary. Treatment often includes empiric antibiotics and possibly surgery, so people who inject drugs and have suggestive symptoms require urgent evaluation.

Most infections are caused by commensal flora (bacteria that naturally exist in the human body), but contaminated drugs, drug adulterants, or drug use paraphernalia may also introduce bacteria. *Staphylococcus aureus* or *Streptococcus* species most frequently cause SSTIs; however, outbreaks of less common organisms, such as *Pseudomonas* or *Clostridium* species, may also occur among commensalism. Methicillin-resistant *Staphylococcus aureus* (MRSA) is particularly concerning due to its virulence and association with more severe infections (e.g., necrotizing fasciitis) (Lloyd-Smith et al. 2010). MRSA often requires intravenous antibiotics and hospitalization. Outbreaks from lethal *Clostridium* species that cause botulism, tetanus, and necrotizing fasciitis occur more frequently among people who inject drugs than in other populations. Although botulism is uncommon, signs and symptoms, such as difficulty swallowing, slurred speech, blurry vision, and muscle paralysis, could be confused with intoxication. Safer injection practices could reduce the risk of these infections.

Pulmonary infections, including pneumonia, tuberculosis (TB), and septic emboli, are also common among people who inject drugs. TB is highly transmissible through respiratory droplets, making outbreaks most common in communal settings that lack proper ventilation. People who inject drugs may be exposed to TB in jails or homeless shelters, and HIV infection is also an important risk factor. Symptoms of TB include cough, fever, night sweats, and weight loss. Routine TB testing is recommended throughout OUD treatment. Pneumonia is also common via several possible mechanisms: bacteria introduced into the bloodstream can hematogenously spread to the lungs; opioids induce stupor and suppress the cough reflex, predisposing to aspiration pneumonia; and associated risks such as smoking or HIV/AIDS may also impair defense mechanisms within the lungs (Heavner et al. 2014). Antibiotic treatment for pneumonia is usually targeted toward common organisms, such as *Streptococcus pneumoniae,* but people who inject drugs are also at risk for fungal infections and HIV-associated opportunistic infections, which must be considered. Septic emboli occur when clots detach from infected heart valves or peripheral veins and become trapped in the lungs. The radiographic appearance of septic emboli is different from community-acquired pneumonia and should trigger assessment for infective endocarditis (Heavner et al. 2014).

Injecting crushed prescription opioids can also introduce novel risks. Tablets, including oxycodone and buprenorphine, use talc (magnesium silicate) as filler. Injecting talc (or other adulterants) can lead to foreign body granulomatosis of the lung, liver, or other organs. Injected particles lodge in pulmonary capillaries, leading to an immune reaction, and subsequently can cause fibrosis, emphysema, and pulmonary hypertension. Patients present with cough, shortness of breath, and increased sputum production, but chest X-ray can be normal, making diagnosis difficult (Heavner et al. 2014). People who inject drugs may perceive prescription opioids to be safer to inject than heroin, but they should be counseled about the risks of talc granulomatosis.

Intranasal Opioid Use

Another common mode of opioid administration is intranasal insufflation (or "sniffing") of powder or dissolved opioids. Less of the drug is bioavailable via intranasal versus intravenous administration; therefore, overdose risk is also lower (Gossop et al. 1996). However, opioid overdoses do occur from intranasal use, and with fentanyl or other highly potent synthetic opioids in the drug supply, overdoses are becoming more common. Intranasal opioid use is a risk factor for HCV infection, but the precise mechanism of HCV transmission is unknown. Intranasal insufflation can lead to other medical comorbidities (see Table 6–1), including asthma exacerbations, sinus problems, hypersensitivity pneumonitis, and nasal septum necrosis or perforation (Peyrière et al. 2013). Sniffing crushed pills can also lead to talc granulomatosis.

Inhalation of Combusted Smoke

Smoking of heroin or other opioids is not as common in the United States as other modes of administration; the practice is more popular in Asia and Western Europe. Powdered heroin may be smoked in cigarettes or heated on foil so that fumes can be inhaled through a tube (a process called "chasing the dragon"). Overdose risk appears to be lower with heroin inhalation than with intravenous use (Gossop et al. 1996), but respiratory illnesses still present serious health risks. Pulmonary diseases associated with inhalation include asthma exacerbations, pneumothorax, pulmonary edema, and early-onset emphysema (Tashkin 2001). These problems stem from smoke causing thermal damage to the throat and lungs or from bronchospasm due to fumes from heroin (or other chemicals) or opioid-induced histamine release (Tashkin 2001). Additionally, inhaled bacteria from contaminated heroin samples may also increase the risk of pneumonia or pulmonary TB (Advisory Council on the Misuse of Drugs 2011).

Extrapulmonary complications are also possible from inhaling opioids. Chasing the dragon has been associated with progressive spongiform leukoencephalopathy, which is a form of neuronal injury in the cerebral cortex and cerebellum; patients may present with slurred speech, ataxia, tremors, or neurobehavioral symptoms. The condition is rare, but 25% of reported cases have been fatal. It is unclear whether the toxic insult is from heroin itself or an unknown contaminant. Additionally, the prevalence of HCV infection is higher among noninjection heroin users than in the general population (though lower than among injection users), which could be due to shared inhalation equipment or other coexistent risk factors (Advisory Council on the Misuse of Drugs 2011). The potential medical comorbidities associated with smoking or inhalation are summarized in Table 6–1.

Some concerns have been expressed about health risks from heating foil and inhaling fumes. Public Health England found no evidence of adverse health effects attributable to the heated foil and approved foil distribution as a harm reduction measure, encouraging people to switch from injecting to inhalation (Advisory Council on the Misuse of Drugs 2011). The United States has not endorsed similar measures, but the lower risks of overdose, HIV and HCV transmission, and other infections may warrant action.

Co-occurring Behaviors

Concomitant Substance Use Disorders

Many people with OUD have other SUDs that can lead to significant medical complications (see Table 6–2). As described in Chapter 7, "Opioid Use Disorder and Psychiatric Comorbidity," alcohol use disorder, tobacco use disorder, and other drug use disorders are more common among people with OUD than in the general population (Saha et al. 2016). Between 2011 and 2013, Americans who reported heroin use in the past year also reported alcohol use (>33%), cocaine use (25%), cannabis use (25%), and illicit prescription opioid use (nearly 50%) (Jones et al. 2015). Morbidity and mortality associated with polysubstance abuse are substantial. Benzodiazepine use disorder is common among people with OUD and dramatically increases overdose risk (Jones et al. 2012). Alcohol use disorder is associated with accidents, gastrointestinal disorders (e.g., peptic ulcer disease), liver disease, cancers, and hypertension, and also increases overdose risk. Cocaine use disorder is linked to cardiovascular disease, particularly stroke and myocardial infarction, as well as chronic kidney disease. Cannabis use disor-

TABLE 6–2. Medical comorbidities by system and co-occurring behavior and direct effects of opioids

Organ system or disease category	Direct effects of opioids	Conditions associated with co-occurring behaviors[a]
Cardiovascular	Possible cardiotoxicity	Atherosclerosis, stroke, myocardial infarction, peripheral vascular disease, hypertension, arrhythmias
Cancer	—	Oral cavity, larynx, lung, cervix, esophagus, pancreas, kidney, stomach, bladder cancers
Endocrine	Hypogonadism, osteoporosis	Diabetes, gout
Hepatic	—	Nonalcoholic fatty liver disease, alcoholic hepatitis
Infectious diseases	Aspiration pneumonia	Sexually transmitted infections, pneumonia
Neurological	Seizure, cognitive impairment, opioid-induced hyperalgesia	Stroke, cognitive impairment
Gastrointestinal	Constipation	Peptic ulcer disease, gastroesophageal reflux, gastritis
Pulmonary	Respiratory depression and failure, pulmonary edema	Chronic obstructive pulmonary disease, pneumonia, pulmonary hypertension, interstitial fibrosis
Renal	Rhabdomyolysis and acute renal failure	Hypertension, chronic kidney disease, hepatorenal syndrome
Sleep	Insomnia, sleep-disordered breathing	Sleep apnea
Trauma	Motor vehicle accident, other injury	Sexual abuse, motor vehicle accident, other injury

[a]Co-occurring behaviors = tobacco use, cocaine use, alcohol use, high-risk sexual behaviors. Dashes indicate no known major comorbidities.
Source. Adapted from Ries et al. 2014.

der, although often considered more benign, may be associated with accidents, respiratory conditions, and adverse cognitive effects.

Tobacco-related illnesses also disproportionately affect people with OUD. Cohort studies suggest that half of people with SUDs die from tobacco-related illnesses, and the death rate of smokers is 4 times greater than that of nonsmokers over long periods of follow-up (Hser et al. 1994). The prevalence of tobacco use may be as high as 83% among patients in methadone maintenance treatment (MMT) programs (Nahvi et al. 2006). Chronic medical conditions stemming from tobacco use, such as cardiovascular disease, stroke, and cancer, are also common among people with OUD. Patients receiving OUD treatment infrequently receive evidence-based smoking cessation interventions despite the high burden of illness. Although pharmacotherapy for tobacco use disorder is less efficacious among people with versus those without OUD, increasing length of treatment or providing adherence supports could lead to better results than standard care. Implementing systematic interventions at OUD treatment programs to increase access to smoking cessation treatments should be a high priority.

Sexual Risk Behaviors

Rates of sexually transmitted infections (STIs) are higher among people who use drugs than among the general population. Intoxication may influence decisions regarding sexual activity, including lack of condom use, which could lead to gonorrhea, syphilis, herpes, chlamydia, HIV, or other STI exposure. Additionally, people who exchange sex for money or drugs are also at elevated risk for STIs, and they may be in threatening situations in which they are unable to control sexual risk behaviors. STI treatment is similar for people with OUD as it is for anyone else; however, there are some interactions between antibiotics and medications used for OUD (e.g., methadone) and common comorbidities (e.g., HIV infection). Assessing the "five Ps"—sexual partners, practices, prevention of pregnancy, protection from STIs, and past history of STIs—elucidates patients' STI risk and can dictate the need for prevention education and interventions (Workowski et al. 2015).

Comorbidities due to Direct Opioid Effects

With any route of administration, the opioid itself can have negative health effects. Comorbidities directly related to opioid effects are given in

Table 6–2. The most serious is respiratory depression, which can lead to death. Other direct opioid effects may be less recognized. Because μ opioid receptors are ubiquitous throughout the body, opioid effects are wide ranging. In the short term, opioid administration can lead to euphoria, analgesia, constipation, nausea, and itching, among other effects. In the long term, chronic opioid exposure can affect bone health, sexual function, cognitive functioning, sleep quality, and sensitivity to pain (Carmona-Bayonas et al. 2017). The direct effects occur whether opioids are prescribed or taken illicitly, but in general they are manageable in clinical practice and are much less life-threatening than the risks of untreated OUD.

Opioids directly affect the endocrine system by suppressing sex hormones. At least half of people using chronic opioids develop clinically significant endocrine dysfunction—namely, hypogonadism, with low levels of testosterone, estrogen, and other sex hormones (Carmona-Bayonas et al. 2017). Clinically, patients may experience sexual and erectile dysfunction, infertility, decreased libido, or amenorrhea. Mental health providers should be aware that these hormonal pathways also affect mood and cognitive well-being. Hypogonadism may contribute to anxiety, depressed mood, worsening fatigue, or cognitive impairment. Patients with chronic opioid exposure may also have bone mineral density loss, likely due to hypogonadism, leading to osteoporosis and increased risk of fractures from falls. Hypogonadism from opioid use is reversible, and testosterone levels are likely to correct if opioids are discontinued. Some symptomatic individuals may be eligible for testosterone replacement therapy; however, testosterone supplementation carries its own health risks. It is unclear if buprenorphine, a partial opioid agonist, has the same endocrine-modulating effects as full opioid agonists, but in comparison with methadone, it may lead to less symptomatic hypogonadism (Carmona-Bayonas et al. 2017).

Opioids may have other potential toxicities. In a large cohort of patients with chronic pain, those receiving long-acting opioids had a 72% increased risk of death from cardiovascular and non-overdose-related causes than those receiving nonopioid medications (Ray et al. 2016). A major concern is sleep-disordered breathing, which can lead to hypoxia, arrhythmias, myocardial ischemia and infarction, and sudden cardiac death. There is a strong association between opioid use and sleep-disordered breathing, primarily central sleep apnea, which occurs in up to 70%–85% of people with chronic opioid use (Van Ryswyk and Antic 2016). Sleep apnea presents with excessive daytime sleepiness and is most common among people who snore or are overweight. Other morbidities associated with sleep apnea include hypertension, lung disease, and cardiovascular disease. Opioids have a dose-dependent effect on sleep apnea; therefore, reducing the dose of opioids can reduce risk, although this may not be indicated for patients on therapeutic methadone doses. Nighttime positive-pressure ventilation is also an effective treatment for sleep apnea (Van Ryswyk and Antic 2016).

There are other hypothesized negative health effects of opioids. The risk of cardiovascular disease, including heart attack and stroke, is elevated among people chronically taking opioids (Dowell et al. 2016). Co-occurring risk factors, such as tobacco use, likely contribute to increased cardiovascular risk, but direct opioid effects may also explain the increased cardiovascular risk. Chronic opioid use may suppress immune function, which has implications for the pathogenesis of HIV/AIDS and risk of bacterial infections (Carmona-Bayonas et al. 2017). Opioids also have a neurotoxic effect on the brain and can cause cognitive impairment, impacting working memory, verbal fluency, and impulsivity (Loeber et al. 2012). During OUD treatment, patients should be asked about symptoms of hypogonadism and sleep apnea and should be assessed for cognitive functioning; positive findings may be a reason for referral to specialty care. Despite these potential risks, stigma about methadone or buprenorphine can lead to exaggerated concerns about opioid side effects. Fear of side effects should not prevent eligible patients from starting OAT, which may be life-saving.

In the United States, opioid prescribing has become commonplace for both acute and chronic pain. The amount of opioids distributed from U.S. pharmacies increased from the equivalent of 96 mg of morphine per person in 1997 to 700 mg of morphine per person in 2007 (Centers for Disease Control and Prevention 2012). It is estimated that 92 million people, or more than one-third of noninstitutionalized adults, took a prescription opioid in 2015; it is also estimated that of these people, 11.5 million misused prescription opioids (e.g., took the medication without a prescription, took a higher dose than was prescribed) and 1.9 million had an OUD due to prescription opioids (Han et al. 2017). A number of studies suggest that a small but significant proportion of people exposed to prescription opioids will develop an

OUD (Edlund et al. 2014). In specialty pain management clinics, the prevalence of OUD has been reported to be between 2% and 14% (Dowell et al. 2016). Chronic pain is reported in 37%–60% of patients enrolled in MMT programs (Center for Substance Abuse Treatment 2005). There is a complex, bidirectional relationship between opioid use and pain. Although most pain patients taking prescription opioids do not misuse their medication or develop OUD, pain is a common antecedent to OUD and also complicates its treatment.

A judicious approach to opioid prescribing may reduce chronic pain patients' risk for developing OUD. As described in Chapter 7, "Opioid Use Disorder and Psychiatric Comorbidity," many chronic pain patients who develop OUD have preceding SUDs and/or comorbid mental health conditions (Dowell et al. 2016). Guidelines recommend screening chronic pain patients for SUDs, mental health conditions, and other OUD risk factors if chronic opioid therapy is being considered. In addition to screening, other risk mitigation strategies, such as using state-based prescription drug monitoring programs and urine drug testing, have been proposed as measures to limit nonmedical use of prescribed opioids (Dowell et al. 2016). Providers can also monitor patients being treated with chronic opioid therapy for early signs of OUD, such as running out of medication early or taking nonprescribed substances to relieve pain. However, additional research is needed to understand the impact of these measures.

Pain is common among individuals with OUD for several reasons: 1) chronic pain may have preceded OUD, 2) accidents or trauma may occur because of OUD, 3) opioid withdrawal can cause pain, and 4) chronic exposure to opioids can lead to opioid-induced hyperalgesia. Although relatively infrequent, iatrogenic addiction does occur with chronic opioid therapy. Edlund and colleagues (2014) found that 0.7%–6.1% of patients who started chronic opioid therapy for pain developed a new-onset OUD within 18 months of their first opioid prescription. Accidents or trauma are more common among those with SUDs, and they can also lead to chronic pain. An important symptom of the opioid withdrawal syndrome is pain, including back pain, abdominal cramping, or more generalized musculoskeletal pain. When people with OUD present for treatment, they are often in opioid withdrawal, and pain symptoms may improve or resolve completely with management of opioid withdrawal. Additionally, opioids themselves may lead to increased pain sensitivity, which is called opioid-induced hyperalgesia.

Although opioid-induced hyperalgesia has been documented in the literature, the proportion of people exposed to chronic opioids who develop increased pain sensitivity is unknown. The adaptations within the nociceptive pain pathway responsible for increased pain sensitivity are also poorly defined (Yi and Pryzbylkowski 2015). Opioid-induced hyperalgesia often becomes apparent when patients being treated with chronic opioid therapy develop widespread pain without a clear medical explanation or when they experience worsened pain despite escalating doses of opioids. In contrast to pain from injury, opioid withdrawal, or physiological tolerance, opioid-induced hyperalgesia pain symptoms will paradoxically improve by reducing the dose of prescribed opioids (Yi and Pryzbylkowski 2015).

Many people with OUD misuse nonprescribed opioids to "self-treat" chronic pain. If they engage in OUD treatment, their chronic pain will also require management (Center for Substance Abuse Treatment 2005; Han et al. 2017). This pain can be difficult to treat but may be responsive to nonopioid therapies. Patients typically benefit from comprehensive multimodal approaches that include pharmacotherapy (or other treatments) for OUD, nonopioid analgesics, nonpharmacological chronic pain treatments (e.g., physical therapy, acupuncture), and psychosocial treatments directed at pain and comorbid mental health conditions (Liebschutz et al. 2014). Providers should avoid prescribing opioid analgesics, which may trigger relapse to OUD; however, prescription opioids may be necessary to control acute pain when severe (e.g., postsurgical pain), and may be appropriate for chronic pain in some scenarios (e.g., for a patient stable in MMT without illicit opioid use who has worsening osteoarthritis and cannot have surgery) (Liebschutz et al. 2014). Multidisciplinary treatment teams with pain, addiction, and mental health specialists may be better equipped to care for patients with OUD and chronic pain than any single provider alone.

The medications used to treat OUD have some utility in chronic pain management (Neumann et al. 2013). Methadone is a full opioid agonist with strong analgesic properties and is sometimes used for chronic pain, with multiple daily doses. However, the once-daily methadone dosing used at MMT programs for OUD treatment does not provide adequate analgesia because the duration of effect for analgesia is shorter than that for suppression of withdrawal (Alford et al. 2006).

Methadone dosing can be adjusted to every 6 or 8 hours to optimize pain control and addiction treatment, but this requires programs to provide take-home doses of methadone, which may not be appropriate for all patients (Center for Substance Abuse Treatment 2005). Small studies suggest that buprenorphine treatment can control both chronic pain and OUD (Neumann et al. 2013), but buprenorphine is a partial agonist at μ opioid receptors and may provide insufficient analgesia for some patients. The opioid antagonist naltrexone will not provide pain relief in patients with OUD and chronic pain, and will in fact make opioid analgesics less effective, requiring higher doses for acute pain.

Medical Comorbidities and Unintentional Opioid Overdose Risk

Patients with various medical and psychiatric comorbidities, especially pain, respiratory conditions, liver disease, and mood disorders, may also have multiple risk factors for opioid overdose. Although the epidemiology of opioid overdose is changing as illicit fentanyl and other synthetic opioids have become increasingly implicated in overdoses, some studies suggest that more than half of opioid overdose decedents have had chronic pain diagnoses (Olfson et al. 2017). Medications commonly prescribed for chronic pain, mental health conditions, or even hypertension have sedating effects, which can lead to respiratory depression when combined with prescribed or illicit opioids. Most notably, co-prescribing a benzodiazepine and an opioid is a major risk factor for opioid overdose (Jones et al. 2012). Also, anticonvulsants used for neuropathic pain, such as gabapentin and pregabalin; antidepressants, such as mirtazapine, trazodone, or amitriptyline; antipsychotics, such as quetiapine; and medications used for sleep, such as hydroxyzine, diphenhydramine, doxepin, and zolpidem, are commonly prescribed together, and the cumulative effects of multiple sedating medications can increase overdose risk (Kim et al. 2017). Chronic obstructive pulmonary disease and obstructive sleep apnea are risk factors for overdose, because underlying lung disease exacerbates the opioid effect of respiratory depression. Chronic liver disease may also predispose to overdose, because if opioid metabolism is impaired, serum drug levels may be elevated. Additionally, with acute illness (e.g., pneumonia), overdose risk can be elevated due to weakened respiratory effort.

Opioid Use Disorder Treatment Considerations for Patients With Medical Comorbidities

Treatment of OUD is similar in patients with and without medical comorbidities, but a few critical adjustments need to be made in the context of medical comorbidities. Methadone can lead to changes in electrical conduction within cardiac tissue, which is detected as prolongation of the QT interval on an electrocardiogram (ECG), and is associated with torsades de pointes, a potentially fatal arrhythmia. QT prolongation is typically asymptomatic, but patients can experience palpitations, seizures, or syncope. Female sex, cardiac disease, hypokalemia (which can occur with diuretics or vomiting), and use of other QT-prolonging drugs are all risk factors for developing torsades de pointes (Stringer et al. 2009). Experts have given different recommendations about screening for QT prolongation, but patients considering MMT should first provide a careful history of personal or familial heart disease, cardiac risk factors, and use of QT-prolonging drugs (e.g., macrolide antibiotics, several antipsychotics, tricyclic antidepressants, cocaine). The most recent recommendations suggest that 1) patients with risk factors for QT prolongation, prior ECG with a QT interval >450 milliseconds, or history suggestive of ventricular arrhythmia should receive an ECG before treatment can begin; 2) patients with a QT interval >500 milliseconds should not initiate MMT; 3) monitoring intervals for follow-up ECGs should be based on baseline ECG findings, methadone dose changes, and risk factors for QT prolongation; and 4) methadone dose should be lowered, or an alternative treatment used, if the QT interval increases to >500 milliseconds during follow-up (Chou et al. 2014).

Another important consideration for methadone or buprenorphine maintenance treatment is the possibility of interactions with other prescribed medications. Methadone interacts with a number of commonly used medications, leading to methadone blood levels that are increased with some drugs (e.g., antibiotics including ciprofloxacin, macrolides, or azoles; quetiapine; benzodiazepines; many selective serotonin reuptake inhibitors; verapamil; cimetidine; omeprazole) or decreased with others (e.g., rifampin, carbamazepine, phenytoin, phenobarbital, HIV medications, cocaine). Buprenorphine has fewer known interactions, but the HIV medication atazanavir can increase buprenorphine levels, leading to sedation, and the antibiotic rifampin can lower buprenorphine levels, leading to withdrawal (McCance-Katz et al. 2010). Communication between providers treating OUD and those treating comorbid medical or psychiatric conditions is critical to prevent negative consequences of drug-drug interactions.

OAT for OUD can potentially cause or exacerbate chronic medical conditions, but the overall risks and benefits of OUD treatment must be considered in total, while taking into account the severity of OUD and high mortality rates from untreated OUD. For example, a patient with severe OUD may have risk factors for osteoporosis (e.g., a postmenopausal woman who is thin and smokes), but the risk of osteoporosis and fracture will rarely outweigh the potential benefits of methadone maintenance in comparison with other treatments. Although OUD treatments carry different risks, MMT continues to be the option with the strongest evidence of a mortality benefit (Sordo et al. 2017). As in making any treatment decision, clinicians should carefully inform patients about the potential risks and benefits, and the treatment plan should reflect their preferences.

Ensuring Adequate Medical Care for People With Opioid Use Disorder

When people with OUD enter treatment, they may have neglected their physical health and preventive care for years. Because of the high burden of medical conditions among people with OUD, facilitating access to medical care is imperative. Comorbid SUDs, mental illnesses, poverty, and other social factors (e.g., prior incarceration) put OUD patients with medical conditions at risk for poor health outcomes. For example, in comparison with other risk groups, people who inject drugs and have HIV have worse access to antiretroviral therapy, lower medication adherence, and higher AIDS mortality rates; however, these disparities can be mitigated with adequate access to care and supportive interventions (Malta et al. 2008). For other chronic medical conditions, such as diabetes or congestive heart failure, fewer outcome data are available specific to people with OUD, but disparities are also likely. Drivers of disparities may lie within the individual (e.g., health behaviors) and/or society at large (e.g., discrimination, health insurance availability); therefore, efforts at many levels are needed to tailor medical care to the needs of people with OUD.

Within the health care system, several important modifications could make medical care more accessible to people with OUD. In general, people with SUDs report experiencing stigma and discrimination in medical settings, which dissuades them from seeking medical care (Shim and Rust 2013). People with SUDs may face other barriers, including provider availability, insurance status, or transportation, especially in rural areas and certain regions of the United States. Finding medical providers who are highly experienced in caring for people with OUD may be challenging, and follow-up after referral is often incomplete. Therefore, integrating medical care and OUD treatment within a single location may address barriers to care and ensure that patients receive both OUD treatment and care for acute and chronic medical conditions.

The Institute of Medicine (2006) has defined *integration* as "any mechanism by which treatment interventions for co-occurring disorders are combined within the context of a primary treatment relationship or service setting" (p. 213). This could include coordinated care, with improved communication between the medical and SUD treatment providers; colocated care, with medical and SUD treatment providers sharing a location but not collaborating on treatment plans; or fully integrated care, with medical and SUD treatment providers sharing a location, treatment plan, and organizational structure. Full integration appears to be a feasible model; OUD treatment may be offered in primary care settings, or primary care may be offered at MMT programs or other SUD treatment programs.

Office-based treatment of OUD, meaning maintenance treatment with buprenorphine or injectable extended-release naltrexone (XR-naltrexone), offers several potential benefits. Medical conditions may be undetected and first recognized only upon the patient's entry into office-based treatment (Rowe et al. 2012). Accessing primary care is also associated with reduced addiction severity (Saitz et al. 2005). A single medical provider or team managing chronic medical conditions and OUD could ensure adequate attention to both medical and OUD outcomes. OUD treatment based in primary care may also have higher retention in treatment when compared with referral to specialty centers (O'Connor et al. 1998). There are many examples of integrated treatment programs, but specifically, combining HIV or HCV care and office-based buprenorphine treatment has a strong rationale.

Primary care may also be integrated into MMT programs or other SUD treatment programs. Some MMT programs offer only methadone administration and the required psychosocial counseling, which is a missed opportunity for HCV, HIV, and STI screening or management of acute and chronic medical conditions. Integrating HIV or HCV care into MMT programs has demonstrated success, especially when nurses can administer daily medications concomitantly with methadone ("directly observed therapy") (Berg et al. 2011). Not all OUD treatment providers will be able to integrate on-site care for medical conditions, but they can offer other supports that may facilitate access to medical care. OUD treatment settings could implement case management, medical referrals, support groups, and health education. Health systems and treatment providers should take a holistic view of health and wellness, simultaneously prioritizing addiction, mental health, and medical care.

Preventive Care for People With Opioid Use Disorder

Medical care for people with OUD should routinely include screening, vaccination, counseling, and chemoprophylaxis, as well as patient-centered care for chronic medical conditions. Patients with OUD should receive age-appropriate preventive care consistent with national guidelines, such as those of the U.S. Preventive Services Task Force (https://www.uspreventiveservicestaskforce.org). Table 6–3 shows additional considerations specific to OUD and related risk factors. Patients with OUD should be offered at least annual screening for hepatitis A, B, and C; TB; and syphilis and other STIs. SUD treatment programs may be the only contact with the health care system for some people with OUD; therefore, ensuring dental care and age-appropriate cancer screening is also important. Vaccines are recommended to prevent hepatitis A and B, tetanus, and pneumococcal pneumonia. Prevention can also include medications. As mentioned above, PrEP is effective in preventing HIV infection among people who inject drugs.

Family planning is another critical aspect of care. Before women of reproductive age become pregnant, contraception should be offered to them, and discussing the fetal risks of tobacco, alcohol, and illicit drugs may be helpful. Condoms can be distributed to reduce STI risk and pre-

TABLE 6–3. Additional preventive care considerations for people with opioid use disorder

Health care service	Recommended interval
Counseling and health education	Every visit
Overdose prevention counseling	
Injection drug use counseling	
Family planning (contraception, etc.)	
Sexual health counseling	
Intimate partner violence screening	
Tobacco cessation counseling	
Screening tests	
Hepatitis A, B, and C	Every 6–12 months
Tuberculosis	Every 6–12 months
Syphilis and other sexually transmitted infections	Every 6–12 months
Vaccinations	
Hepatitis A[a] and B[b]	See vaccination schedule
Tetanus	Every 10 years
Pneumococcal[c]	See vaccination schedule

Note.   People with OUD should receive all age-appropriate preventive measures per national guidelines. See U.S. Preventive Services Task Force for recommendations (https://www.uspreventiveservicestaskforce.org).
[a]Two doses: 0 and 6 months.
[b]Three doses: 0, 1–2, and 4–6 months.
[c]Only if person is older than age 65 years, is HIV positive, or has other chronic medical conditions.

vent unwanted pregnancies. Although starting methadone or buprenorphine treatment during pregnancy may be stigmatized, these treatments are safe, effective, and beneficial to both the mother and the fetus.

Counseling should be provided that emphasizes overdose prevention and harm reduction. All patients should be advised about factors that increase overdose risk, such as using multiple sedating drugs, using while alone, using opioids of unknown strength, and using after a period of abstinence when tolerance is reduced (e.g., following hospitalization, detoxification, incarceration). When people with OUD are not interested in stopping drug use, harm reduction counseling can focus on practices (e.g., using sterile syringes) that reduce health risks. Discussed in great detail in Chapter 12, "Harm Reduction: Caring for People Who Misuse Opioids," a tenet of harm reduction is to "meet people where they are," which means discussing drug use in a nonjudgmental manner and directing care to their own specific concerns. Whether medical care is provided in primary care, specialty settings, or integrated programs, communication strategies—including shared decision making, acknowledging and discussing substance use openly, setting limits, and maintaining hope and optimism—can strengthen patient-provider relationships and may improve adherence to medical treatments.

Key Chapter Points

▶ Medical comorbidities associated with OUD can be categorized as those associated with route of opioid administration (injection drug use, intranasal insufflation, or inhalation of smoke), addiction-related behaviors (concomitant substance use disorders [SUDs] or sexual risk behaviors), and direct opioid effects.

▶ Hepatitis C virus (HCV) infection is common among people with OUD and increasingly prevalent among young people who inject drugs. New direct-acting antiviral HCV treatments are better tolerated, simpler, and more effective (commonly curative) than past regimens. Patients who continue to use drugs can still be successfully treated for HCV infection and should be referred for evaluation and treatment.

▶ HIV infection has decreased among people who inject drugs; however, recent HIV outbreaks demonstrate the importance of screening and treatment, pre-exposure prophylaxis, and access to syringe exchange programs and other preventive measures to reduce HIV transmission.

▶ People with OUD commonly have co-occurring SUDs, such as alcohol, cocaine, or tobacco use disorders, which increase their risk of cardiovascular disease, liver disease, pulmonary disease, and cancer. Tobacco use is a leading cause of preventable illness and death, and evidence-based smoking cessation treatments should be offered early and often during OUD treatment.

▶ Direct effects of opioids include hypogonadism, leading to osteoporosis and sexual dysfunction; sleep-disordered breathing; neurocognitive impairment; and possibly cardiovascular toxicity and immunosuppression.

▶ People with OUD should be routinely offered screenings for infectious diseases (HCV, HIV, sexually transmitted infections, TB) and cancers, vaccinations (hepatitis A and B, tetanus, pneumococcal pneumonia), overdose prevention counseling, family planning services, and pre-exposure prophylaxis for HIV prevention.

References

Advisory Council on the Misuse of Drugs: Report into the physical effects of smoking heroin/crack cocaine and the risks of infections. December 21, 2011. Available at: https://www.gov.uk/government/uploads/system/uploads/attachment_data/file/119169/acmd-foil-report-2011.pdf. Accessed April 2, 2018.

Alford DP, Compton P, Samet JH: Acute pain management for patients receiving maintenance methadone or buprenorphine therapy. Ann Intern Med 144(2):127–134, 2006 16418412

American Association for the Study of Liver Diseases, Infectious Diseases Society of America: HCV testing and linkage to care. September 21, 2017. Available at: https://www.hcvguidelines.org/evaluate/testing-and-linkage. Accessed April 2, 2018.

Amon JJ, Garfein RS, Ahdieh-Grant L, et al: Prevalence of hepatitis C virus infection among injection drug users in the United States, 1994–2004. Clin Infect Dis 46(12):1852–1858, 2008 18462109

Antiretroviral Therapy Cohort Collaboration: Survival of HIV-positive patients starting antiretroviral therapy between 1996 and 2013: a collaborative analysis of cohort studies. Lancet HIV 4(8):e349–e356, 2017 28501495

Bahorik AL, Satre DD, Kline-Simon AH, et al: alcohol, cannabis, and opioid use disorders, and disease burden in an integrated health care system. J Addict Med 11(1):3–9, 2017 27610582

Berg KM, Litwin A, Li X, et al: Directly observed antiretroviral therapy improves adherence and viral load in drug users attending methadone maintenance clinics: a randomized controlled trial. Drug Alcohol Depend 113(2–3):192–199, 2011 20832196

Carmona-Bayonas A, Jiménez-Fonseca P, Castañón E, et al: Chronic opioid therapy in long-term cancer survivors. Clin Transl Oncol 19(2):236–250, 2017 27443415

Center for Substance Abuse Treatment: Associated medical problems in patients who are opioid addicted, in Medication-Assisted Treatment for Opioid Addiction in Opioid Treatment Programs. Substance Abuse and Mental Health Services Administration, 2005. Available at: https://www.ncbi.nlm.nih.gov/books/NBK64167/. Accessed April 2, 2018.

Centers for Disease Control and Prevention: 1993 revised classification system for HIV infection and expanded surveillance case definition for AIDS among adolescents and adults. MMWR Recomm Rep 41(RR-17):1–19, 1992 1361652

Centers for Disease Control and Prevention: CDC grand rounds: prescription drug overdoses—a U.S. epidemic. MMWR Morb Mortal Wkly Rep 61(1):10–13, 2012 22237030

Centers for Disease Control and Prevention: HIV and injection drug use. November 2016a. Available at: https://www.cdc.gov/hiv/pdf/risk/cdc-hiv-idu-fact-sheet.pdf. Accessed April 2, 2018.

Centers for Disease Control and Prevention: HIV surveillance report, 2015. 2016b. Available at: http://www.cdc.gov/hiv/library/reports/hiv-surveillance.html. Accessed April 2, 2018.

Chak E, Talal AH, Sherman KE, et al: Hepatitis C virus infection in USA: an estimate of true prevalence. Liver Int 31(8):1090–1101, 2011 21745274

Choopanya K, Martin M, Suntharasamai P, et al; Bangkok Tenofovir Study Group: Antiretroviral prophylaxis for HIV infection in injecting drug users in Bangkok, Thailand (the Bangkok Tenofovir Study): a randomised, double-blind, placebo-controlled phase 3 trial. Lancet 381(9883):2083–2090, 2013 23769234

Chou R, Cruciani RA, Fiellin DA, et al; American Pain Society; Heart Rhythm Society: Methadone safety: a clinical practice guideline from the American Pain Society and College on Problems of Drug Dependence, in collaboration with the Heart Rhythm Society. J Pain 15(4):321–337, 2014 24685458

Ciccarone D, Unick GJ, Cohen JK, et al: Nationwide increase in hospitalizations for heroin-related soft tissue infections: associations with structural market conditions. Drug Alcohol Depend 163:126–133, 2016 27155756

Cicero TJ, Ellis MS, Surratt HL, et al: The changing face of heroin use in the United States: a retrospective analysis of the past 50 years. JAMA Psychiatry 71(7):821–826, 2014 24871348

Degenhardt L, Larney S, Randall D, et al: Causes of death in a cohort treated for opioid dependence between 1985 and 2005. Addiction 109(1):90–99, 2014 23961881

Dowell D, Haegerich TM, Chou R: CDC guideline for prescribing opioids for chronic pain—United States, 2016. MMWR Recomm Rep 65(1):1–49, 2016 26987082

Edlund MJ, Martin BC, Russo JE, et al: The role of opioid prescription in incident opioid abuse and dependence among individuals with chronic noncancer pain: the role of opioid prescription. Clin J Pain 30(7):557–564, 2014 24281273

Feinberg J, Keeshin S: Management of newly diagnosed HIV infection. Ann Intern Med 167(1):ITC1–ITC16, 2017 28672393

Fernandes RM, Cary M, Duarte G, et al: Effectiveness of needle and syringe programmes in people who inject drugs: an overview of systematic reviews. BMC Public Health 17(1):309, 2017 28399843

Gossop M, Griffiths P, Powis B, et al: Frequency of non-fatal heroin overdose: survey of heroin users recruited in non-clinical settings. BMJ 313(7054):402, 1996 8761230

Han B, Compton WM, Blanco C, et al: Prescription opioid use, misuse, and use disorders in U.S. adults: 2015 National Survey on Drug Use and Health. Ann Intern Med 167(5):293–301, 2017 28761945

Harm Reduction Coalition: H is for heroin. 2001. Available at: http://harm reduction.org/drugs-and-drug-users/drug-tools/h-is-for-heroin/. Accessed April 2, 2018.

Heavner JJ, Saukkonen JJ, Akgun KM: Respiratory tract disorders related to alcohol and other drug use, in The ASAM Principles of Addiction Medicine, 5th Edition. Edited by Ries RK, Fiellin DA, Miller SC, et al. Philadelphia, PA, Wolters Kluwer, 2014, pp 1057–1076

Hser YI, McCarthy WJ, Anglin MD: Tobacco use as a distal predictor of mortality among long-term narcotics addicts. Prev Med 23(1):61–69, 1994 8016035

Institute of Medicine: Improving the Quality of Health Care for Mental and Substance-Use Conditions. Washington, DC, National Academies Press, 2006

Jones CM, Logan J, Gladden RM, et al: Vital signs: demographic and substance use trends among heroin users—United States, 2002–2013. MMWR Morb Mortal Wkly Rep 64(26):719–725, 2015 26158353

Jones CM, Christensen A, Gladden RM: Increases in prescription opioid injection abuse among treatment admissions in the United States, 2004–2013. Drug Alcohol Depend 176:89–95, 2017 28531769

Jones JD, Mogali S, Comer SD: Polydrug abuse: a review of opioid and benzodiazepine combination use. Drug Alcohol Depend 125(1–2):8–18, 2012 22857878

Kim A: Hepatitis C virus. Ann Intern Med 165(5):ITC33–ITC48, 2016 27595226

Kim TW, Walley AY, Heeren TC, et al: Polypharmacy and risk of non-fatal overdose for patients with HIV infection and substance dependence. J Subst Abuse Treat 81:1–10, 2017 28847449

Larney S, Peacock A, Mathers BM, et al: A systematic review of injecting-related injury and disease among people who inject drugs. Drug Alcohol Depend 171:39–49, 2017 28013096

Liebschutz J, Beers D, Lange A: Managing chronic pain in patients with opioid dependence. Curr Treat Options Psychiatry 1(2):204–223, 2014 24892008

Lloyd-Smith E, Hull MW, Tyndall MW, et al: Community-associated methicillin-resistant Staphylococcus aureus is prevalent in wounds of community-based injection drug users. Epidemiol Infect 138(5):713–720, 2010 20202284

Loeber S, Nakovics H, Kniest A, et al: Factors affecting cognitive function of opiate-dependent patients. Drug Alcohol Depend 120(1–3):81–87, 2012 21802223

Ly KN, Hughes EM, Jiles RB, et al: Rising mortality associated with hepatitis C virus in the United States, 2003–2013. Clin Infect Dis 62(10):1287–1288, 2016 26936668

Malta M, Strathdee SA, Magnanini MM, et al: Adherence to antiretroviral therapy for human immunodeficiency virus/acquired immune deficiency syndrome among drug users: a systematic review. Addiction 103(8):1242–1257, 2008 18855813

Martin NK, Vickerman P, Dore GJ, et al: The hepatitis C virus epidemics in key populations (including people who inject drugs, prisoners and MSM): the use of direct-acting antivirals as treatment for prevention. Curr Opin HIV AIDS 10(5):374–380, 2015 26248124

McCance-Katz EF, Sullivan LE, Nallani S: Drug interactions of clinical importance among the opioids, methadone and buprenorphine, and other frequently prescribed medications: a review. Am J Addict 19(1):4–16, 2010 20132117

Nahvi S, Richter K, Li X, et al: Cigarette smoking and interest in quitting in methadone maintenance patients. Addict Behav 31(11):2127–2134, 2006 16473476

Neumann AM, Blondell RD, Jaanimägi U, et al: A preliminary study comparing methadone and buprenorphine in patients with chronic pain and coexistent opioid addiction. J Addict Dis 32(1):68–78, 2013 23480249

O'Connor PG, Oliveto AH, Shi JM, et al: A randomized trial of buprenorphine maintenance for heroin dependence in a primary care clinic for substance users versus a methadone clinic. Am J Med 105(2):100–105, 1998 9727815

Olfson M, Wall M, Wang S, et al: Service use preceding opioid-related fatality. Am J Psychiatry Nov 28, 2017 [Epub ahead of print] 29179577

Peters PJ, Pontones P, Hoover KW, et al; Indiana HIV Outbreak Investigation Team: HIV infection linked to injection use of oxymorphone in Indiana, 2014–2015. N Engl J Med 375(3):229–239, 2016 27468059

Peyrière H, Léglise Y, Rousseau A, et al: Necrosis of the intranasal structures and soft palate as a result of heroin snorting: a case series. Subst Abus 34(4):409–414, 2013 24159913

Ray WA, Chung CP, Murray KT, et al: Prescription of long-acting opioids and mortality in patients with chronic noncancer pain. JAMA 315(22):2415–2423, 2016 27299617

Ries RK, Fiellin DA, Miller SC, Saitz R: Medical and surgical complications of addiction, in The ASAM Principles of Addiction Medicine, 5th Edition. Edited by Ries RK, Fiellin DA, Miller SC, et al. Philadelphia, PA, Wolters Kluwer, 2014, pp 1067–1089

Rowe TA, Jacapraro JS, Rastegar DA: Entry into primary care-based buprenorphine treatment is associated with identification and treatment of other chronic medical problems. Addict Sci Clin Pract 7:22, 2012 23186008

Saha TD, Kerridge BT, Goldstein RB, et al: Nonmedical prescription opioid use and DSM-5 nonmedical prescription opioid use disorder in the United States. J Clin Psychiatry 77(6):772–780, 2016 27337416

Saitz R, Horton NJ, Larson MJ, et al: Primary medical care and reductions in addiction severity: a prospective cohort study. Addiction 100(1):70–78, 2005 15598194

Shim R, Rust G: Primary care, behavioral health, and public health: partners in reducing mental health stigma. Am J Public Health 103(5):774–776, 2013 23488498

Smith ME, Robinowitz N, Chaulk P, et al: High rates of abscesses and chronic wounds in community-recruited injection drug users and associated risk factors. J Addict Med 9(2):87–93, 2015 25469653

Sordo L, Barrio G, Bravo MJ, et al: Mortality risk during and after opioid substitution treatment: systematic review and meta-analysis of cohort studies. BMJ 357:j1550, 2017 28446428

Stringer J, Welsh C, Tommasello A: Methadone-associated Q-T interval prolongation and torsades de pointes. Am J Health Syst Pharm 66(9):825–833, 2009 19386945

Substance Abuse and Mental Health Services Administration: The CBHSQ Report: Opioid Misuse Increases Among Older Adults. July 25, 2017. Available at: https://www.samhsa.gov/data/sites/default/files/report_3186/Spotlight-3186.html. Accessed April 2, 2018.

Tashkin DP: Airway effects of marijuana, cocaine, and other inhaled illicit agents. Curr Opin Pulm Med 7(2):43–61, 2001 11224724

Turner KM, Hutchinson S, Vickerman P, et al: The impact of needle and syringe provision and opiate substitution therapy on the incidence of hepatitis C virus in injecting drug users: pooling of UK evidence. Addiction 106(11):1978–1988, 2011 21615585

Van Handel MM, Rose CE, Hallisey EJ, et al: County-level vulnerability assessment for rapid dissemination of HIV or HCV infections among persons who inject drugs, United States. J Acquir Immune Defic Syndr 73(3):323–331, 2016 27763996

Van Ryswyk E, Antic NA: Opioids and sleep-disordered breathing. Chest 150(4):934–944, 2016 27262224

Workowski KA, Bolan GA; Centers for Disease Control and Prevention: Sexually transmitted diseases treatment guidelines, 2015. MMWR Recomm Rep 64(RR-03):1–137, 2015 26042815

Yi P, Pryzbylkowski P: Opioid induced hyperalgesia. Pain Med 16 (suppl 1):S32–S36, 2015 26461074

Zibbell JE, Iqbal K, Patel RC, et al; Centers for Disease Control and Prevention: Increases in hepatitis C virus infection related to injection drug use among persons aged ≤30 years— Kentucky, Tennessee, Virginia, and West Virginia, 2006–2012. MMWR Morb Mortal Wkly Rep 64(17):453–458, 2015 25950251

7

Opioid Use Disorder and Psychiatric Comorbidity

Marc W. Manseau, M.D., M.P.H.
Michael T. Compton, M.D., M.P.H.

Clinical Vignette: Tyler's Escalating Pill Use

Tyler is a 34-year-old with bipolar disorder diagnosed at age 21. He has a long history of intermittent psychiatric care at a public mental health clinic, where his psychiatrists have prescribed lithium at times and valproate at other times. Over the years, the clinicians have deemed both medications to be highly effective, but his adherence with the medications—in fact, his engagement in care generally—has been very limited. Although Tyler has never experienced a major depressive episode, he has had four instances of mania, each of which precipitated a psychiatric hospitalization. The first two hospital stays were for less than 10 days, but his third one (just over 1 year ago) was protracted (32 days) because of psychotic features (mood-congruent grandiose delusions). Although his mother, father, and older sister have remained supportive and encouraging of treatment, Tyler is highly resistant to his family's help and has been almost completely alienated from them in recent months. Outside of manic episodes, he is gregarious, energetic, and highly social, at times appearing hypomanic.

Prior to being diagnosed with bipolar disorder, Tyler had been seen by a psychiatrist and therapist for several years during middle school and was diagnosed with oppositional defiant disorder. He began drinking alcohol in the ninth grade and escalated his use to nearly every day before dropping out of school in the beginning of his senior year. His drink of choice has always been vodka, typically mixed with cola or fruit juice, and poured into the container of those beverages to avoid being noticed as drinking alcohol. He tried smoking marijuana on several occasions in eighth grade, but he never escalated his use as he found it made him "lazy and boring." He experimented occasionally with ketamine and ecstasy (3,4-methylenedioxymethamphetamine) in high school, but he always preferred the effects of alcohol ("crazy funny and in the limelight") to those of illicit drugs. He has never received any treatment for alcohol use disorder (AUD), although he clearly meets diagnostic criteria for it.

During his fourth (most recent) manic episode, and while intoxicated, Tyler was involved in a car accident, resulting in both legal charges and a fractured rib and fractured arm (his left ulna). Acetaminophen-oxycodone was prescribed for 10 days, during which time he reduced his drinking. In the intervening 6 months, he has used the pain pills daily, initially by getting refills ("I just tell the docs I still have bad pain"), and later by finding street purchases through his connections with former friends who deal in various prescribed addictive medications. His use has increased substantially in the past 3 weeks, and he now presents to the emergency department with withdrawal symptoms and a desire to "get detoxed so I can go back to vodka instead of these expensive pills that make me numb."

Tyler's circumstances raise a number of questions for the evaluating health care provider. What psychiatric and substance use disorders are most associated with opioid use disorder (OUD), both in terms of increasing risk for OUD and as a consequence of OUD? What are the recent trends in comorbidity, regarding both prescription opioid misuse and heroin and related illicit drugs? How does the presence of a comorbid psychiatric disorder and OUD impact course and outcomes of both disorders? What is the best way to approach treatment of individuals with comorbid OUD and mental illnesses?

Introduction

In 2015, as epidemiologists, clinicians, and public health experts were struggling to understand the dramatic recent increases in opioid misuse, addiction, and overdose death in North America and specifically the United States, a study was published with striking findings: between

1999 and 2013, middle-aged non-Hispanic whites in the United States experienced an increase in mortality, representing the only reversal of decades of progress in mortality in the industrialized world (Case and Deaton 2015). Further, this population-level mortality rate increase was explained primarily by increases in drug and alcohol poisonings (which are largely driven by opioid-related overdoses; Rudd et al. 2016), suicide, and chronic liver diseases and cirrhosis. The study also reported decreases in self-reported physical and mental health, reductions in daily functioning, and increases in chronic pain, pointing to population-wide increases in emotional and physical distress.

Then, in the summer of 2017, another landmark paper reported that the 16% of Americans with a psychiatric disorder receive over half of the opioid prescriptions filled each year. In addition, whereas 5% of adults without mental disorders use prescription opioids, 18.7% of adults with mental disorders use them, and even after the researchers controlled for sociodemographic characteristics, health status, and health services use, persons with psychiatric illness were still shown to be more than twice as likely to use prescription opioids (Davis et al. 2017). These important studies directly lead to urgent questions about the connections between opioid use and misuse and psychiatric illness. We need to better understand whether psychiatric symptoms and disorders increase the likelihood that people will be exposed to opioids. We also need to determine whether health care providers are (inadvertently) prescribing opioids to treat symptoms of mental illnesses and emotional distress in addition to physical pain, and whether having a mental illness increases the chances that prescription opioid use will progress to nonmedical prescription opioid use. Additionally, better research is needed on opioid use and misuse among people with psychiatric disorders, and the extent to which use in that segment of the population is driving the opioid addiction and overdose epidemic.

In this chapter, we explore these and other issues related to comorbidity between OUD and psychiatric disorders. We begin with a general review of comorbidity between substance use disorders (SUDs) and mental illnesses. We then summarize important findings on comorbidity between illicit opioids, such as heroin, and psychiatric disorders. Next, we explore the emerging literature on the relationship between both mental illnesses and SUDs and nonmedical prescription opioid use. As discussed in depth in Chapter 2, "Prescription Opioids," nonmedical prescription opioid use is a key driver of the current opioid epidemic, so understanding its relationship to psychopathology will shed light on the underlying causes of this recent trend. We then address the consequences of comorbidity, first looking at the impact of psychiatric illness on overdose death, and then examining the effects of comorbidity on the course and outcomes of both OUD and psychiatric disorders. Finally, we provide guidance on the treatment approach to individuals with comorbid psychiatric illness and OUD.

Comorbidity Between Substance Use Disorders and Psychiatric Disorders

Combinations of comorbid psychiatric disorders and SUDs are also called co-occurring disorders (CODs). CODs are common, because individuals with mental illnesses are much likelier to experience addiction, and vice versa (Compton et al. 2007). The Substance Abuse and Mental Health Services Administration (2017) estimated that about 3.4% of all adults in the United States experienced CODs in 2016. Among individuals with mental illnesses, 22.5% experienced a co-occurring SUD (Figure 7–1), whereas 33.8% of those with serious mental illnesses (SMIs) such as schizophrenia or bipolar disorder also had an addiction. Large, population-based, representative studies such as the Epidemiologic Catchment Area study have reported even higher rates of CODs, with around 30% of individuals with mental illnesses having an SUD, and between one-half and two-thirds of those with SMIs having a COD (Regier et al. 1990). The most common substances used by individuals with SMI, in descending order of prevalence, are tobacco, alcohol, cannabis, and cocaine; use of multiple substances with multiple comorbid SUDs is common (Manseau and Bogenschutz 2016; Selzer and Lieberman 1993; Soyka et al. 1993). Tobacco use is often overlooked, and tobacco use disorder is not included as an SUD in the comorbidity numbers reported above. However, tobacco use is the leading cause of preventable death in individuals with mental illnesses (Bandiera et al. 2015). People with psychiatric disorders are at least twice as likely to smoke as those without mental illness, and they smoke almost half the total number of cigarettes in the United States (Lasser et al. 2000). Among individuals with SMIs, tobacco use rates have been estimated to be almost two-thirds in individuals with schizophrenia and almost one-half in persons with bipolar disorder (Dickerson et al. 2013).

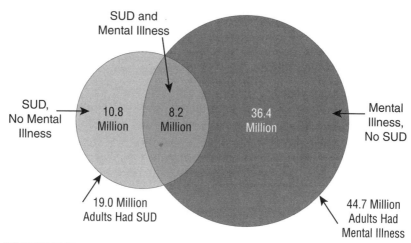

SUD and Mental Illness

SUD, No Mental Illness → 10.8 Million

8.2 Million

36.4 Million

Mental Illness, No SUD

19.0 Million Adults Had SUD

44.7 Million Adults Had Mental Illness

FIGURE 7–1. Past-year substance use disorders and mental illness among adults in the United States age 18 or older: 2016.

SUD=substance use disorder.

Source. Reprinted from Substance Abuse and Mental Health Services Administration 2017.

CODs tend to produce worse outcomes, including more severe psychiatric symptoms, higher rates of violence and suicidality, worse overall functioning, higher rates of homelessness and legal problems, worse behavioral health treatment engagement, and more intensive health care services use (Bennett and Gjonbalaj 2007; Manseau and Bogenschutz 2016; Swofford et al. 2000; Talamo et al. 2006). In addition, comorbid SUDs, including but not limited to tobacco use, place individuals with mental illness at increased risk of a host of physical health problems as well as death (Schulte and Hser 2014). Owing to these strong associations with an array of negative outcomes, CODs present significant challenges to clinicians and place substantial burdens on the health care and social services systems (Odlaug et al. 2016).

Addictions researchers have posited several theories to explain the association between psychiatric illnesses and SUDs; the theories have varying amounts of evidence to support them and are not mutually exclusive. First, the *precipitation model* suggests that drug or alcohol use causes symptoms of mental illnesses. This theory requires that substance use precede psychiatric symptoms and the development of a psychiatric disorder. For example, use of cannabis can cause psychotic symptoms and has been implicated in the etiology of psychotic disorders (Manseau and Goff 2015) and an earlier onset of psychotic disorders (Compton et al. 2009; Kelley et al. 2016).

Second, the *self-medication hypothesis* proposes that individuals with psychiatric disorders use drugs in an attempt (successful or not) to alleviate symptoms and/or psychotropic medication side effects. This explanation requires that an initiation of or increase in drug use follows the development of the psychiatric disorder in time. This theory is conceptually compelling, but little research has shown this to be a major factor in the etiology of CODs, although it may hold partially true in explaining the relationships between use of certain substances and specific psychiatric illnesses (Khantzian 1997). For instance, there is some literature to suggest that individuals with schizophrenia may smoke cigarettes to temporarily reverse cognitive symptoms using nicotine (Conway 2009; Featherstone and Siegel 2015) and/or to reduce side effects from antipsychotic medications.

Third, the *shared vulnerability model*, which does not depend on any specific temporal sequencing, explains the association between mental disorders and SUDs through a third common underlying factor. This third shared factor could be biological, such as genetic vulnerability; psychological, such as personality traits; or environmental/social, such as exposure to trauma or adversity during upbringing (Kendler et al. 2003). Studies demonstrating a common underlying genetic link between tobacco use and major depressive disorder (MDD) provide important evidence for the shared vulnerability model (Lyons et al. 2008).

The complex relationships between AUD and mood disorders demonstrate the concept that the theories of CODs are not mutually exclusive. Although there is evidence that alcohol-induced depressive disorders are separate and distinct entities from unipolar MDD, AUD and MDD frequently co-occur. Likewise, for bipolar disorder, there is evidence both that AUD can cause bipolar episodes at either pole of the mood spectrum and that there is shared genetic vulnerability for bipolar disorder and AUD (Raimo and Schuckit 1998).

Possibly because CODs involving opioid use are less common than those involving use of other substances, the literature on psychiatric comorbidity with OUD has been less robust. However, because of concerning recent trends, researchers have been turning increasing attention to the topic of OUD and psychiatric comorbidity. Their findings have uncovered a nuanced relationship between psychiatric symptoms, diagnosable mental illnesses, opioid use, and OUD. Prior work has demonstrated a consistent relationship between certain psychiatric disorders and heroin addiction (Brooner et al. 1997; Carpentier et al. 2009; Strain 2002), and more recent research adds to this body of knowledge with an understanding of the interplay between chronic pain, psychiatric symptomatology, and opioid use (Amari et al. 2011). For instance, there is a well-established bidirectional association between chronic pain and depressive symptoms, making opioids less effective in treating pain and increasing the risk of developing an OUD in those with depression (Howe and Sullivan 2014; Mason et al. 2016; Wasan et al. 2015). Possibly because of this complex interplay between pain, depression, and response to opioids, psychiatric comorbidity—and depression in particular—has been recognized as a major risk factor for prescribed opioid use progressing to nonmedical prescription opioid use (Katz et al. 2013; Novak et al. 2009). Some mediating factors potentially explaining the association between OUD and depression include, but are not limited to, the findings that opioid use can lead to sleep-disordered breathing, as well as to endocrine disruptions such as hypogonadism (as discussed in Chapter 6, "Opioid Use Disorder and Medical Comorbidity"), both of which can increase risk for depression (i.e., precipitation). Nonmedical prescription opioid use is in turn a predisposing factor for a host of adverse outcomes, including initiation of heroin use and opioid-related overdose (Bogdanowicz et al. 2015). For these and other reasons, the growing literature on comorbidity between psychiatric disorders and OUD is elucidating some of the driving forces behind the recent opioid epidemic.

Comorbidity Between Opioid Use Disorder Primarily Involving Heroin and Psychiatric Disorders

Prior to the current opioid epidemic, most of the literature on psychiatric comorbidity with OUD involved populations with heroin addiction, and most studies included samples in OUD treatment, such as methadone maintenance treatment (MMT). Estimates for rates of comorbid psychiatric disorders vary widely across studies, due to differences in study design, sample selection, and psychiatric assessment methods

(Brooner et al. 1997; Carpentier et al. 2009; Strain 2002). However, even with this variation, reports have consistently demonstrated elevated rates of several psychiatric disorders. Table 7–1 summarizes the data from studies regarding rates of psychiatric disorders among individuals with a history of heroin-related OUD (second column from left) and rates for individuals using nonmedical prescription opioids (right-hand column). Between those columns, for easy comparison with either column, are rates of the listed psychiatric disorders among adults in the general U.S. population, from the 2016 National Survey on Drug Use and Health (Substance Abuse and Mental Health Services Administration 2017) and the National Epidemiologic Survey on Alcohol and Related Conditions (NESARC; Hasin and Grant 2015). Heroin use has consistently been associated with elevated rates of mood disorders, including MDD; anxiety disorders, including social and specific phobias, generalized anxiety disorder (GAD), and posttraumatic stress disorder (PTSD); and personality disorders, especially antisocial personality disorder among men (Brooner et al. 1997; Carpentier et al. 2009; Kidorf et al. 2004; Peles et al. 2007; Roncero et al. 2016; Rosen et al. 2011; Strain 2002). Women with heroin addiction may experience higher rates of depression and anxiety than men (Rosen et al. 2008). Individuals with heroin addiction also experience higher rates of nonopioid substance misuse and SUDs, including tobacco use, alcohol use, cannabis use, and cocaine use disorders (Brooner et al. 1997; Carpentier et al. 2009; Kidorf et al. 2004; Roncero et al. 2016; Rosen et al. 2011; Strain 2002; Zirakzadeh et al. 2013). There is evidence that multiple SUDs tend to cluster in individuals with OUD (Strain et al. 1991).

The literature is less consistent regarding the association between heroin dependence and SMI. Although there are reports of elevated rates of OUD within samples of individuals with bipolar disorder (Hunt et al. 2016a, 2016b), it seems that rates of OUD among those with schizophrenia are the same as or even lower than in the general population and that individuals with schizophrenia may have lower rates of heroin use when compared with the larger population in addiction treatment (Brooner et al. 1997; Chiappelli et al. 2018; Kidorf et al. 2004; Soyka et al. 1993; Strain 2002). However, some treatment samples do include a relatively high proportion of individuals with SMIs, likely given the nature of the specific treatment modalities from which they were drawn (e.g., dual-diagnosis treatment programs) (Marienfeld and Rosenheck 2015).

TABLE 7–1. Psychiatric comorbidity with primarily heroin-related opioid use disorder and nonmedical prescription opioid use

Disorder	Rates in individuals with heroin-related opioid use disorder (%)	Rates in general U.S. adult population (%)	Rates in individuals with nonmedical prescription opioid use (%)
Any mood disorder	13.4–54	NA	10.6–59.7
Major depressive disorder	3–54	5.3–13.2	10.5–51.5
Dysthymia	3.4–6.4	1.4–3.2	18.6
Bipolar disorder	0.4–7	2.0–3.3	17.3–20.1
Any anxiety disorder	5–60	11.1–17.2	8.9–39
Generalized anxiety disorder	0.1–29.7	2.1–4.1	10.4–12.3
Phobias	2.3–45.3	2.8–9.4	12.7–18.5
Panic disorder	1.5–13.6	2.1–5.1	6.6–18.3
Posttraumatic stress disorder	3.1–27.8	4.5–6.4	14.6–19.8
Obsessive–compulsive disorder	0.3–15	NA	NA
Personality disorders	9–68	NA	3.0–49.7
Antisocial personality disorder	17.6–55	3.6	30.3
Eating disorders	0.7–10	NA	NA
Psychotic disorders	0.1–10	NA	NA

TABLE 7–1. Psychiatric comorbidity with primarily heroin-related opioid use disorder and nonmedical prescription opioid use *(continued)*

Disorder	Rates in individuals with heroin-related opioid use disorder (%)	Rates in general U.S. adult population (%)	Rates in individuals with nonmedical prescription opioid use (%)
Any substance use disorder	84.5	7.5	NA
Tobacco	73.5–94	23.5	NA
Alcohol	2.4–68.4	5.6	21.8–63
Cannabis	7.5–83.4	1.5	19.6–50.7
Cocaine	5.3–84.5	0.3	18.4–30.9
Sedative	1.7–44.6	0.2–0.7	9.9–32.9

Note. NA=data not available.

Source. Data from Hasin and Grant 2015; Substance Abuse and Mental Health Services Administration 2017.

Researchers have not thoroughly explored the reasons for increased rates of certain psychiatric disorders among persons with heroin addiction. There is little evidence in the literature for heroin use precipitating psychiatric symptoms or disorders. However, given the short half-life and difficulty of obtaining heroin, individuals with heroin addiction frequently go through periods of acute opioid withdrawal. Chronic opioid dependence also leads to chronic withdrawal phenomena, unless adequately treated with a medication-assisted treatment (MAT) such as opioid agonist treatment (OAT; i.e., methadone or buprenorphine) (Satel et al. 1993). Table 7–2 lists coinciding diagnostic criteria from the *Diagnostic and Statistical Manual of Mental Disorders,* Fifth Edition (DSM-5; American Psychiatric Association 2013) for opioid withdrawal syndrome, MDD, and GAD. There is significant overlap of both psychiatric and physical symptoms between the three sets of criteria, which could partially explain the high frequency of depressive and anxious symptoms reported by individuals with heroin addiction.

There is likewise little evidence for the self-medication hypothesis, although some innovative work has demonstrated that a subset of persons with bipolar disorders may be more likely to use opioids, including heroin, and that consistent OAT may have a mood-stabilizing effect above and beyond mood stabilization with traditional psychotropic medications (Maremmani et al. 2006). Although the possibility of shared genetic vulnerability between heroin addiction and psychiatric illnesses has not been thoroughly investigated, there is obvious potential for shared psychosocial vulnerability (e.g., similar psychological difficulties, exposure to similar background circumstances). Given the fact that comorbid nonopioid SUDs are common in heroin addiction, it is also possible that these represent common third factors to explain psychiatric comorbidity. For instance, if an individual with heroin addiction has comorbid alcohol or cocaine use disorder, either could cause significant depressive symptoms. In addition, persons with SUDs in general, as well as individuals from previous generations with heroin addiction specifically, are more likely to be affected by a host of adverse social conditions, including racism, poverty, unemployment, deprived neighborhoods, increased exposure to violence and other traumatic experiences, and the effects of the criminalization of and societal stigma toward drug addiction. This is especially true for individuals in MMT programs, from which many study samples have been recruited. These

TABLE 7–2. Overlap between symptoms of opioid withdrawal syndrome, major depressive disorder, and generalized anxiety disorder

Opioid withdrawal	Major depressive disorder	Generalized anxiety disorder
Dysphoric mood/anxiety	Depressed mood most of the day, nearly every day, as indicated by either subjective report (e.g., feels sad, empty, or hopeless) or observation made by others (e.g., appears tearful). (**Note:** In children and adolescents, can be irritable mood.)	Excessive anxiety and worry (apprehensive expectation), occurring more days than not for at least 6 months, about a number of events or activities (such as work or school performance). Irritability
Nausea or vomiting	Significant weight loss when not dieting or weight gain (e.g., a change of more than 5% of body weight in a month), or decrease or increase in appetite nearly every day. (Note: In children, consider failure to make expected weight gain.)	
Restlessness or sweating[a] (Pupillary dilation, piloerection, or sweating in DSM-5)	Psychomotor agitation or retardation nearly every day (observable by others, not merely subjective feelings of restlessness or being slowed down).	Restlessness, feeling keyed up or on edge

TABLE 7–2. Overlap between symptoms of opioid withdrawal syndrome, major depressive disorder, and generalized anxiety disorder *(continued)*

Opioid withdrawal	Major depressive disorder	Generalized anxiety disorder
Insomnia	Insomnia or hypersomnia nearly every day	Sleep disturbance (difficulty falling or staying asleep, or restless, unsatisfying sleep).
	Fatigue or loss of energy nearly every day	
	Diminished ability to think or concentrate, or indecisiveness, nearly every day (either by subjective account or as observed by others)	Difficulty concentrating or mind going blank
Muscle aches	Fatigue or loss of energy nearly every day	Muscle tension
		Being easily fatigued

[a]Included in Clinical Opiate Withdrawal Scale (COWS; Wesson and Ling 2003).
Source.   Adapted from American Psychiatric Association: *Diagnostic and Statistical Manual of Mental Disorders*, 5th Edition. Arlington, VA, American Psychiatric Association, 2013. Copyright © 2013 American Psychiatric Association. Used with permission.

social determinants of mental health are well-known risk factors for the development of many psychiatric disorders, including depressive and anxiety disorders as well as comorbid nonopioid SUDs (Compton and Shim 2015).

The case of the consistently demonstrated association between heroin addiction and antisocial personality disorder provides an especially interesting example of the potential role of social factors in driving comorbidity. As shown in Box 7–1, a diagnosis of antisocial personality disorder requires only three of the A criteria, and all but one of them (lack of remorse) could potentially be met by drug-use and drug-seeking behaviors (failure to obey laws; lying, deception, or manipulation; impulsive behaviors; blatant disregard for the safety of self and others; a pattern of irresponsibility) and/or by acute or chronic opioid withdrawal symptoms (irritability and aggression; impulsive behaviors). In addition, owing to (often chronically) increased exposure to the adverse social conditions described above, individuals with a history of heroin addiction may have learned certain behaviors or attitudes over time that technically match diagnostic criteria for antisocial personality disorder but that were relatively adaptive in the settings in which individuals learned them (e.g., violent neighborhoods, unstable households, the criminal justice system) (Alterman and Cacciola 1991). This last point could cause an individual with a deprived or traumatic background to meet Criterion C for antisocial personality disorder (childhood conduct disorder) in addition to Criterion A.

BOX 7–1.   Diagnostic Criteria, Antisocial Personality Disorder

---

A. A pervasive pattern of disregard for and violation of the rights of others, occurring since age 15 years, as indicated by three (or more) of the following:

1. Failure to conform to social norms with respect to lawful behaviors, as indicated by repeatedly performing acts that are grounds for arrest.
2. Deceitfulness, as indicated by repeated lying, use of aliases, or conning others for personal profit or pleasure.
3. Impulsivity or failure to plan ahead.
4. Irritability and aggressiveness, as indicated by repeated physical fights or assaults.

5. Reckless disregard for safety of self or others.
6. Consistent irresponsibility, as indicated by repeated failure to sustain consistent work behavior or honor financial obligations.
7. Lack of remorse, as indicated by being indifferent to or rationalizing having hurt, mistreated, or stolen from another.

B. The individual is at least age 18 years.

C. There is evidence of conduct disorder with onset before age 15 years.

D. The occurrence of antisocial behavior is not exclusively during the course of schizophrenia or bipolar disorder.

Source. Reprinted from American Psychiatric Association: *Diagnostic and Statistical Manual of Mental Disorders*, 5th Edition. Arlington, VA, American Psychiatric Association, 2013. Copyright © 2013 American Psychiatric Association. Used with permission.

Comorbidity Between Opioid Use Disorder Primarily Involving Prescription Medications and Psychiatric Disorders

The current opioid epidemic seems to have begun with dramatic increases in prescription opioid availability, leading to significantly rising nonmedical prescription opioid use. Much of the literature examining psychiatric comorbidity with nonmedical prescription opioid use and related OUD is based on data from population-representative surveys, such as NESARC and the Medical Expenditure Panel Survey. Although the nonmedical prescription opioid epidemic seems to have subsequently driven a new heroin epidemic, this trend remains relatively new, and the scientific literature on recent psychiatric comorbidity with heroin use is still sparse.

The right column of Table 7–1 summarizes the literature on rates of psychiatric disorders in individuals with nonmedical prescription opioid use and/or related OUD. Even though the study designs and methods are quite different and more advanced than those used in most of the heroin-related literature, the general findings are remarkably similar. Individuals with nonmedical prescription opioid use and related OUD are more likely than the general population to experience depressive and bipolar disorders, at least several anxiety disorders, personality disorders (again, especially antisocial personality disorder in men), and nonopioid SUDs (Fischer et al. 2012, 2016; Goldner et al. 2014; Grella et al. 2009;

Martins et al. 2009; Mason et al. 1998; Schepis and Hakes 2011). The combination of personality disorders and other psychiatric illnesses may confer particularly high risk for nonmedical prescription opioid use (Katz et al. 2013). Women with OUD may be more likely than men to have mood and anxiety disorders, including PTSD, and nonopioid SUDs tend to increase the risk of other psychiatric comorbidity (Grella et al. 2009; Smith et al. 2016). There is no evidence that psychosis spectrum disorders are more common in individuals with nonmedical prescription opioid use. Where this body of literature differs most from the older, heroin-related research is in its examination of explanatory connections between OUD and mental illnesses.

There is evidence that exposure to opioids, and nonmedical prescription opioid use in particular, can precipitate psychiatric illness, particularly mood and anxiety disorders. Martins and colleagues (2009) demonstrated this using NESARC data. In a study analyzing data from Wave 1 of NESARC, collected in 2001–2002, the researchers demonstrated that preexisting nonmedical opioid use was associated with a significantly increased risk of incident psychiatric disorders after adjusting for demographic factors and alcohol or other drug use, including mood disorders in general (adjusted hazard ratio [AHR]=3.2), anxiety disorders in general (AHR=2.8), MDD (AHR=3.1), bipolar disorder (AHR=3.6), GAD (AHR=2.8), and panic disorder (AHR=3.6). They also demonstrated even stronger associations between preexisting opioid dependence resulting from nonmedical prescription opioid use and incident psychiatric disorders, including mood disorders in general (AHR=4.9), anxiety disorders in general (AHR=6.1), MDD (AHR=5.2), bipolar disorder (AHR=5.0), GAD (AHR=4.1), and panic disorder (AHR=8.5). In a study using data from Waves 1 and 2 of NESARC (Martins et al. 2012), the same team partially replicated their earlier findings by demonstrating that baseline lifetime nonmedical prescription opioid use in Wave 1 was associated with incidence in Wave 2 of any mood disorder (adjusted odds ratio [AOR]=1.8), MDD (AOR=1.4), bipolar disorder (AOR=2.0), any anxiety disorder (AOR=1.4), and GAD (AOR=1.5). However, in this study, baseline lifetime OUD was not associated with incidence of any psychiatric disorders in adjusted models. In a similar study using data from Waves 1 and 2 of NESARC, Schepis and Hakes (2011) demonstrated that any lifetime and past-year nonmedical prescription opioid use were both associated with incidence of psychiatric disorders, including any psychiatric disorder, nonopioid SUDs, depressive disorders, bipolar disorder, and anxiety disorders. Incident AUD was only associated with lifetime nonmedical prescription opioid use and not past-year use. Lifetime and past-year nonmedical prescription opioid use were also both associated with recurrence of AUD and nonopioid SUDs among those with these diagnoses at baseline. In 2013, a report from the same team demonstrated a dose-response relationship between nonmedical prescription opioid use and the same psychiatric disorders (Schepis and Hakes 2013).

There is also evidence that mere exposure to prescription opioids, even if used exactly as prescribed, can precipitate psychiatric disorders, particularly depression. The mechanisms by which exposure to prescription opioids might cause depression are currently mostly speculative, although explanations involving changes in neuroplasticity or neurotransmission with chronic opioid exposure have been proposed (Fischer et al. 2016), and frequent alternating periods of opioid intoxication and withdrawal could also play a role (see Table 7–2). Using medical record data from 49,770 patients with no recent history of depression or prescription opioid use at the U.S. Department of Veterans Affairs (VA) health care system, Scherrer and colleagues (2014) showed that the risk of developing depression increased as the duration of opioid analgesic exposure lengthened. The same team conducted a similar analysis using two large samples at the VA and a private health system and demonstrated that new-onset depression was related to duration of opioid exposure but not dose, suggesting that pain levels might not fully explain the relationship between opioid exposure and the development of depression (Scherrer et al. 2016b). Using smaller samples from the same two health systems, Scherrer and colleagues (2016a) also showed that prescription opioid exposure was related to depression recurrence in patients whose depression had remitted. Prescription opioid use may also be associated with more severe symptoms in those who already have other psychiatric disorders. For instance, there is evidence that prescription opioid use, and particularly problematic use in combination with other substances such as sedatives and cocaine, is associated with more severe PTSD symptoms, especially among women and younger people (Meier et al. 2014).

There is also some support for the self-medication hypothesis to explain the relationship between nonmedical prescription opioid use and psychiatric disorders, suggesting a bidirectional relationship. In the same studies using NESARC data described above (Martins et al. 2009, 2012), the authors demonstrated an increased risk of nonmedical prescription opioid initiation and related OUD in individuals with preexisting psychiatric disorders. In the study using only data from Wave 1 of NESARC (Martins et al. 2012), the increased risk of nonmedical prescription opioid initiation ranged from an AHR of 2.2 for anxiety disorders in general and GAD to an AHR of 3.1 for bipolar disorder. For nonmedical prescription opioid–related OUD, the increase in risk ranged from an AHR of 4.6 for MDD to an AHR of 10.8 for GAD. In the report on data from Waves 1 and 2 of NESARC (Martins et al. 2012), all lifetime mood disorders and GAD were significantly associated with increased risks of incident nonmedical prescription opioid use, with AORs ranging from 1.5 for MDD to 2.0 for bipolar disorder. Mood disorders in general (AOR=2.1), MDD (AOR=1.7), dysthymia (AOR=2.2), and panic disorder (AOR=2.3) were associated with an increased risk of incident OUD. It is important to note that even though preexisting psychiatric disorders have been shown to often precede nonmedical prescription opioid use, this evidence does not alone prove the validity of the self-medication hypothesis or even guarantee a causal link, but it does show that psychiatric illnesses are important risk factors for nonmedical prescription opioid use and related OUD.

The most important evidence for the shared vulnerability model is likely provided by the complex connection between psychiatric disorders, particularly depression; opioid exposure; and chronic pain. Patients with chronic pain are more likely to be depressed and more likely to have recently started taking prescribed opioids (Howe and Sullivan 2014; Sullivan et al. 2006). Studies have shown that opioid-naïve individuals with psychiatric and/or substance use (including tobacco and cannabis) comorbidity are more likely to progress to persistent opioid use (Bateman et al. 2016; Kim et al. 2017) and nonmedical prescription opioid use (Olfson et al. 2018a; Wasan et al. 2015) and to experience other adverse opioid-related outcomes following prescription of opioids for pain (Howe and Sullivan 2014). In addition, psychiatric comorbidity with chronic pain has been associated with progressively decreased opioid analgesia and the resultant need for higher opioid doses (Wasan et al. 2015), and depression has been shown to moderate the relationship between pain and progression to nonmedical prescription opioid use (Mason et al. 2016). In a compelling example of the relationships among psychiatric illness, pain, and opioid-related outcomes, Seal and colleagues (2012) reported the results of a retrospective cohort study involving 141,029 veterans who had served in Iraq and Afghanistan and who received at least one non–cancer-related pain diagnosis within a year of entering the VA health care system. Their analysis showed that patients with mental health diagnoses, especially PTSD, were at an increased risk of receiving prescription opioids, of high-risk opioid use, and of a host of adverse clinical outcomes, including opioid-related accidents and overdoses, self-inflicted injuries, and violence-related injuries. In this way, chronic pain may serve as a third common factor linking both psychiatric illnesses and opioid exposure to negative outcomes, including OUD, and may therefore be creating an adverse selection process whereby patients with mental disorders and nonopioid SUDs are more likely to be prescribed opioids, which end up inadvertently providing temporary relief for psychiatric symptoms but which eventually cause harm (Howe and Sullivan 2014).

Opioid-Related Overdose Deaths and All-Cause Mortality Among Individuals With Psychiatric Disorders

Psychiatric comorbidity increases mortality in OUD, both all-cause mortality and overdose deaths. In an examination of mortality rates among individuals with OUD in the United Kingdom, Bogdanowicz and colleagues (2015) found that comorbid personality disorders or AUD increased all-cause mortality, after controlling for sociodemographic factors, severity of drug use, risk behaviors, and physical health. They also found that comorbid AUD specifically increased overdose-related deaths, that personality disorders or AUD increased hepatic-related deaths, and that comorbid SMI was not associated with increased mortality in adjusted models. Olfson and colleagues (2018b) analyzed Medicaid claims data to show that individuals who died of opioid-related overdoses in the United States, and especially those with chronic pain diagnoses, commonly received prescriptions for benzodiazepines and were diagnosed with drug-related, depressive, or anxiety disorders in the year preceding their death, although diagnosis of OUD was relatively uncommon near the time of death; this finding suggests that the combination of chronic pain and psychiatric illness and/or non-opioid SUDs may be driving opioid-related overdoses even in the absence of formally diagnosed OUD.

As Figure 7–2 shows, overdoses related to the combination of opioids and benzodiazepines have been increasing for more than a decade, with a recent acceleration. In 2015, about 23% of those who died of an opioid overdose also tested positive for a benzodiazepine; by 2017, that proportion had increased to 30% of opioid overdose deaths (National Institute on Drug Abuse 2018). The combination of benzodiazepines and opioids is unsafe, because both can suppress breathing and their respiratory depression actions can be synergistic. The risk of overdose death in individuals prescribed opioids and benzodiazepines simultaneously (or in people with nonmedical use of these medications) is significantly elevated (Dasgupta et al. 2016; Gomes et al. 2011; Park et al. 2015). Unfortunately, many people are prescribed both drug classes simultaneously (Sun et al. 2017), likely because benzodiazepines are highly effective in relieving acute anxiety and insomnia. Owing to the relatively high risk of death, the Centers for Disease Control and Prevention issued new guidelines in 2016 recommending that clinicians avoid prescribing benzodiazepines and opioids simultaneously when possible, and the U.S. Food and Drug Administration (FDA) added black box warnings to the labels of both drug classes warning about the dangers of using them together (Dowell et al. 2016).

There tends to be an assumption that most overdose deaths are accidental; however, given high levels of comorbidity between psychiatric illnesses and OUD and given the findings that those with comorbidity have an increased risk of overdose death, it is necessary to consider whether a significant proportion of opioid-related overdose deaths are at least partially intentional (i.e., related to self-harm or suicide). When an individual dies of a drug overdose, the medical examiner or coroner determines whether the overdose was intentional, unintentional, or undetermined and writes the determination on the death certificate (National Institute on Drug Abuse 2017). Research has shown that rates of overdose deaths classified as intentional are relatively low (no more than 30%) and that there is great variability across states in the United States in terms of how overdose deaths are classified. The variability is much too great to be explained by interstate differences in suicide rates and is more likely related to geographic differences in medical examiners' pro-

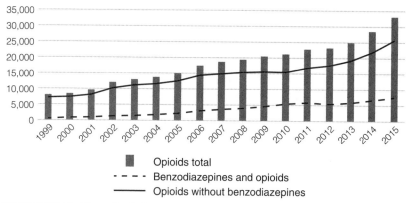

FIGURE 7–2. Opioid overdose deaths involving benzodiazepines.

Source. Reprinted from National Institute on Drug Abuse 2018.

cesses (Rockett et al. 2015). A study by West and colleagues (2015), analyzing over 184,000 calls to poison control centers in the United States, found that about two-thirds of the calls involved at least some suicidal intent, which rose to 75% of calls by those who died from the poisoning between the ages of 20 and 65 years and to 86% by those who died who were age 60 and older. These findings highlight the urgent public health need for more research on the connections between opioid-related overdose deaths and suicide and for greater standardization in the processes that medical examiners and coroners use to classify drug-poisoning deaths.

Impact of Comorbidity on Course and Treatment Outcomes

In general, psychiatric and nonopioid substance use comorbidity with OUD is associated with a more severe illness course and worse outcomes. As noted in earlier sections of this chapter, nonmedical prescription opioid use leads to an increase in the recurrence of depression (Scherrer et al. 2016a), psychiatric comorbidity is associated with a host of negative opioid-related and nonopioid-related outcomes among patients receiving opioids for chronic pain (Seal et al. 2012), and people with psychiatric illnesses and nonopioid SUDs are at elevated risk of opioid-related overdose (Bogdanowicz et al. 2015). In samples of patients in MMT programs, psychiatric and substance use comorbidity has been shown to be associated with lower quality of life (Carpentier et al. 2009; Teoh Bing Fei et al. 2016), and attention-deficit/hyperactivity disorder has been shown to predict greater addiction severity and more psychiatric comorbidity in general (Carpentier et al. 2011). In another study of patients in MMT, both the number of comorbid psychiatric diagnoses and the severity of psychiatric comorbidity were shown to correlate with ongoing concurrent drug abuse, family problems, and unemployment (Mason et al. 1998). Psychiatric and nonopioid substance use comorbidity has also been shown to be associated with more medical comorbidity and psychosocial problems in MMT patients (Roncero et al. 2016). In a sample of individuals with heroin addiction, psychiatric comorbidity was shown to increase the risk of drug-related hospitalization, but successful treatment with either methadone or long-acting injectable extended-release naltrexone (XR-naltrexone) improved outcomes over time (Ngo et al. 2011).

In terms of treatment-related outcomes, comorbid cannabis use, cigarette smoking, psychiatric comorbidity, and benzodiazepine use have been associated with nonadherence with buprenorphine by pill count but not by urine screening, suggesting that psychiatric and substance use comorbidity leads to partial adherence, but not complete nonadherence, due to, for instance, diversion of the medication (Fareed et al. 2014). In a study within the VA health care system, patients with SMI who were also in MMT were more complex with greater health services use than patients with SMI who did not have OUD (Marienfeld and Rosenheck 2015). In patients receiving OAT, comorbid AUD has been shown to lead to poorer opioid-related treatment outcomes, including nonadherence; there is no evidence that OAT leads to reductions in alcohol use for individuals with both AUD and OUD (Soyka 2015). In an 11-year follow-up study of individuals who used heroin, reduction in current heroin use was associated with decreases in risk taking (i.e., needle sharing), crime, and injection-related health problems, as well as improvements in general physical and mental health; however, MDD was associated with an increased likelihood of continued heroin use and poorer outcomes in every domain studied (Teesson et al. 2015).

Even though psychiatric comorbidity is commonly associated with poorer outcomes, the literature is not completely consistent on this topic. For instance, in samples of treatment-resistant individuals who use heroin, both those with general psychiatric comorbidity and those with bipolar I disorder had *better* outcomes (survival in treatment, ability to stabilize within 1 year of treatment, global functioning scores) than those without any psychiatric comorbidity, although those with psychiatric comorbidity required higher methadone doses to stabilize their OUD (Maremmani et al. 2008; Maremmani et al. 2013). Findings such as these suggest that individuals with comorbid psychiatric illness and OUD can do well in treatment, as long as treatment is tailored to meet their unique needs.

Treatment Approach to Comorbid Opioid Use Disorder and Psychiatric Disorders

In general, the best treatment approach for individuals with CODs is to integrate the treatment as much as possible. Rather than older models of treatment, such as the sequential model (i.e., treat either the SUD or the psychiatric disorder first) or the parallel model (i.e., treat both CODs simultaneously but in separate programs), a "no wrong door" approach is most supported by evidence and most likely to achieve success (Green et al. 2007). An integrated treatment approach to CODs means that psychiatric disorders and SUDs are treated by the same clinician or in a single program by a team of clinicians with expertise in both sets of disorders; treatment plans are person centered and individualized to the needs of the patient. For CODs that involve SMIs, the evidence-based treatment model is called integrated dual diagnosis treatment (IDDT; McGovern et al. 2014). In IDDT, pharmacotherapy for psychiatric symptoms is guided by best practices for working with individuals with SUDs (e.g., treat psychiatric symptoms through substance use treatment, avoid potentially addictive or unsafe medications such as benzodiazepines), and MAT for substance use is encouraged when options are available and appropriate. Psychosocial interventions include (but are not limited to) motivation interventions including motivational interviewing, harm reduction, cognitive-behavioral therapy, relapse prevention, family work, and 12-step facilitation, some of which have been modified for working with individuals with SMI.

The general approach to CODs applies to treatment of comorbid psychiatric disorders and OUD but with a few additional considerations. First, MAT with either OAT or XR-naltrexone is the standard of care for OUD because MAT is associated with much lower rates of negative outcomes, including continued opioid use, physical health complications, and overdose death, and there is evidence that MAT produces good outcomes in populations with psychiatric comorbidity (Saunders et al. 2015). Therefore, clinicians treating CODs including OUD must be able to deliver MAT. Second, because the most common form of MAT, methadone, can only be dispensed in specially licensed and regulated opioid treatment programs (OTPs), this is where psychosocial treatment and harm reduction options are often located, and it may be difficult for clinicians and programs prescribing buprenorphine and XR-naltrexone to develop and maintain capacity to deliver a robust array of psychosocial treatments, not to mention the social services that populations with OUD often need. However, it is important for clinicians to resist the temptation to refer patients away for separate psychiatric or SUD services, as there is evidence that referring patients with OUD out of addictions programs for separate psychiatric care often fails (King et al. 2014) and that patients with CODs involving OUD do better in integrated care than in nonintegrated services (Brooner et al. 2013).

Finally, there are a few important medication considerations when treating patients with MAT and psychotropic medications. Even though benzodiazepines are not considered safe when prescribed along with opioids, as described above (see section "Opioid-Related Overdose Deaths and All-Cause Mortality Among Individuals With Psychiatric Disorders"), in September 2017 the FDA issued a Drug Safety Communication "advising that the opioid addiction medications buprenorphine and methadone should not be withheld from patients taking benzodiazepines or other drugs that depress the central nervous system (CNS). The combined use of these drugs increases the risk of serious side effects; however, the harm caused by untreated opioid addiction can outweigh these risks. Careful medication management by health care professionals can reduce these risks" (U.S. Food and Drug Administration 2017). In addition, clinicians should be aware of potential drug-drug interactions between MAT and psychiatric medications. Chapters 9, "Opioid Withdrawal Management and Transition to Treatment," and 10, "Medication-Assisted Treatment for Opioid Use Disorder," go into great detail on the pharmacology of MAT options, and clinicians should consult a *Physicians' Desk Reference* or an equivalent resource when prescribing psychiatric medications in combination with MAT medications. However, an example of a common potential complication worth mentioning here is the ability of both methadone and many psychiatric medications (particularly antipsychotic drugs) to cause prolongation of the QT interval on the electrocardiogram. Therefore, clinicians prescribing psychiatric medications with QT-prolongation potential to patients taking methadone should periodically obtain electrocardiograms. In addition, methadone confers the highest risk of overdose of the OUD MAT options. Therefore, although clinicians should not withhold methadone if it is deemed the best option, they should use caution and monitor carefully when prescribing other sedating medications for a patient taking methadone, or when treating a patient who uses other substances that elevate the risk of overdose, such as alcohol. For patients with AUD, naltrexone is likely the most effective MAT option and confers no inherent additional risk of overdose. Therefore, for patients who have comorbid OUD and AUD, XR-naltrexone may be a good option, especially because there is little evidence that OAT reduces drinking in individuals with AUD (Soyka 2015). However, naltrexone's label includes warnings about potential mood changes and suicidal thinking, for which individuals with comorbid psychiatric disorders and OUD may already be at elevated risk. Again, this should not be a reason in and of itself to withhold this MAT option if it is the most appropriate for a patient, but clinicians should be aware of these potential complications and monitor carefully for them.

Figure 7–3 presents a version of the four-quadrant model for treating CODs, modified for treatment of co-occurring psychiatric disorders and OUD. The four-quadrant model was originally developed to assist mental health systems in developing appropriate treatment options and in guiding treatment setting placement for individuals with CODs (National Association of State Mental Health Program Directors and National Association of State Alcohol and Drug Abuse Directors 1998). Patients with less severe psychiatric illness and addiction fall into quadrant I; patients with more severe psychiatric illness (i.e., SMI) and less severe addiction are in quadrant II; patients with more severe addiction and less severe mental illness are in quadrant III; and patients with a combination of severe addiction and SMI are in quadrant IV. Programs and clinicians serving patients in quadrants I through III need to be COD "capable," which means that they have the ability, basic skills, and willingness to address both the mental health and substance use problems that their patients present with. Patients in quadrant IV require fully integrated programs, such as IDDT programs, which have

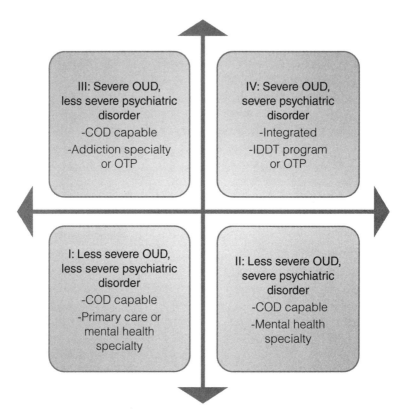

FIGURE 7–3. An adaptation of the four-quadrant model for treating co-occurring psychiatric and opioid use disorders.

COD=co-occurring disorder; IDDT=integrated dual diagnosis treatment; OTP=opioid treatment program; OUD=opioid use disorder.
Source. Adapted from National Association of State Mental Health Program Directors and National Association of State Alcohol and Drug Abuse Directors 1998.

the capacity to address both the SMI and more severe SUDs in a robust and comprehensive manner.

For patients with OUD, those falling into quadrant I can likely be adequately treated in a primary care or mental health specialty setting, with buprenorphine or XR-naltrexone and appropriate psychiatric care. Patients in quadrant II will likely require treatment in a mental health specialty setting geared toward managing individuals with SMI, but this setting also must be capable of providing MAT for OUD. Patients in quadrant III will likely benefit from more intensive addiction treatment in an addiction specialty setting or an OTP that is capable of providing psychiatric treatment. Finally, patients in quadrant IV will need an IDDT program that is capable of providing MAT or an OTP that has developed robust psychosocial treatments for individuals with CODs.

Key Chapter Points

▶ Co-occurring disorders (CODs) are common and are associated with an array of poor outcomes; as such, they present significant clinical and public health challenges. Three general theories to explain co-occurrence are the precipitation, self-medication, and shared vulnerability models.

▶ Certain psychiatric disorders and substance use disorders (SUDs) are more common among individuals with OUD, including depressive disorders, bipolar disorders, anxiety disorders, personality disorders, and nonopioid SUDs. These CODs tend to be comorbid with both heroin-related and nonmedical prescription opioid–related OUD. There is evidence for all three general theories in explaining CODs involving OUD.

▶ The literature related to nonmedical prescription opioid use shows that preexisting exposure to opioids can increase incident psychiatric disorders and that preexisting psychiatric disorders and nonopioid SUDs can increase the risk of developing subsequent nonmedical prescription opioid use. Chronic pain is likely an important shared vulnerability explaining the relationship between psychiatric disorders—especially depression—and OUD, and clinicians may be inadvertently prescribing opioids to individuals with mental disorders to temporarily relieve psychiatric symptoms or emotional distress.

▶ CODs involving OUD are associated with elevated risks of multiple poor outcomes, including increased psychiatric symptoms, poor adherence and response to addiction treatment, and increased mortality, including overdose deaths. Intentional opioid-related overdose deaths (i.e., suicides by overdose) may be underreported, and the phenomenon requires more research.

▶ Integrated psychiatric and addiction treatment that includes medication-assisted treatment (MAT) is the best approach for

CODs involving OUD. Depending on the severity of both the addiction and the psychiatric illness, integrated treatment can be delivered in a range of settings, including primary care, mental health specialty settings, and addictions specialty settings. Methadone must be dispensed in official opioid treatment programs (OTPs). Individuals with a combination of serious mental illness and severe addiction would likely be most successful in an OTP or a mental health program that offers integrated dual diagnosis treatment and MAT.

References

Alterman AI, Cacciola JS: The antisocial personality disorder diagnosis in substance abusers: problems and issues. J Nerv Ment Dis 179(7):401–409, 1991 1869868

Amari E, Rehm J, Goldner E, et al: Nonmedical prescription opioid use and mental health and pain comorbidities: a narrative review. Can J Psychiatry 56(8):495–502, 2011 21878161

American Psychiatric Association: Diagnostic and Statistical Manual of Mental Disorders, 5th Edition. Arlington, VA, American Psychiatric Association, 2013

Bandiera FC, Anteneh B, Le T, et al: Tobacco-related mortality among persons with mental health and substance abuse problems. PLoS One 10(3):e0120581, 2015 25807109

Bateman BT, Franklin JM, Bykov K, et al: Persistent opioid use following cesarean delivery: patterns and predictors among opioid-naïve women. Am J Obstet Gynecol 215(3):353.e1–353.e18, 2016 26996986

Bennett ME, Gjonbalaj S: The problem of dual diagnosis, in Adult Psychopathology and Diagnosis, 5th Edition. Edited by Hersen MTS, Beidel D. New York, Wiley, 2007, pp 34–77

Bogdanowicz KM, Stewart R, Broadbent M, et al: Double trouble: psychiatric comorbidity and opioid addiction—all-cause and cause-specific mortality. Drug Alcohol Depend 148:85–92, 2015 25578253

Brooner RK, King VL, Kidorf M, et al: Psychiatric and substance use comorbidity among treatment-seeking opioid abusers. Arch Gen Psychiatry 54(1):71–80, 1997 9006403

Brooner RK, Kidorf MS, King VL, et al: Managing psychiatric comorbidity within versus outside of methadone treatment settings: a randomized and controlled evaluation. Addiction 108(11):1942–1951, 2013 23734943

Carpentier PJ, Krabbe PF, van Gogh MT, et al: Psychiatric comorbidity reduces quality of life in chronic methadone maintained patients. Am J Addict 18(6):470–480, 2009 19874168

Carpentier PJ, van Gogh MT, Knapen LJ, et al: Influence of attention deficit hyperactivity disorder and conduct disorder on opioid dependence severity and psychiatric comorbidity in chronic methadone-maintained patients. Eur Addict Res 17(1):10–20, 2011 20881401

Case A, Deaton A: Rising morbidity and mortality in midlife among white non-Hispanic Americans in the 21st century. Proc Natl Acad Sci USA 112(49):15078–15083, 2015 26575631

Chiappelli J, Chen S, Hackman A, Eliot-Hong L et al: Evidence for differential opioid use disorder in schizophrenia in an addiction treatment population. Schizophr Res 194:26–31, 2018 28487076

Compton MT, Shim RS (eds): The Social Determinants of Mental Health. Washington, DC, American Psychiatric Publishing, 2015

Compton MT, Kelley ME, Ramsay CE, et al: Association of pre-onset cannabis, alcohol, and tobacco use with age at onset of prodrome and age at onset of psychosis in first-episode patients. Am J Psychiatry 166(11):1251–1257, 2009 19797432

Compton WM, Thomas YF, Stinson FS, et al: Prevalence, correlates, disability, and comorbidity of DSM-IV drug abuse and dependence in the United States: results from the National Epidemiologic Survey on Alcohol and Related Conditions. Arch Gen Psychiatry 64(5):566–576, 2007 17485608

Conway JL: Exogenous nicotine normalises sensory gating in schizophrenia: therapeutic implications. Med Hypotheses 73(2):259–262, 2009 19328631

Dasgupta N, Funk MJ, Proescholdbell S, et al: Cohort study of the impact of high-dose opioid analgesics on overdose mortality. Pain Med 17(1):85–98, 2016 26333030

Davis MA, Lin LA, Liu H, et al: Prescription opioid use among adults with mental health disorders in the United States. J Am Board Fam Med 30(4):407–417, 2017 28720623

Dickerson F, Stallings CR, Origoni AE, et al: Cigarette smoking among persons with schizophrenia or bipolar disorder in routine clinical settings, 1999–2011. Psychiatr Serv 64(1):44–50, 2013 23280457

Dowell D, Haegerich TM, Chou R: CDC guideline for prescribing opioids for chronic pain—United States, 2016. MMWR Recomm Rep 65(1):1–49, 2016 26987082

Fareed A, Eilender P, Ketchen B, et al: Factors affecting noncompliance with buprenorphine maintenance treatment. J Addict Med 8(5):345–350, 2014 25072677

Featherstone RE, Siegel SJ: The role of nicotine in schizophrenia. Int Rev Neurobiol 124:23–78, 2015 26472525

Fischer B, Lusted A, Roerecke M, et al: The prevalence of mental health and pain symptoms in general population samples reporting nonmedical use of prescription opioids: a systematic review and meta-analysis. J Pain 13(11):1029–1044, 2012 23040158

Fischer B, Murphy Y, Kurdyak P, et al: Depression—a major but neglected consequence contributing to the health toll from prescription opioids? Psychiatry Res 243:331–334, 2016 27434203

Goldner EM, Lusted A, Roerecke M, et al: Prevalence of Axis-1 psychiatric (with focus on depression and anxiety) disorder and symptomatology among non-medical prescription opioid users in substance use treatment: systematic review and meta-analyses. Addict Behav 39(3):520–531, 2014 24333033

Gomes T, Mamdani MM, Dhalla IA, et al: Opioid dose and drug-related mortality in patients with nonmalignant pain. Arch Intern Med 171(7):686–691, 2011 21482846

Green AI, Drake RE, Brunette MF, et al: Schizophrenia and co-occurring substance use disorder. Am J Psychiatry 164(3):402–408, 2007 17329463

Grella CE, Karno MP, Warda US, et al: Gender and comorbidity among individuals with opioid use disorders in the NESARC study. Addict Behav 34(6–7):498–504, 2009 19232832

Hasin DS, Grant BF: The National Epidemiologic Survey on Alcohol and Related Conditions (NESARC) Waves 1 and 2: review and summary of findings. Soc Psychiatry Psychiatr Epidemiol 50(11):1609–1640, 2015 26210739

Howe CQ, Sullivan MD: The missing "P" in pain management: how the current opioid epidemic highlights the need for psychiatric services in chronic pain care. Gen Hosp Psychiatry 36(1):99–104, 2014 24211157

Hunt GE, Malhi GS, Cleary M, et al: Comorbidity of bipolar and substance use disorders in national surveys of general populations, 1990–2015: systematic review and meta-analysis. J Affect Disord 206:321–330, 2016a 27426694

Hunt GE, Malhi GS, Cleary M, et al: Prevalence of comorbid bipolar and substance use disorders in clinical settings, 1990–2015: systematic review and meta-analysis. J Affect Disord 206:331–349, 2016b 27476137

Katz C, El-Gabalawy R, Keyes KM, et al: Risk factors for incident nonmedical prescription opioid use and abuse and dependence: results from a longitudinal nationally representative sample. Drug Alcohol Depend 132(1–2):107–113, 2013 23399466

Kelley ME, Wan CR, Broussard B, et al: Marijuana use in the immediate 5-year premorbid period is associated with increased risk of onset of schizophrenia and related psychotic disorders. Schizophr Res 171(1–3):62–67, 2016 26785806

Kendler KS, Prescott CA, Myers J, et al: The structure of genetic and environmental risk factors for common psychiatric and substance use disorders in men and women. Arch Gen Psychiatry 60(9):929–937, 2003 12963675

Khantzian EJ: The self-medication hypothesis of substance use disorders: a reconsideration and recent applications. Harv Rev Psychiatry 4(5):231–244, 1997 9385000

Kidorf M, Disney ER, King VL, et al: Prevalence of psychiatric and substance use disorders in opioid abusers in a community syringe exchange program. Drug Alcohol Depend 74(2):115–122, 2004 15099655

Kim SC, Choudhry N, Franklin JM, et al: Patterns and predictors of persistent opioid use following hip or knee arthroplasty. Osteoarthritis Cartilage 25(9):1399–1406, 2017 28433815

King VL, Brooner RK, Peirce J, et al: Challenges and outcomes of parallel care for patients with co-occurring psychiatric disorder in methadone maintenance treatment. J Dual Diagn 10(2):60–67, 2014 24976801

Lasser K, Boyd JW, Woolhandler S, et al: Smoking and mental illness: a population-based prevalence study. JAMA 284(20):2606–2610, 2000 11086367

Lyons M, Hitsman B, Xian H, et al: A twin study of smoking, nicotine dependence, and major depression in men. Nicotine Tob Res 10(1):97–108, 2008 18188750

Manseau M, Bogenschutz M: Substance use disorders and schizophrenia. Focus 14:333–342, 2016

Manseau MW, Goff DC: Cannabinoids and schizophrenia: risks and therapeutic potential. Neurotherapeutics 12(4):816-824, 2015 26311150

Maremmani AG, Rovai L, Bacciardi S, et al: The long-term outcomes of heroin dependent-treatment-resistant patients with bipolar 1 comorbidity after admission to enhanced methadone maintenance. J Affect Disord 151(2):582–589, 2013 23931828

Maremmani I, Perugi G, Pacini M, et al: Toward a unitary perspective on the bipolar spectrum and substance abuse: opiate addiction as a paradigm. J Affect Disord 93(1–3):1–12, 2006 16675028

Maremmani I, Pacini M, Lubrano S, et al: Long-term outcomes of treatment-resistant heroin addicts with and without DSM-IV axis I psychiatric comorbidity (dual diagnosis). Eur Addict Res 14(3):134–142, 2008 18552489

Marienfeld C, Rosenheck RA: Psychiatric services and prescription fills among veterans with serious mental illness in methadone maintenance treatment. J Dual Diagn 11(2):128–135, 2015 25781867

Martins SS, Keyes KM, Storr CL, et al: Pathways between nonmedical opioid use/dependence and psychiatric disorders: results from the National Epidemiologic Survey on Alcohol and Related Conditions. Drug Alcohol Depend 103(1–2):16–24, 2009 19414225

Martins SS, Fenton MC, Keyes KM, et al: Mood and anxiety disorders and their association with non-medical prescription opioid use and prescription opioid-use disorder: longitudinal evidence from the National Epidemiologic Study on Alcohol and Related Conditions. Psychol Med 42(6):1261–1272, 2012 21999943

Mason BJ, Kocsis JH, Melia D, et al: Psychiatric comorbidity in methadone maintained patients. J Addict Dis 17(3):75–89, 1998 9789161

Mason MJ, Golladay G, Jiranek W, et al: Depression moderates the relationship between pain and the nonmedical use of opioid medication among adult outpatients. J Addict Med 10(6):408–413, 2016 27559846

McGovern MP, Lambert-Harris C, Gotham HJ, et al: Dual diagnosis capability in mental health and addiction treatment services: an assessment of programs across multiple state systems. Adm Policy Ment Health 41(2):205–214, 2014 23183873

Meier A, Lambert-Harris C, McGovern MP, et al: Co-occurring prescription opioid use problems and posttraumatic stress disorder symptom severity. Am J Drug Alcohol Abuse 40(4):304–311, 2014 24809229

National Association of State Mental Health Program Directors, National Association of State Alcohol and Drug Abuse Directors: National dialogue on co-occurring mental health and substance abuse disorders. June 16–17, 1998. Available at: https://www.nasmhpd.org/sites/default/files/National%20Dialogue.pdf. Accessed February 24, 2018.

National Institute on Drug Abuse: Intentional vs. unintentional overdose deaths. February 2017. Available at: https://www.drugabuse.gov/related-topics/treatment/intentional-vs-unintentional-overdose-deaths. Accessed February 25, 2018.

National Institute on Drug Abuse: Benzodiazepines and opioids. March 2018. Available at: https://www.drugabuse.gov/drugs-abuse/opioids/benzodiazepines-opioids. Accessed February 25, 2018.

Ngo HT, Tait RJ, Hulse GK: Hospital psychiatric comorbidity and its role in heroin dependence treatment outcomes using naltrexone implant or methadone maintenance. J Psychopharmacol 25(6):774–782, 2011 20360157

Novak SP, Herman-Stahl M, Flannery B, et al: Physical pain, common psychiatric and substance use disorders, and the non-medical use of prescription analgesics in the United States. Drug Alcohol Depend 100(1–2):63–70, 2009 19010611

Odlaug BL, Gual A, DeCourcy J, et al: Alcohol dependence, co-occurring conditions and attributable burden. Alcohol Alcohol 51(2):201–209, 2016 26246514

Olfson M, Wall MM, Liu SM, et al: Cannabis use and risk of prescription opioid use disorder in the United States. Am J Psychiatry 175(1):47–53, 2018a 28946762

Olfson M, Wall M, Wang S, et al: Service use preceding opioid-related fatality. Am J Psychiatry 175(6):538–544, 2018b 29179577

Park TW, Saitz R, Ganoczy D, et al: Benzodiazepine prescribing patterns and deaths from drug overdose among U.S. veterans receiving opioid analgesics: case-cohort study. BMJ 350:h2698, 2015 26063215

Peles E, Schreiber S, Naumovsky Y, et al: Depression in methadone maintenance treatment patients: rate and risk factors. J Affect Disord 99(1–3):213–220, 2007 17055063

Raimo EB, Schuckit MA: Alcohol dependence and mood disorders. Addict Behav 23(6):933–946, 1998 9801727

Regier DA, Farmer ME, Rae DS, et al: Comorbidity of mental disorders with alcohol and other drug abuse: results from the Epidemiologic Catchment Area (ECA) study. JAMA 264(19):2511–2518, 1990 2232018

Rockett IR, Hobbs GR, Wu D, et al: Variable classification of drug-intoxication suicides across U.S. states: a partial artifact of forensics? PLoS One 10(8):e0135296, 2015 26295155

Roncero C, Barral C, Rodríguez-Cintas L, et al: Psychiatric comorbidities in opioid-dependent patients undergoing a replacement therapy programme in Spain: the PROTEUS study. Psychiatry Res 243:174–181, 2016 27416536

Rosen D, Smith ML, Reynolds CF III: The prevalence of mental and physical health disorders among older methadone patients. Am J Geriatr Psychiatry 16(6):488–497, 2008 18515693

Rosen D, Hunsaker A, Albert SM, et al: Characteristics and consequences of heroin use among older adults in the United States: a review of the literature, treatment implications, and recommendations for further research. Addict Behav 36(4):279–285, 2011 21237575

Rudd RA, Seth P, David F, et al: Increases in drug and opioid-involved overdose deaths—United States, 2010–2015. MMWR Morb Mortal Wkly Rep 65(5051):1445–1452, 2016 28033313

Satel SL, Kosten TR, Schuckit MA, et al: Should protracted withdrawal from drugs be included in DSM-IV? Am J Psychiatry 150(5):695–704, 1993 8097618

Saunders EC, McGovern MP, Lambert-Harris C, et al: The impact of addiction medications on treatment outcomes for persons with co-occurring PTSD and opioid use disorders. Am J Addict 24(8):722–731, 2015 26388539

Schepis TS, Hakes JK: Non-medical prescription use increases the risk for the onset and recurrence of psychopathology: results from the National Epidemiological Survey on Alcohol and Related Conditions. Addiction 106(12):2146–2155, 2011 21631624

Schepis TS, Hakes JK: Dose-related effects for the precipitation of psychopathology by opioid or tranquilizer/sedative nonmedical prescription use: results from the National Epidemiologic Survey on Alcohol and Related Conditions. J Addict Med 7(1):39–44, 2013 23222127

Scherrer JF, Svrakic DM, Freedland KE, et al: Prescription opioid analgesics increase the risk of depression. J Gen Intern Med 29(3):491–499, 2014 24165926

Scherrer JF, Salas J, Copeland LA, et al: Increased risk of depression recurrence after initiation of prescription opioids in noncancer pain patients. J Pain 17(4):473–482, 2016a 26884282

Scherrer JF, Salas J, Copeland LA, et al: Prescription opioid duration, dose, and increased risk of depression in 3 large patient populations. Ann Fam Med 14(1):54–62, 2016b 26755784

Schulte MT, Hser YI: Substance use and associated health conditions throughout the lifespan. Public Health Rev 35(2), 2014 28366975

Seal KH, Shi Y, Cohen G, et al: Association of mental health disorders with prescription opioids and high-risk opioid use in U.S. veterans of Iraq and Afghanistan. JAMA 307(9):940–947, 2012 22396516

Selzer JA, Lieberman JA: Schizophrenia and substance abuse. Psychiatr Clin North Am 16(2):401–412, 1993 8332568

Smith KZ, Smith PH, Cercone SA, et al: Past year non-medical opioid use and abuse and PTSD diagnosis: interactions with sex and associations with symptom clusters. Addict Behav 58:167–174, 2016 26946448

Soyka M: Alcohol use disorders in opioid maintenance therapy: prevalence, clinical correlates and treatment. Eur Addict Res 21(2):78–87, 2015 25413371

Soyka M, Albus M, Kathmann N, et al: Prevalence of alcohol and drug abuse in schizophrenic inpatients. Eur Arch Psychiatry Clin Neurosci 242(6):362–372, 1993 8323987

Strain EC: Assessment and treatment of comorbid psychiatric disorders in opioid-dependent patients. Clin J Pain 18(4)(suppl):S14–S27, 2002 12479251

Strain EC, Brooner RK, Bigelow GE: Clustering of multiple substance use and psychiatric diagnoses in opiate addicts. Drug Alcohol Depend 27(2):127–134, 1991 2055161

Substance Abuse and Mental Health Services Administration: Key substance use and mental health indicators in the United States: results from the 2016 National Survey on Drug Use and Health (NSDUH Series H-52, HHS

Publ No SMA 17–5044). Rockville, MD, Center for Behavioral Health Statistics and Quality. September 2017. Available at: https://store. samhsa.gov/shin/content//SMA17-5044/SMA17-5044.pdf. Accessed February 24, 2018.

Sullivan MD, Edlund MJ, Zhang L, et al: Association between mental health disorders, problem drug use, and regular prescription opioid use. Arch Intern Med 166(19):2087–2093, 2006 17060538

Sun EC, Dixit A, Humphreys K, et al: Association between concurrent use of prescription opioids and benzodiazepines and overdose: retrospective analysis. BMJ 356:j760, 2017 28292769

Swofford CD, Scheller-Gilkey G, Miller AH, et al: Double jeopardy: schizophrenia and substance use. Am J Drug Alcohol Abuse 26(3):343–353, 2000 10976661

Talamo A, Centorrino F, Tondo L, et al: Comorbid substance-use in schizophrenia: relation to positive and negative symptoms. Schizophr Res 86(1–3):251–255, 2006 16750347

Teesson M, Marel C, Darke S, et al: Long-term mortality, remission, criminality and psychiatric comorbidity of heroin dependence: 11-year findings from the Australian Treatment Outcome Study. Addiction 110(6):986–993, 2015 25619110

Teoh Bing Fei J, Yee A, Habil MH: Psychiatric comorbidity among patients on methadone maintenance therapy and its influence on quality of life. Am J Addict 25(1):49–55, 2016 26692463

U.S. Food and Drug Administration: FDA Drug Safety Communication: FDA urges caution about withholding opioid addiction medications from patients taking benzodiazepines or CNS depressants: careful medication management can reduce risks. September 26, 2017. Available at: https:// www.fda.gov/Drugs/DrugSafety/ucm575307.htm. Accessed February 25, 2018.

Wasan AD, Michna E, Edwards RR, et al: Psychiatric comorbidity is associated prospectively with diminished opioid analgesia and increased opioid misuse in patients with chronic low back pain. Anesthesiology 123(4):861–872, 2015 26375824

Wesson DR, Ling W: The Clinical Opiate Withdrawal Scale (COWS). J Psychoactive Drugs 35(2):253–259, 2003 12924748

West NA, Severtson SG, Green JL, et al: Trends in abuse and misuse of prescription opioids among older adults. Drug Alcohol Depend 149:117–121, 2015 25678441

Zirakzadeh A, Shuman C, Stauter E, et al: Cigarette smoking in methadone maintained patients: an up-to-date review. Curr Drug Abuse Rev 6(1):77–84, 2013 23506370

8

Assessment and Care of Patients With Opioid Use Disorder

Snehal Bhatt, M.D.

Bellelizabeth Foster, M.D.

Vanessa Jacobsohn, M.D.

Paul Romo, M.D.

Tyler Seybert, M.D.

Roxanne Russell, M.D.

Clinical Vignette: Mr. Sandoval's Addiction to Prescription Opioids

Ted Sandoval is a 48-year-old American Indian man with a 15-year history of prescription opioid addiction. Mr. Sandoval came in to see Dr. Sam, a new consulting addiction psychiatrist at the local community clinic. Mr. Sandoval felt fortunate to be happily married with two children, well respected in his community, and the owner of a construction company, before developing his addiction to opioids. His occupation led to a series of job-related injuries, including a serious injury to his knee 16 years ago that required surgical repair. Postoperative management included oxycodone-acetaminophen 10/325 mg every 4 hours as needed

211

for pain control. He noted that his pain continued even after this intervention, and he experienced reduced mobility, which limited his ability to work. This led to his losing his construction contracts and ultimately to the closing of his business. After this, he experienced the onset of depressed mood, along with more generalized pain throughout his body as his mood deteriorated. He had continued access to opioid pain medications during this time through his primary care provider. Although he was interested in alternative modalities of treatment, such as physical therapy and acupuncture, these were not available to him locally.

Within 1 year of the surgery, Mr. Sandoval found that he required escalating doses of opioid medications to control his pain and prevent opioid withdrawal symptoms. At that point, he began to see multiple providers in a larger city, from whom he received several different prescriptions for opioid pain medications. His use progressed over the years to peak at total daily doses of tramadol 200 mg/day, hydrocodone 40 mg/day, and oxycodone 90 mg/day, along with diazepam 30 mg/day. Importantly, even at these doses, he was running out too soon, subsequently experiencing debilitating withdrawal symptoms, and then purchasing illicit opioids "off the street." Mr. Sandoval reported to Dr. Sam that he was "addicted" to his pain medications and that they were "ruining" his life. He now struggled financially, felt unable to work due to repeated cycles of opioid intoxication and withdrawal, experienced more pain than ever before, and was concerned that he was no longer active in his community, which diminished his respect as an elder. He also felt shame at having to see multiple physicians for his medications. Mr. Sandoval reported to Dr. Sam that he had been attempting to get help with his opioid use for a "long time" but had had no success due to his long distance from any available treatment. He had tried to stop opioid medications on his own many times but found himself repeatedly relapsing due to severe cravings and withdrawal symptoms.

Mr. Sandoval denied other psychiatric or substance use history. He only reported using tobacco and peyote ceremonially. Medically, he reported a history of chronic pain and knee surgery, along with non–insulin-dependent diabetes mellitus, hypertension, and hyperlipidemia, for which he took metformin, lisinopril, and atorvastatin, respectively. He grew up in a traditional family on the reservation, and his childhood was tumultuous at times due to poverty and his father's alcohol use. In fact, he stated that his stepfather largely raised him but he felt "unwanted." He reported feeling a sense of abandonment, along with emotional and physical abuse by his stepfather.

A full evaluation resulted in a diagnosis of severe opioid use disorder (OUD). Dr. Sam discussed treatment options with Mr. Sandoval, including inpatient versus outpatient treatment, along with detoxification versus maintenance treatment. They also discussed options for medication-assisted treatment (MAT) with methadone, buprenorphine, or long-acting injectable extended-release naltrexone (XR-naltrexone), although there were no methadone outpatient treatment programs in the vicinity. Dr. Sam did not travel to the clinic regularly and, as a result, was unable to follow Mr. Sandoval at this facility on an ongoing basis. The one inpatient facility the patient could readily access provided detoxification only. On the basis of his evaluation, Dr. Sam assessed that outpatient maintenance treatment, which was also Mr. Sandoval's preference, was most appropriate clinically. Dr. Sam carried out an outpatient induction onto buprenorphine, and Mr. Sandoval rapidly stabilized on buprenorphine-naloxone (Suboxone) 16/4 mg/day. The clinic treatment team made arrangements for him to be seen at an academic clinic about 50 miles away for ongoing office-based buprenorphine treatment. The local clinic was able to provide individual drug counseling, along with traditional healing, on-site, and Mr. Sandoval showed interest in both of these modalities of care. After obtaining informed consent, his treatment team also contacted his medical providers, who discontinued all opioid pain medications.

Six years later, Mr. Sandoval, now 54 years of age, remains engaged in office-based treatment with buprenorphine. He reports that although traveling 50 miles for his medication is not ideal because of the cost of gasoline, it is a "blessing" compared with the suffering he experienced as a result of his addiction. He has been able to achieve monthly prescription privileges by providing urine drug screens that are negative for substances of abuse, by regularly attending his appointments, and by being free of any aberrant drug-related behaviors (e.g., all random pill counts have been accurate). After initially engaging in drug counseling at his local clinic, he is now connected with a psychotherapist at the academic clinic, where he is treated with acceptance and commitment therapy for his chronic pain diagnosis. He schedules appointments with this therapist to coincide with when he goes in for a medication refill. He continues to participate in traditional healing ceremonies through the local clinic, which employs a traditional healer. He has also become increasingly active in American Indian community meetings. He reports that involvement in these treatments has allowed him to view his illness within a larger cultural context; additionally, he reports deriving strength and motivation for his well-being through connecting with his culture and community and improving his relationships with family members.

Mr. Sandoval reports that when he goes to the academic clinic for his refills, he also sees a psychiatrist for his underlying depression at the same facility. Since he achieved sobriety, he has been better able to attend primary care appointments, which continue to be at his local clinic. He reports that he has signed appropriate consents, and all of his providers "talk to each other to make sure they are all on the same page." His depression has been in remission, and there have been improvements in his blood glucose control, weight, and blood pressure. He reports that he has a pending appointment at the university pain clinic; he is hopeful that they may be able to offer him other treatment options for his ongoing chronic pain.

This case highlights several important questions about living with addiction, having a diagnosis of OUD, biopsychosocial formulation, treatment planning, and navigating through treatment systems, as well as the concept of recovery. The remainder of this chapter will explore these questions in depth: What are some risk factors for developing OUD? In the setting of chronic pain treatment with opioid medications, how does the provider monitor for emerging aberrant behaviors and misuse of prescribed medications? How does the provider identify and diagnose patients with OUD? How does the provider comprehensively assess patients with OUD and then most effectively provide psychoeducation and engage them in the treatment planning process? How does the provider determine which treatment modalities might be most appropriate for a patient (i.e., deciding on inpatient vs. outpatient treatment, considering detoxification vs. maintenance treatment, choosing the best fit with psychosocial treatment approaches, selecting the most appropriate option for MAT)? What is the subjective experience of a person living with OUD and seeking treatment? What is the concept of recovery in the realm of substance use disorders (SUDs)? How does the provider help patients achieve recovery?

Screening for Opioid Use Disorder

An estimated 2.1 million individuals met criteria for OUD in 2016, although the vast majority of this population did not receive specialty treatment for their illness (Substance Abuse and Mental Health Services Administration. 2017). On the other hand, a majority of the population with OUD comes into contact with a primary care provider each year. As a result, medical settings can identify and help those individuals with OUD who may otherwise never see an addiction specialist. Substance use can sometimes be missed as part of a patient evaluation due to assumptions (e.g., "This patient doesn't seem like an addict, so I don't need to ask") or because of provider discomfort with discussing this topic. Screening is the first step in identifying and diagnosing any

SUD or detecting problem substance use. Screening can serve several important functions; it can 1) help identify a problem early and prevent escalation to addiction, 2) inform how a particular substance may interact with a person's medications and overall medical care, and 3) identify patients who have already developed an addiction so they can be provided with or referred to more intensive treatment. All patients should be screened for SUDs. Universal screening eliminates the risk of bias in assessment and lowers the likelihood of underdiagnosing substance use problems (Sullivan and Fleming 1997).

A number of validated screening tools are available to providers free of cost. These screening tools have often been modified from their original versions to reduce their administration time and complexity. One example of this is the Drug Abuse Screening Test (DAST), which in its original iteration is a 28-item screening tool that takes approximately 5–8 minutes to administer; however, a shortened, 10-item, self- or clinician-administered version has been validated (Yudko et al. 2007). This tool assesses drug use in the past 12 months and comes with associated recommendations. Another example of a screening tool is the National Institute on Drug Abuse's NIDA-Modified ASSIST, which is designed to screen for drug use in general medical settings. Importantly, this tool is made available online (www.drugabuse.gov/nmassist/), so that clinicians can easily work through this screening tool with their patients. This tool has been further adapted by the American Psychiatric Association (APA) to expand the target population from adults to include adolescents (ages 11–17 years), as well as children. The APA has made this adaptation available to clinicians free of cost (www.psychiatry.org/psychiatrists/practice/dsm/educational-resources/assessment-measures#Disorder).

Patients with chronic pain who are treated with opioid pain medications present a particular challenge for many physicians, who must balance the benefits of providing adequate pain control with the risks of SUD and overdose. Importantly, most patients receiving treatment for chronic pain with opioids do not become addicted, but a relatively high percentage—about 20%–30%—display aberrant drug-related behaviors during the course of their treatment (Bailey and Vowles 2017; Vowles et al. 2015). Responsible opioid prescribing begins with knowing the individual risk factors for addiction and overdose, as summarized in Table 8–1.

Another aspect of responsible opioid prescribing is the use of validated screening tools that assess the potential risk of developing addic-

TABLE 8–1. Risk factors for misusing prescribed opioids and for overdose

Risk factors for misusing prescribed opioids[a]	Risk factors for overdose among those taking prescription opioids[b]
Lifetime history of a substance use disorder	High opioid dose (>100 mg morphine equivalents)
Increased functional impairment due to pain	History of overdose
	Sleep apnea
Psychiatric comorbidity	Hepatic or renal impairment
Use of psychotropic medications	Concurrent use of other central
Young age (16–45) or age >65	nervous system depressants, such as alcohol or benzodiazepines
	Long-acting or extended-release formulations

[a]Boscarino et al. 2010. [b]Darke and Ross 2002; Zedler et al. 2014.

tion to prescribed opioids. Several such tools exist and are available in the public domain. The best studied of these tools is the Screener and Opioid Assessment for Patients with Pain—Revised (SOAPP-R; Butler et al. 2008), a 24-item, self-administered scale that takes into account factors such as mood symptoms, family history, and legal history. It is designed to stratify which patients require more monitoring and has associated monitoring and treatment recommendations. Another validated tool is the Continuing Opioid Misuse Measure (COMM; Butler et al. 2010), a 17-item, self-administered scale that evaluates medication overuse behaviors over the past 30 days, which is designed to identify misuse of currently prescribed medications.

Clinicians must be aware of the limitations of these predictive screening tools when using them. Recently published guidelines by the Centers for Disease Control and Prevention (Dowell et al. 2016) on prescribing opioids for chronic pain management point out that the evidence supporting the use of these screening tools is "sparse." Bailey and Vowles (2017) suggested that these screening tools have a low positive predictive value; in other words, while a negative screening test may demonstrate a high likelihood that the patient will not go on to misuse prescribed opioids, a positive screening test is much less useful. Screening tools should not be used to deprive patients of pain management or opioid therapy but rather to identify those who are at risk for addiction. They should be used as a guide to help determine the frequency and intensity of monitoring during the course of treatment and, ultimately, to develop the most efficacious and safest treatment strategy for a particular patient. Indeed, the clinical interview and clinician judgment are still the gold standards for diagnosis and risk assessment and management.

A final aspect of safe opioid prescribing is ongoing monitoring for any emerging aberrant behaviors (Webster and Webster 2005). Table 8–2 lists some behaviors that clinicians most commonly see. It is essential for clinicians to directly and objectively address any of these behaviors. If, during the course of chronic pain evaluation and treatment, a patient scores in the high-risk range on a screening test or displays aberrant drug-related behaviors, it is necessary to refer the patient for a more thorough evaluation of possible OUD.

Initial Assessment of Opioid Use Disorder

The clinical assessment is a key component of successful treatment planning for OUD. Clinicians must develop a clear understanding of the patient's motivation for treatment and recovery goals. This assessment involves more than completing a series of questions; it must elicit information leading to the most appropriate and safest treatment plan for the patient. It is critical to use motivational interviewing principles and techniques to ensure that the patient is empowered to take the lead in his or her recovery. Once the patient can express in his or her own words a desire for change, the initial interview can help encourage the patient to move from desire to commitment and to develop a specific plan for recovery.

The assessment is also key to the development of a therapeutic alliance between the patient and his or her provider. In addition, it allows the patient to connect with care for comorbid medical, psychiatric, and substance use issues. It is crucial to identify risk factors that may complicate, as well as strengths that may assist, the recovery process and the overall health of the individual. In the outpatient setting, the following procedures are helpful and at times required prior to initiating treat-

TABLE 8–2. Aberrant behaviors related to substance misuse

Mild aberrant behaviors	Moderate aberrant behaviors	Severe aberrant behaviors
Requests for higher doses	Use of prescribed medication to treat symptoms other than pain	Continual dose escalation
Requests for specific formulations	Stockpiling prescriptions	Seeking prescriptions from outside providers or emergency departments
Occasional reported loss of prescription	Significant energy spent ensuring supply	Stealing medications
Occasional dose escalation without permission	Multiple unsanctioned dose escalations	Consistently buying medications off the street
	Recurrent reported prescription losses	Diverting/selling medications
	Decline in functioning from baseline	Forging prescriptions
	Concurrent use of other substances	Injecting oral medications

ment. At patient check-in, the nurse or medical assistant should do the following:

- Establish a nonjudgmental treatment environment that fosters patient trust.
- Review consent for treatment with the patient and have him or her sign it.
- Check vital signs.
- Administer a Clinical Opiate Withdrawal Scale (COWS; Wesson and Ling 2003).
- Check point-of-care urine toxicology drug dip when available.
- Perform an electrocardiogram (if methadone is being considered).
- Communicate critical information to the clinician.

The clinician should then complete a history and physical, key aspects of which are shown in Table 8–3.

The initial assessment should provide sufficient information to allow the clinician to generate an appropriate SUD diagnosis using criteria in the *Diagnostic and Statistical Manual of Mental Disorders*, Fifth Edition (DSM-5; American Psychiatric Association 2013); if the patient has an OUD, the assessment should allow the clinician to determine the severity of the disorder. At the conclusion of the first visit, the clinician should be sure to write a prescription for the opioid antagonist naloxone (for overdose reversal) if the patient does not already have this at home. It is crucial that all patients with OUD have access to naloxone, as multiple studies have shown that it safely reverses an opioid overdose and saves lives (Katzman et al. 2018). Additionally, the clinician should provide basic overdose education, including how to properly administer naloxone, and stress the importance of calling 911 after the administration of naloxone. An opioid overdose tool kit that includes patient education on proper use of naloxone, along with additional links to useful resources, is available through the Substance Abuse and Mental Health Services Administration (SAMHSA) (https://store.samhsa.gov/system/files/sma18-4742.pdf).

Developing a Biopsychosocial Formulation

The biopsychosocial formulation is a clinical tool that allows a clinician to reflect on the data gathered during the initial assessment and under-

TABLE 8–3. Key components of the initial assessment of opioid use disorder

Component	Purpose	Major topics to assess
History of the present illness	Evaluation of the patient's current opioid use and perspectives on use, treatment, and plans for the future	Motivation to seek treatment Experiences with opioid use patterns and problems, including intoxication and withdrawal Goals of treatment

Substance use history	Evaluation of prior patterns of substance use and treatment experiences	Inquire about all drugs of abuse:
		    First use
		    Most recent use
		    Heaviest use
		    Consequences of use
		    Attempts at cessation
		    Motivation to abstain or reduce use

History of overdose	Risk assessment and harm reduction	Personal history of overdose Witness to overdose death Naloxone use and access

TABLE 8–3. Key components of the initial assessment of opioid use disorder *(continued)*

Component	Purpose	Major topics to assess
Psychiatric review of systems	Evaluation of current psychiatric symptoms	Depression
		Anxiety
		Mania
		Psychosis
		Suicidal ideation
		Violent ideation
Medical review of systems	Evaluation of current medical symptoms	Chest pain or shortness of breath
		Heart palpitations
		Fever
		Abdominal pain
		Symptoms of withdrawal
Past psychiatric history	Evaluation for co-occurring psychiatric illness	Psychiatric hospitalizations
		Suicide attempts
		History of self-harm/cutting
		Aggressive behavior
		Psychiatric diagnoses
		Psychotropic medication trials
		History of traumatic experiences

TABLE 8–3. Key components of the initial assessment of opioid use disorder *(continued)*

Component	Purpose	Major topics to assess
Past medical history, past surgical history, family history	Screening for ongoing chronic illness and predisposition for chronic illness	Lung, heart, liver, or kidney disease Infectious diseases Traumatic brain injuries Medical devices Family history of chronic illness
Medications, herbal supplements, and allergies	Consideration of current medical and psychiatric diagnoses and treatments	Current prescribed medications Current over-the-counter medications Current herbal supplements Medication and food allergies
Social history	Gathering contextual information for insight into risk and protective factors for substance use and treatment outcomes	Domestic violence assessment Housing Finances Transportation Relationships Education
Health care maintenance	Coordination of comprehensive health care	Insurance Primary care provider Vaccinations

TABLE 8–3. Key components of the initial assessment of opioid use disorder *(continued)*

Component	Purpose	Major topics to assess
Physical examination	Evaluation for ongoing or undiagnosed medical conditions; assessment for intoxication or withdrawal severity	Neurological exam Cardiovascular exam Abdominal exam Skin exam for abscesses Clinical Opiate Withdrawal Scale (COWS) Current intoxication
Laboratory testing and electrocardiogram	Evaluation for ongoing or undiagnosed medical conditions; screening for undisclosed substance use	Screening Human immunodeficiency virus Hepatitis viruses Sexually transmitted infections Tuberculosis Urine toxicology Complete blood count Metabolic panel Liver function tests QTc prolongation
Prescription drug monitoring program	Screening for concurrent prescriptions of opioids or medications posing a high risk of interaction with treatment methods	Ongoing prescriptions for opioids, benzodiazepines, and other prescription drugs with potential for misuse

stand the influence of a wide variety of factors regarding the patient's presentation and experience. These factors can be placed broadly into three categories: biological, psychological, and social. Factors in each of these categories can serve to 1) predispose an individual to developing an SUD, 2) precipitate the disorder, 3) perpetuate the disorder, or 4) protect the individual from adverse outcomes related to the SUD. This framework allows clinicians to understand the network of factors influencing the course of an individual's substance use, his or her motivation to change, and the anticipated treatment trajectory.

Predisposing Factors

In the clinical vignette, the patient, Mr. Sandoval, reported a family history of alcohol abuse in his father. This is an important biological predisposing factor. Multiple twin studies have shown a shared genetic influence across a variety of substances (Agrawal et al. 2012).

The impact of social factors, such as childhood abuse and neglect, on the development of an OUD has been well established (Dube et al. 2003). Although initiating and sustaining a discussion concerning childhood abuse, neglect, and household dysfunction may be difficult for the clinician and patient, it can foster empathy and reveal underlying psychological conflicts. Mr. Sandoval's reported social history of emotional and physical childhood abuse is an indication to investigate further for underlying posttraumatic stress disorder (PTSD), generalized anxiety, depression, or somatic disorders.

Although this portion of the psychosocial assessment provides an important window into the effects of early experiences, it is crucial to remain conscientious of boundaries and to ensure confidentiality during the discussion of such sensitive topics. During the first interview with the patient, the subject of neglect, abuse, and violence in childhood may initially evoke a guarded response toward the interviewer. To support the patient and continue to develop a therapeutic relationship, the clinician needs to remind the patient that he or she does not need to share beyond his or her level of comfort. Additionally, utilizing nonthreatening language to approach delicate subjects is a useful way to transition into the discussion. For example, employing the term *mistreatment* when screening for childhood abuse and neglect can cast a wider net and encourage the patient to initially share the amount of detail that he or she desires. However, depending on the patient's initial response and comfort with sharing, the clinician may decide to ask a more detailed set of questions to reveal the extent of the childhood adversity (Read et al. 2007). It is crucial to empower the patient with reminders of autonomy throughout sensitive portions of the initial assessment.

Precipitating Factors

Mr. Sandoval had multiple sources of pain that eventually led to his opioid exposure. It is critical to assess and discuss historical or ongoing challenges with pain during the biopsychosocial assessment. Pain is the leading motivating factor for past-year illicit prescription opioid use among U.S. adults (Lipari et al. 2017), and its effects on psychosocial functioning can be tremendous. Chronic noncancer pain may increase the risk of psychiatric, social, and health problems in patients with OUD, potentially impacting the course of treatment (Dennis et al. 2015). For these reasons, the biopsychosocial formulation should incorporate the impact of pain on the individual's interpersonal relationships, occupational functioning, and self-image.

Perpetuating Factors

The most common reason for continued use of opioids is opioid withdrawal. Although the physical symptoms of opioid withdrawal are an important motivating factor for continued use, the psychosocial impact of opioid withdrawal is equally important. Exploring the patient's experiences with opioid withdrawal in the context of his or her interactions with relatives, friends, or strangers can reveal underlying emotions relevant to the treatment. In the case of Mr. Sandoval, the increased severity of pain during withdrawal led him to seek opioid prescriptions from multiple physicians, which led to feelings of shame. Similarly, fear of the symptoms and decline in functioning associated with withdrawal is a common cause of continued opioid use.

Lack of access to adequate and appropriate OUD treatment, whether due to geography, insurance, transportation, or finances, is another common perpetuating factor. It is also important to consider barriers to recovery pertaining to transportation, occupation, ongoing legal cases, exposure to substance use at home, finances, chronic illness, and lack of coordinated health care. Once clinicians identify these barriers, they should address them through treatment; this may require connecting the patient to outside resources.

Protective Factors

The previously mentioned components of the biopsychosocial formulation focus primarily on difficult experiences and current hardships in an individual's life. Closing the assessment with a discussion of protective factors, including motivations for seeking treatment, can be an effective way to transition the conversation toward recovery and hope.

In the vignette, Mr. Sandoval was able to name a few protective factors: no misuse of other substances, being married, involvement in cultural traditions, and willingness to engage in treatment. These components form a foundation on which to build positive change. Commending the patient's first step of seeking treatment is a helpful starting point. Continuing the conversation by discussing positive relationships with family, friends, and/or coworkers can uncover a network of support that may bolster engagement in recovery. Additional areas that may strengthen motivation may be children, exercise and fitness, desire to improve physical health, religion and spirituality, and a meaningful job. Predisposing, precipitating, perpetuating, and protective factors related to Mr. Sandoval are shown in Table 8–4.

Example of a Biopsychosocial Formulation

Ted Sandoval is a 48-year-old American Indian man with a 15-year history of prescription opioid dependence. The patient has a long history of inadequately treated chronic pain in his right knee, resulting in decreased mobility and inability to work. He has developed increasing tolerance to opioid analgesics. Mr. Sandoval's family history is significant for a paternal history of heavy alcohol use. Additionally, the patient reports having experienced childhood abuse and neglect, both physical and emotional, by his stepfather. The patient's substance use, chronic pain, and decline in physical functioning have resulted in financial distress and reduced participation in cultural traditions. Because of a lack of access to treatment options for pain and OUD, Mr. Sandoval has had difficulty seeking treatment for his growing addiction to prescription opioids. At the same time, Mr. Sandoval is hopeful and highly motivated to engage in treatment.

Treatment Planning

The treatment planning process begins during the initial assessment, when the patient voices his or her preferences, goals, and hopes, all of which are key to developing an individualized treatment plan.

TABLE 8–4. Biopsychosocial formulation for Mr. Sandoval

	Biological	Psychological	Social
Predisposing factors	Family history of addiction	Depression Possible posttraumatic stress disorder	History of trauma History of neglect
Precipitating factors	Chronic pain	Tolerance to opioids	Poor access to health care Opioid availability
Perpetuating factors	Chronic pain Opioid withdrawal	Depression Depression Fear of pain Fear of withdrawal	Opioid availability Poor access to opioid use disorder treatment Lack of coordinated care Inability to work
Protective factors	Absence of other substance use disorders	Hope Motivation to seek treatment Willingness to engage in treatment	Being married Having children Community participation Involvement in traditions/spiritual practices

Levels of Care

After the initial assessment, the clinician must determine whether the patient meets DSM-5 criteria for intoxication. If he or she is intoxicated, the clinician must decide what immediate treatment is indicated (hospitalization vs. close outpatient monitoring). Certain medical conditions can present with altered mental status that may mimic intoxication and could be potentially life threatening. Clinicians must triage for hospitalization for any of the following: hypoxemia (blood oxygen saturation [SpO_2] < 90%), respiratory depression (< 12 breaths per minute), hypotension (systolic blood pressure < 90 mm Hg), tachycardia (pulse > 120 beats per minute), head injury, symptomatic hypoglycemia, or an uncertain cause of altered mental status. If the patient is ready to leave the clinic, the clinician must determine and document that the patient's state of intoxication does not pose a risk to self or to others. Intervention options for intoxication include observation until the risk is no longer present, transfer to a higher level of care, or having a friend or family member transport the patient home (Donroe and Tetrault 2017).

The treatment planning process can also utilize the American Society of Addiction Medicine (ASAM; Herron and Brennan 2015) criteria for treatment, which are meant to optimize resource utilization and patient outcomes by appropriately matching patients to levels of care. The ASAM criteria are readily available, are easy to explain to patients, and incorporate each individual's treatment needs. A patient's treatment needs are evaluated along six dimensions: current and past potential for intoxication/withdrawal, health history/medical conditions, mental health, readiness to change, relapse/continued use, and social supports/recovery. Five levels of care are recognized: early intervention, outpatient treatment, intensive outpatient treatment, residential or inpatient treatment, and medically managed intensive inpatient treatment.

With regard to Mr. Sandoval, Dr. Sam should use the ASAM criteria to determine the appropriate level of care, taking into account the patient's preferences. Involving Mr. Sandoval in this discussion will empower him, while helping him fully understand the treatment recommendations and steps in recovery. In this particular case, Mr. Sandoval met ASAM Level 1 outpatient criteria and had a preference for outpatient treatment.

Inpatient Versus Outpatient

When a patient has attempted outpatient treatment and has experienced repeated relapses, transitioning to an intensive outpatient model or an inpatient rehabilitation model may be indicated. Although some patients may benefit from extended periods of residential care (i.e., more than 28 days), recent randomized trials have not found benefits of longer stays (Herron and Brennan 2015). In general, it is unlikely that one's first attempt at recovery would take place at an inpatient rehabilitation facility; however, certain co-occurring psychiatric, medical, or social issues could make it necessary. In such a case, the patient's recovery would then require a step-down to outpatient care once the patient was clinically stable.

Detoxification Versus Maintenance

MAT with buprenorphine or methadone is the gold standard for OUD and has the most evidence for efficacy among all available treatments. Therefore, MAT is a strongly recommended treatment modality. It is also recommended that maintenance MAT be continued for as long as the patient is benefiting from the treatment. Clinicians should explicitly discuss the goals of treatment with patients. These may include reduction in opioid use, being better equipped for employment or furthering one's education, improving relationships, and enhancing mental and physical health. Clinicians should reinforce hope for recovery during these discussions.

When a patient is unable or unwilling to try opioid agonist–based MAT, such as a patient who is living in a homeless shelter that does not permit opioid replacement therapy, a few alternatives to this line of treatment are available. There is growing evidence that ongoing treatment with XR-naltrexone is an effective form of MAT for OUD (Lee et al. 2018; Tanum et al. 2017). With regard to detoxification, rates of relapse following detoxification alone are very high (Ball and Corty 1988; Ling et al. 2009). Therefore, detoxification alone is unlikely to lead to positive long-term outcomes, and rates of unintentional overdose are subsequently elevated due to a loss of tolerance. Patients need to be educated about these risks. Similarly, psychosocial treatments without medications are not as effective as MAT for OUD and should only be considered after a thorough discussion.

If a patient declines MAT following this conversation, further discussion of the patient's goals should follow in an empathetic and nonjudgmental manner, and patient autonomy should be respected. The clinician should continue to be the patient's advocate, collaborator, and educator. Some interventions at this point may include the following:

- Education regarding the risk of overdose and prescribing naloxone with instructions on how to use it
- Education regarding the transmission of human immunodeficiency virus (HIV) and hepatitis C virus (HCV) and reviewing locations of needle exchange programs, if available
- Testing for infectious diseases and referring for treatment when needed
- Inviting the patient to return for further discussion, keeping the door open to other treatment options.

If the patient opts to begin MAT, deciding among the options should be a collaborative process. A number of factors may influence this decision. In addition to patient preference, practical considerations such as treatment availability, distance from an opioid treatment program, and insurance coverage may be pertinent. Good candidates for antagonist treatment with XR-naltrexone may include patients with a high degree of motivation for abstinence, people engaged in professions in which agonist treatment would be controversial (e.g., pilots, physicians), and patients who are tapering off agonist treatment but want the comfort of a "safety net."

Regardless of the medication that the patient and clinician choose, clinicians should introduce and recommend psychosocial interventions. Clinicians must therefore learn about local resources and understand that psychosocial treatments, when used in conjunction with MAT, can be effective in reducing opioid use and improving outcomes. Patients with underlying psychiatric illnesses in particular may benefit greatly from adjunctive psychotherapy. For example, for a patient with OUD and PTSD, engagement in evidence-based treatment for PTSD would be an essential element of the overall treatment plan. Finally, clinicians should consider discussing mutual-help group engagement when clinically appropriate.

Navigating Treatment Services

National data underscore the need for increased treatment access and retention for OUD. Once an individual has been linked to treatment, it is crucial to retain that person in treatment to reduce disability, morbidity, and mortality. The individual, his or her family, and the community at large benefit from access to care and continued engagement in treatment.

According to systematic reviews of multiple studies, MAT with methadone or buprenorphine is most likely to decrease problematic opioid use and keep people engaged in treatment. However, initiating these treatments can be difficult. Mattick et al. (2009, 2014) showed that at least half of the patients who intended to begin treatment with buprenorphine never started treatment. The authors concluded that reducing barriers to medication, such as starting buprenorphine immediately after a visit to the hospital or emergency department, may increase the likelihood that patients will actually start the medication. Oftentimes, patients with OUD present to an emergency department or medical inpatient setting following an overdose event. Results from recent studies support the practice of initiating buprenorphine in these settings and immediately connecting patients with ongoing outpatient treatment. Delaying the initiation of MAT until the patient attends an outpatient appointment can increase risk of relapse, especially in areas with limited resources and long wait times for clinics specializing in addiction (D'Onofrio et al. 2015; Liebschutz et al. 2014).

Another factor that can determine an individual's likelihood of entering and remaining in treatment is his or her ability to pay for services. National Survey on Drug Use and Health data from 2008 to 2014 show that since implementation of the Patient Protection and Affordable Care Act of 2010 (P.L. 111-148), the number of people receiving treatment for SUDs in general has increased substantially (McKenna 2017). However, the majority of people with OUD continue to go without treatment.

A variety of opioid treatment models emerging throughout the United States have the goal of increasing access to care. One success story in navigating treatment services is the Vermont hub-and-spoke model of care for OUD (Brooklyn and Sigmon 2017). This model integrates centers of addiction expertise ("hubs") with a network of providers in regional catchment areas ("spokes"). Each opioid treatment program is designated as the hub where staff can assess patients' needs and determine the most appropriate placement for treatment: methadone or buprenorphine at the hub or office-based buprenorphine treatment at a spoke, an outpatient site in that region. Points of entry to the hub include self-referrals, hospitals and emergency departments, the department of corrections, and community health programs. Inductions occur at the hubs, and patients can either be promptly transferred to the spokes or remain for further treatment at the hubs. This model of care ensures the most appropriate initial match for patient needs and allows for transfer of care to and from the hubs and spokes according to patients' needs and preferences in the course of recovery. Addiction specialists at the hubs also serve as consultants for providers and staff at the spokes. As a result of this integrated system of care, Vermont has significantly increased its capacity to provide treatment for OUD.

Another example of a successful approach is the Massachusetts Collaborative Care Model, in which nurse care managers work in collaboration with physicians at federally qualified health centers to perform intake and ongoing management of patients with OUD. A pilot study of this program showed increased retention in treatment, more than 90% negative urine toxicology screens at 1 year of treatment, and a significant increase in the number of physicians obtaining waivers to prescribe buprenorphine (Korthuis et al. 2017).

Other treatment models have explored offering OUD treatment in conjunction with primary care and psychiatric services to optimize access to needed services, while leveraging resources and ensuring continuity of care. In an integrated model, primary care clinics—in addition to caring for acute and chronic medical conditions—can serve as the point of access for addiction and psychiatric services. Likewise, addiction treatment clinics can offer full-spectrum care to their patients by including on-site primary care and psychiatric care. Regardless of the site of care, collaboration of treatment services is likely to enhance patient retention in treatment and therefore improve outcomes.

One example of this approach is the Buprenorphine HIV Evaluation and Support collaborative model, funded by the Health Resources and Services Administration, in which primary care providers at nine HIV treatment sites provided office-based buprenorphine to more than 300 patients. An evaluation of this collaborative showed that opioid use in the past 30 days decreased from 84% to 42%, and treatment retention at 1 year was 49% (Korthuis et al. 2017). Another example of such integration of care is the "one-stop shop" approach, which was developed in response to an outbreak of HIV in a rural community in Indiana. In this model, patients can access treatment for OUD, HIV infection, HCV infection, other health conditions, and psychiatric disorders all at the same site (Korthuis et al. 2017). Where it is not possible to include all services at one site, models such as the University of New Mexico's Project ECHO (Extension for Community Healthcare Outcomes; Komaromy et al. 2016) connect patients to specialty care within their home clinics. Through a combination of education and multidisciplinary case consultations using teletechnology, ECHO helps local providers feel comfortable prescribing buprenorphine to their patients.

Living With Addiction

Many people, including professionals, hold preconceived ideas about patients with OUD. Some may imagine a person of a particular race or certain economic status or an individual often stereotypically portrayed in movies as a "junkie." However, when clinicians increase their ability to detect opioid misuse and addiction, they will encounter a broad spectrum of people who do not fit into stereotypes. Because addiction is a common disorder, and addictive substances are virtually ubiquitous in society, people from all sociodemographic backgrounds are vulnerable to addiction.

DSM-5 provides a system with which to diagnose OUD, and it bases severity of the disorder on how many criteria are met at a given time. However, the diagnostic criteria do not provide the full clinical picture. For this, it is essential to appreciate a patient's subjective experience. This is not to say that a clinician must know firsthand what it is like to experience opioid intoxication, withdrawal, or living with addiction. Being in recovery oneself does not necessarily make a clinician better, but the ability to empathize and form a therapeutic alliance is a widely accepted component of effective patient care and retention in treatment (Meier et al. 2006).

Although the number of DSM-5 criteria that a given patient meets will place his or her illness along a spectrum of severity, each criterion also has its own depth and intensity in terms of functional impairment, effects on quality of life, and impact on a patient's social network. Factors such as a person's background, values, strengths, desires, resources, and goals influence a patient's personal experience with a given criterion.

It is useful to take each criterion for OUD, apply it to the individual patient, and try to appreciate how it affects that particular individual's life.

One of the diagnostic criteria for OUD is a persistent desire or unsuccessful effort to cut down or control opioid use. This may manifest in many ways. One patient may be dedicated to engaging in treatment and reducing opioid use, but she may find this difficult to achieve because her spouse with OUD continues to use substances and encourages or coerces the patient to continue to use. In this case, the addiction is woven into the fabric of the relationship, and the patient's efforts at cessation are undermined in part because the partner remains in the precontemplation stage of change. Another patient, who desires to control his use because of external ramifications, may compulsively inject "a bebe"—a small amount of heroin—despite knowing that a positive urine toxicology sample may result in incarceration. This smaller relapse may lead to feelings of guilt, shame, and anger, resulting in a full-blown relapse despite his desire to control opioid use. It is not difficult to imagine how painful it is and how helpless a patient with a persistent desire to quit might feel when he or she continues to engage in behaviors that lead to impairment and adverse consequences.

As many providers may know, most actual experiences of addiction to opioids are filled with themes of tragedy for the patients, their loved ones, and their communities. It is important and humbling to remember that all people who are exposed to substances of abuse, including opioids, are vulnerable to addiction. This knowledge may help clinicians approach each patient struggling with addiction with empathy and without judgment. For clinicians to do this successfully, it is important that they reflect on their own biases, or they risk contributing to the stigma and alienation that many patients already feel.

Addiction and Stigma

Among several identified barriers to treatment, such as lack of providers and resources, stigma remains a pervasive barrier to accessing care and pursuing recovery. According to recent work, stigma can be categorized into three main types (Corrigan et al. 2017): public stigma, label avoidance, and self-stigma. Together, these forms of stigma interfere with patient care.

Public stigma comprises prejudices and stereotypes held toward individuals with SUD by the general population and the health care community. Some commonly held beliefs about individuals with SUDs include perceptions that they are dangerous, possess moral weakness or character flaws, are not trustworthy, or are criminals. These stigmatizing attitudes can lead to discrimination through laws and policies directed at people with addiction, and also affect opinions about public policy. For example, Olsen et al. (2003), summarizing six studies from the United States, Australia, and Britain, reported that respondents felt that people with SUDs should receive less priority in health care. As one might imagine, these attitudes and their eventual effects on policies can make day-to-day life for someone with an SUD incredibly difficult. They can also make true recovery an incredibly hard-to-reach goal.

The health care community is not immune from stigmatizing patients with SUD. For example, a review of 28 studies (van Boekel et al. 2013) reported that health care professionals perceived violence, manipulation, and poor motivation as factors impeding health care delivery to patients with SUDs. Additionally, these attitudes by professionals adversely affected patients' sense of empowerment and, critically, led to worse outcomes. The authors also reported that health care professionals had inadequate education, training, and support to treat individuals with addictions. Strikingly, a recent study demonstrated that psychiatry residents' attitudes toward patients with SUDs might worsen through the course of their training (Avery et al. 2017).

Some interfaces with the health care system can be particularly stigmatizing to a patient trying to access care. As subtle as it seems, even a provider referring to a urine toxicology test as "dirty" instead of as "positive for specific substances" may have profound adverse effects on a vulnerable patient seeking medical assistance (Olsen and Sharfstein 2014). When a patient expends great effort to conceal his or her substance misuse, it is a misconception to classify the behavior solely as intentionally deceptive. The pressure of public stigma may be great enough that the patient will be fearful of seeking health care services or revealing that he or she has an SUD. This is when label avoidance comes into play.

The net effect of public stigma pushes people with SUDs to the outskirts of society, into subcultures or groups where substance use is acceptable, or forces them to conceal their disorder for as long as possible, delaying treatment. Indeed, as Kulesza et al. (2014) report, stigma related to substance use has been associated with poorer mental health, worse physical health, decreased employment, poor housing, a breakdown of social support systems, reduced treatment seeking, and worse substance use outcomes.

When an individual with an SUD internalizes public stigma, this leads to the phenomenon of self-stigma. An individual with self-stigma accepts the public stigma, manifesting lower self-efficacy and self-esteem, often going on to fulfill the self-destructive tendencies itemized in the OUD criteria (Corrigan et al. 2017). A person may suffer further impairment by demonstrating the "why try" effect, which manifests as learned helplessness and lowers the likelihood that an individual will receive treatment in any form. For patients with this state of mind, the temporary relief provided by opioid intoxication will only perpetuate and intensify their lack of control, driving them deeper into addiction.

The burden of stigma remains elevated despite recent national coverage of the opioid epidemic and efforts to neutralize addiction discrimination. Reduction of stigma may lead to improved social networks and self-efficacy for patients, thereby positively influencing long-term trajectories and enhancing recovery. Health care providers, community advocates, family members, and individuals must therefore be prepared to meet patients wherever they are in the cycle of recovery and to instill hope and optimism that recovery from opioid addiction is real and tangible.

Recovery Among Individuals With Opioid Use Disorder

It is important to keep in mind that recovery from SUDs, including OUD, is possible. A systematic review and meta-analysis (Fleury et al. 2016) examined 21 studies published between 2000 and 2015 with a follow-up period of at least 3 years. The authors reported that for all SUDs, 35%–54.4% of individuals achieved remission, defined as no longer meeting diagnostic criteria for abuse or dependence for a minimum of 6 months. Among the four studies looking specifically at OUD, 27.5%–54% of individuals eventually achieved remission.

Robust research supports the idea that addictions are chronic diseases with courses often marked by multiple cycles of relapse and remission. Indeed, McLellan et al. (2000) showed that heritability, treatment adherence, and relapse rates for SUDs are similar to those of chronic medical illnesses such as asthma, hypertension, and type 2 diabetes.

A number of studies examining the longitudinal course of OUD support the chronic disease model of opioid addiction by demonstrating that remission is generally achieved after multiple attempts over a number of years that are punctuated by multiple episodes of relapse and remission (Fleury et al. 2016; Nosyk et al. 2013). Darke et al. (2007), analyzing data from the Australian Treatment Outcome Study, reported that although the percentage of patients who had achieved continuous abstinence from heroin since baseline went down from 14% at 12 months to 8% at 36 months, rates of past-12-month abstinence rose steadily from 14% at 12 months to 40% at 36 months. Additionally, by the 36-month follow-up, 61% of the patients had achieved at least 12 months of cumulative abstinence, indicating that although patients cycle in and out of treatment, an increasing proportion of patients are able over time to achieve a significant period of sobriety. In that study, cumulative exposure to treatment, including MAT and excluding detoxification alone, was associated with improved outcomes. A rich body of literature now supports the notion that continued treatment and longer cumulative treatment are associated with more favorable outcomes (Darke et al. 2007; Eastwood et al. 2017; Fleury et al. 2016; Flynn et al. 2003; Nosyk et al. 2013; Skinner et al. 2011). In fact, Simpson (2004) reported that the positive relationship between treatment retention and outcomes has been replicated in every major national evaluation study.

Increasingly, the paradigm has shifted to a focus not only on the duration of remission but on the concept of recovery. This framework places cessation of use within a larger context of physical, emotional, relational, and spiritual health. The concept of "wellbriety," used among American Indian and Alaska Native communities in recovery, similarly defines recovery as sobriety plus improved global health or quality of life. Indeed, research has demonstrated that recovery is associated with improved quality of life (Nosyk et al. 2013). Remission is therefore not the end itself, but a means to an end, which has been described as a "reclaiming of the self" that was lost to addiction (White 2008).

SAMHSA defines *recovery* as a process of change through which individuals improve their health and wellness, live self-directed lives, and strive to reach their full potential. The four dimensions of recovery are health, home, purpose, and community.

- *Health:* overcoming or managing symptoms, including those arising from SUDs; making healthy, informed choices that support sobriety and well-being

Ample research supports the idea that reducing substance use is associated with improved mental health, physical health, and coping abilities. In community-based samples, less substance use is associated with lower rates of chronic health and psychiatric problems (Mokdad et al. 2004). Additionally, remission also appears to reduce mortality (Scott et al. 2011). Methadone and buprenorphine maintenance treatments have been similarly associated with substantial reductions in all-cause and overdose mortality in people dependent on opioids (Sordo et al. 2017).

- *Home:* having a stable and safe place to live

    Housing is a key predictor of achieving and sustaining remission (Scott et al. 2005). Residents in a sober housing program linked with an outpatient treatment program demonstrated decreases in substance use and arrests, along with an increase in employment (Polcin 2009). Stable housing can be achieved through a variety of models, including peer-run, self-supported, sober housing, and community-based housing linked to a variety of treatment and case management services (Substance Abuse and Mental Health Services Administration 2011).

- *Purpose:* participating in meaningful daily activities, such as a job, volunteering, school, and family caregiving; having the independence, income, and resources to participate in society

    Employment helps individuals reintegrate into society and also enhances their sense of self-worth. It allows an individual to improve his or her living situation, reduce psychosocial stressors, and earn the income needed to pursue life goals, and it instills motivation and hope for the future. Unemployed individuals are more likely to have SUDs compared with their employed counterparts (Substance Abuse and Mental Health Services Administration 2011).

    Employment has consistently been shown to positively affect recovery in people with SUDs. Studies have demonstrated that employment status predicts long-, medium-, and short-term remission from opioid use (Eastwood et al. 2017; Flynn et al. 2003; Nosyk et al. 2013; Skinner et al. 2011). Research has shown that therapeutic workplaces, which provide abstinence-contingent access to long-term paid employment, improve abstinence rates, along with adherence to MAT (Aklin et al. 2014; Holtyn et al. 2014). Likewise, studies show that remission from SUDs positively impacts employment status. Dennis et al. (2007) demonstrated that increased duration of abstinence was significantly associated with increased days working, greater income from employment, and fewer days of financial problems.

Similarly, education is an important aspect of recovery. Higher educational attainment is associated with lower rates of SUDs (Substance Abuse and Mental Health Services Administration 2011). Skinner et al. (2011) demonstrated that educational attainment was related to improved remission from OUD. Indeed, SAMHSA recommends supported education as an important tool for recovery from SUDs.

Finally, not engaging in criminal activities is an integral part of living a purposeful life. There is robust evidence showing that achieving remission from SUDs leads to rapid decreases in illegal activity (Dennis et al. 2007). Summarizing this dimension of recovery, Flynn et al. (2003) showed that people in recovery were significantly more likely than those not in recovery to participate in school, work, and family activities, as well as meaningful hobbies.

- *Community:* having relationships and social networks that provide support, friendship, love, and hope

Individuals do not recover in isolation; instead, they need to become meaningfully integrated within the community at large. Dennis et al. (2007) demonstrated that duration of abstinence was associated with an increased number of clean and sober friends, along with social and spiritual support. Flynn et al. (2003) reported that individuals in long-term recovery from opioids were 3 times more likely than those not in recovery to perceive personal growth in socializing and relating to others, recognizing and expressing feelings, and conducting themselves with maturity. They were also 3 times more likely to report that their social networks did not include people with SUDs. Importantly, those in recovery could "almost always talk to their family or friends about their problems, rely on them for encouragement to stop using drugs, receive help from them for problems, and count on family/friends for help in emergencies" (p. 183).

In addition to these four dimensions of recovery, higher levels of self-efficacy are associated with greater success in recovery (Worley 2017). Importantly, social support appears to promote enhanced self-efficacy (Stevens et al. 2015). Flynn et al. (2003) reported that individuals in recovery were significantly more likely to perceive themselves as showing personal growth—leading constructive and fulfilling lives, being able to handle responsibilities, taking care of their health, and becoming "productive members of society"—all markers of enhanced personal resolve and self-efficacy.

Finally, the literature documents the role of spirituality in recovery, which generally appears to be positive (Kaskutas et al. 2014; Schoenthaler et al. 2015; Walton-Moss et al. 2013). Therefore, holistic and recovery-oriented evaluation and management of a person with an SUD should include a spiritual assessment and, if appropriate, a discussion about strengthening spirituality during the recovery process. It is important to point out that spirituality is a personal attribute and does not need to be associated with a particular faith (Worley 2017).

Role of Medication-Assisted Treatment in Recovery

Medications for OUD are proven to be effective at reducing opioid use; additionally, they have been linked to reductions in many risk factors and poor health outcomes, including cocaine use, crime, high-risk behaviors, and HIV and HCV infection, as well as fewer deaths from overdose (Flynn et al. 2003). Importantly, rates of relapse following detoxification from methadone and buprenorphine remain unacceptably high. Indeed, MAT is an essential component of recovery from OUD. At the same time, stigma continues to surround the use of these medications. White (2007) suggests that denying medically and socially stabilized methadone patients the status of recovery can be tremendously stigmatizing. Fortunately, the legitimacy of recovery with the use of medications is being increasingly recognized by professional organizations and recovery advocates.

Recovery Is a Spectrum

As discussed earlier in this section, OUD is a chronic illness, often characterized by multiple recovery attempts over many years with increasing durations of remission. Recovery is a spectrum, and certain individuals may be able to improve their overall well-being without completely abstaining from substances. As a result, White (2007) suggests that the term "partial recovery" may be applied to these individuals; by contrast, an "enriched or transcendent state of recovery"—a state of "amplified health, performance, and social contribution superior to one's pre-addiction life"

(p. 234)—is also possible. In this case, individuals derive strength and meaning from their recovery journey in order to reach a heightened state of functioning.

Ten Guiding Principles of Recovery

SAMHSA has put forth the following guiding principles of recovery (Substance Abuse and Mental Health Services Administration 2012, pp. 4–7):

1. Hope is the "catalyst of the recovery process."
2. Individuals have unique goals and follow unique paths to recovery. "Self-determination" and "self-direction" are critical in the recovery process.
3. Recovery occurs via numerous highly personal pathways. They may include medications, social support, or faith-based approaches.
4. Recovery is holistic. It permeates every aspect of an individual's life.
5. Recovery is supported by peers and allies.
6. Recovery is supported through relationships and social networks.
7. Recovery is culturally based and influenced. Recovery pathways therefore need to be culturally informed.
8. Recovery is supported by addressing trauma. Services should be trauma informed in order to foster safety, trust, personal choice, empowerment, and collaboration.
9. Recovery involves individual, family, and community strengths and responsibilities. Although individuals have a responsibility for their own self-care and recovery process, families can provide essential support, and communities can help create systems that address discrimination and promote inclusion.
10. Recovery is based on respect. It is essential to protect the rights of people in recovery. It is also essential to acknowledge that recovery requires courage, self-acceptance, the creation of a positive and meaningful sense of identity, and the regaining of self-belief.

Clinical Implications for Physicians

As physicians move from managing addictions within an acute stabilization model to a model of sustained recovery, the role of the physician becomes broader. It is no longer limited to providing acute treatment; instead, the physician must also be involved in carrying out brief interventions, providing ongoing care with evidence-based pharmacological and nonpharmacological interventions, and coordinating care across systems. The physician must additionally be involved in continued follow-up and relapse prevention for patients in recovery (El-Guebaly 2012). The recovery model stresses that the optimal treatment includes integration of OUD treatment with psychiatric care, primary care, and treatment of related conditions such as chronic pain and infectious diseases. Moreover, recovery involves helping patients to enlist a supportive network of family members, friends, and mutual-help groups. It also involves successful integration of peer support and case management services, including initiatives such as supported employment and education, as well as supportive housing to facilitate reintegration into society. Indeed, under the recovery model, treatment is an essential gateway that begins a process of long-term engagement and ultimately leads to long-term benefits that affect every aspect of an individual's life.

Key Chapter Points

▶ All patients with chronic pain who are candidates for treatment with opioid pain medications should be evaluated for the potential of medication misuse and development of OUD. This is best carried out through a combination of validated screening tools, knowledge of individual risk factors for opioid misuse, and ongoing monitoring for aberrant behaviors.

▶ A comprehensive clinical assessment, leading to a biopsychosocial formulation, remains the gold standard for diagnosing OUD. This assessment should be carried out in a collaborative, empathetic, and nonjudgmental manner, and patient autonomy should be supported whenever possible.

▶ Medication-assisted treatment is a gold standard for the treatment of OUD. Therefore, medication-assisted treatment should be the recommended course of treatment for as long as the patient is benefiting from it. Regardless of the medication chosen, psychosocial interventions should be explored.

▶ Integrating treatment for substance use disorders with primary care, psychiatric care, case management, and specialty medical care, as well as proactively collaborating across different levels of care, improves outcomes.

▶ It is essential to appreciate the highly personal and profound individual experiences of living with an addiction. This attitude can help nurture the therapeutic relationship and impact treatment outcomes. Stigma remains a modifiable risk factor that directly affects care and patient experiences when they engage in treatment.

▶ Recovery is a process of change through which individuals improve their health and wellness, live self-directed lives, and strive to reach their full potential. Hope is the cornerstone of recovery. Clinicians should always strive to be advocates for their patients' recovery process.

References

Agrawal A, Verweij KJ, Gillespie NA, et al: The genetics of addiction—a translational perspective. Transl Psychiatry 2:e140, 2012 22806211

Aklin WM, Wong CJ, Hampton J, et al: A therapeutic workplace for the long-term treatment of drug addiction and unemployment: eight-year outcomes of a social business intervention. J Subst Abuse Treat 47(5):329–338, 2014 25124257

American Psychiatric Association: Diagnostic and Statistical Manual of Mental Disorders, 5th Edition. Arlington, VA, American Psychiatric Association, 2013

Avery J, Han BH, Zerbo E, et al: Changes in psychiatry residents' attitudes towards individuals with substance use disorders over the course of residency training. Am J Addict 26(1):75–79, 2017 27749984

Bailey RW, Vowles KE: Using screening tests to predict aberrant use of opioids in chronic pain patients: caveat emptor. J Pain 18(12):1427–1436, 2017 28669863

Ball JC, Corty E: Basic issues pertaining to the effectiveness of methadone maintenance treatment. NIDA Res Monogr 86:178–191, 1988 3140030

Boscarino JA, Rukstalis M, Hoffman SN, et al: Risk factors for drug dependence among out-patients on opioid therapy in a large U.S. health-care system. Addiction 105(10):1776–1782, 2010 20712819

Brooklyn JR, Sigmon SC: Vermont hub-and-spoke model of care for opioid use disorder: development, implementation, and impact. J Addict Med 11(4):286–292, 2017 28379862

Butler SF, Fernandez K, Benoit C, et al: Validation of the revised Screener and Opioid Assessment for Patients with Pain (SOAPP-R). J Pain 9(4):360–372, 2008 18203666

Butler SF, Budman SH, Fanciullo GT, Jamison RN, et al: Cross validation of the current opioid misuse measure to monitor chronic pain patients on opioid therapy. Clin J Pain 26(9):770–776, 2010 20842012

Corrigan P, Schomerus G, Shuman V, et al: Developing a research agenda for understanding the stigma of addictions, part I: lessons from the mental health stigma literature. Am J Addict 26(1):59–66, 2017 27779803

Darke S, Ross J: Suicide among heroin users: rates, risk factors and methods. Addiction 97(11):1383–1394, 2002 12410779

Darke S, Ross J, Mills KL, et al: Patterns of sustained heroin abstinence amongst long-term, dependent heroin users: 36 months findings from the Australian Treatment Outcome Study (ATOS). Addict Behav 32(9):1897–1906, 2007 17289282

Dennis BB, Bawor M, Naji L, et al: Impact of chronic pain on treatment prognosis for patients with opioid use disorder: a systematic review and meta-analysis. Subst Abuse 9:59–80, 2015 26417202

Dennis ML, Foss MA, Scott CK: An eight-year perspective on the relationship between the duration of abstinence and other aspects of recovery. Eval Rev 31(6):585–612, 2007 17986709

D'Onofrio G, O'Connor PG, Pantalon MV, et al: Emergency department-initiated buprenorphine/naloxone treatment for opioid dependence: a randomized clinical trial. JAMA 313(16):1636–1644, 2015 25919527

Donroe JH, Tetrault JM: Recognizing and caring for the intoxicated patient in an outpatient clinic. Med Clin North Am 101(3):573–586, 2017 28372714

Dowell D, Haegerich TM, Chou R: CDC guideline for prescribing opioids for chronic pain—United States, 2016. MMWR Recomm Rep 65(1):1–49, 2016 26987082

Dube SR, Felitti VJ, Dong M, et al: Childhood abuse, neglect, and household dysfunction and the risk of illicit drug use: the adverse childhood experiences study. Pediatrics 111(3):564–572, 2003 12612237

Eastwood B, Strang J, Marsden J: Effectiveness of treatment for opioid use disorder: a national, five-year, prospective, observational study in England. Drug Alcohol Depend 176:139–147, 2017 28535456

El-Guebaly N: The meanings of recovery from addiction: evolution and promises. J Addict Med 6(1):1–9, 2012 22124289

Fleury MJ, Djouini A, Huynh C, et al: Remission from substance use disorders: a systematic review and meta-analysis. Drug Alcohol Depend 168:293–306, 2016 27614380

Flynn PM, Joe GW, Broome KM, et al: Recovery from opioid addiction in DATOS. J Subst Abuse Treat 25(3):177–186, 2003 14670523

Herron AJ, Brennan TK (eds): The ASAM Essentials of Addiction Medicine, 2nd Edition. Philadelphia, PA, Lippincott Williams & Wilkins, 2015

Holtyn AF, Koffarnus MN, DeFulio A, et al: Employment-based abstinence reinforcement promotes opiate and cocaine abstinence in out-of-treatment injection drug users. J Appl Behav Anal 47(4):681–693, 2014 25292399

Kaskutas LA, Borkman TJ, Laudet A, et al: Elements that define recovery: the experiential perspective. J Stud Alcohol Drugs 75(6):999–1010, 2014 25343658

Katzman JG, Takeda MY, Bhatt SR, et al: An innovative model for naloxone use within an OTP setting: a prospective cohort study. J Addict Med 12(2):113–118, 2018 29227321

Komaromy M, Duhigg D, Metcalf A, et al: Project ECHO (Extension for Community Healthcare Outcomes): A new model for educating primary care providers about treatment of substance use disorders. Subst Abus 37(1):20–24, 2016 26848803

Korthuis PT, McCarty D, Weimer M, et al: Primary care-based models for the treatment of opioid use disorder: a scoping review. Ann Intern Med 166(4):268–278, 2017 27919103

Kulesza M, Ramsey S, Brown R, et al: Stigma among individuals with substance use disorders: does it predict substance use and does it diminish with treatment? J Addict Behav Ther Rehabil 3(1):1000115, 2014 25635257

Lee J, Nunes EV, Novo P, et al: Comparative effectiveness of extended release naltrexone versus buprenorphine-naloxone for opioid relapse prevention (X:BOT): a multicentre, open label, randomised controlled trial. Lancet 391(10118):309–318, 2018 29150198

Liebschutz JM, Crooks D, Herman D, et al: Buprenorphine treatment for hospitalized, opioid-dependent patients: a randomized clinical trial. JAMA Intern Med 174:1369–1376, 2014 25090173

Ling W, Hillhouse M, Domier C, et al: Buprenorphine tapering schedule and illicit opioid use. Addiction 104(2):256–265, 2009 19149822

Lipari RN, Williams M, Van Horn SL: Why do adults misuse prescription drugs? The CBHSQ report. Substance Abuse and Mental Health Services Administration, July 27, 2017. Available at: https://www.samhsa.gov/data/sites/default/files/report_3210/ShortReport-3210.html. Accessed April 3, 2018.

Mattick RP, Breen C, Kimber J, Davoli M, et al: Methadone maintenance therapy versus no opioid replacement therapy for opioid dependence. Cochrane Database Syst Rev 8(3):CD002209 2009 19588333

Mattick RP, Breen C, Kimber J, Davoli M, et al: Buprenorphine maintenance versus placebo or methadone maintenance for opioid dependence. Cochrane Database Syst Rev 6(2):CD002207 2014 24500948

McKenna RM: Treatment use, sources of payment, and financial barriers to treatment among individuals with opioid use disorder following the national implementation of the ACA. Drug Alcohol Depend 179:87–92, 2017 28763780

McLellan AT, Lewis DC, O'Brien CP, et al: Drug dependence, a chronic medical illness: implications for treatment, insurance, and outcomes evaluation. JAMA 284(13):1689–1695, 2000 11015800

Meier PS, Donmall MC, McElduff P, et al: The role of the early therapeutic alliance in predicting drug treatment dropout. Drug Alcohol Depend 83(1):57–64, 2006 16298088

Mokdad AH, Marks JS, Stroup DF, et al: Actual causes of death in the United States, 2000. JAMA 291(10):1238–1245, 2004 15010446

Nosyk B, Anglin MD, Brecht M-L, et al: Characterizing durations of heroin abstinence in the California Civil Addict Program: results from a 33-year observational cohort study. Am J Epidemiol 177(7):675–682, 2013 23445901

Olsen JA, Richardson J, Dolan P, et al: The moral relevance of personal characteristics in setting health care priorities. Soc Sci Med 57(7):1163–1172, 2003 12899901

Olsen Y, Sharfstein JM: Confronting the stigma of opioid use disorder—and its treatment. JAMA 311(14):1393–1394, 2014 24577059

Polcin DL: A model for sober housing during outpatient treatment. J Psychoactive Drugs 41(2):153–161, 2009 19705677

Read J, Hammersley P, Rudegeair T: Why, when, and how to ask about childhood abuse. Adv Psychiatr Treat 13:101–110, 2007

Schoenthaler SJ, Blum K, Braverman ER, et al: NIDA-Drug Addiction Treatment Outcome Study (DATOS) relapse as a function of spirituality/religiosity. J Reward Defic Syndr 1(1):36–45, 2015 26052556

Scott CK, Foss MA, Dennis ML: Pathways in the relapse-treatment-recovery cycle over 3 years. J Subst Abuse Treat 28 (suppl 1):S63–S72, 2005 15797640

Scott CK, Dennis ML, Laudet A, et al: Surviving drug addiction: the effect of treatment and abstinence on mortality. Am J Public Health 101(4):737–744, 2011 21330586

Simon CB, Tsui JI, Merrill JO, et al: Linking patients with buprenorphine treatment in primary care: predictors of engagement. Drug Alcohol Depend 181:58–62, 2017 29035705

Simpson DD: A conceptual framework for drug treatment process and outcomes. J Subst Abuse Treat 27(2):99–121, 2004 15450644

Skinner ML, Haggerty KP, Fleming CB, et al: Opiate-addicted parents in methadone treatment: long-term recovery, health, and family relationships. J Addict Dis 30(1):17–26, 2011 21218307

Sordo L, Barrio G, Bravo MJ, et al: Mortality risk during and after opioid substitution treatment: systematic review and meta-analysis of cohort studies. BMJ 357:j1550, 2017 28446428

Stevens E, Jason LA, Ram D, et al: Investigating social support and network relationships in substance use disorder recovery. Subst Abus 36(4):396–399, 2015 25259558

Substance Abuse and Mental Health Services Administration: Leading Change: A Plan for SAMHSA's Roles and Actions 2011–2014 (HHS Publ No SMA-11-4629). Rockville, MD, Substance Abuse and Mental Health Services Administration, 2011

Substance Abuse and Mental Health Services Administration: SAMHSA's Working Definition of Recovery (Pub ID: PEP12-RECDEF). Rockville, MD, Substance Abuse and Mental Health Services Administration, 2012

Substance Abuse and Mental Health Services Administration: Key substance use and mental health indicators in the United States: Results from the 2016 National Survey on Drug Use and Health. (HHS Publication No. SMA 17-5044, NSDUH Series H-52). Rockville, MD, Center for Behavioral Health Statistics and Quality, Substance Abuse and Mental Health Services Administration, 2017 Available at https://www.samhsa.gov/data/sites/default/files/NSDUH-FFR1-2016/NSDUH-FFR1-2016.htm. Accessed April 3, 2018.

Sullivan E, Fleming M: A Guide to Substance Abuse Services for Primary Care Clinicians (Treatment Improvement Protocol [TIP] Series, No 24, SMA-97-3139). Rockville, MD, Center for Substance Abuse Treatment, 1997

Tanum L, Solli KK, Latif ZE, et al: Effectiveness of injectable extended-release naltrexone vs daily buprenorphine-naloxone for opioid dependence: a randomized clinical noninferiority trial. JAMA Psychiatry 74(12):1197–1205, 2017 29049469

van Boekel LC, Brouwers EP, van Weeghel J, et al: Stigma among health professionals towards patients with substance use disorders and its consequences for healthcare delivery: systematic review. Drug Alcohol Depend 131(1–2):23–35, 2013 23490450

Vowles KE, McEntee ML, Julnes PS, et al: Rates of opioid misuse, abuse, and addiction in chronic pain: a systematic review and data synthesis. Pain 156(4):569–576, 2015 25785523

Walton-Moss B, Ray EM, Woodruff K: Relationship of spirituality or religion to recovery from substance abuse: a systematic review. J Addict Nurs 24(4):217–226, quiz 227–228, 2013 24335768

Webster LR, Webster RM: Predicting aberrant behaviors in opioid-treated patients: preliminary validation of the Opioid Risk Tool. Pain Med 6(6):432–442, 2005 16336480

Wesson DR, Ling W: The Clinical Opiate Withdrawal Scale (COWS). J Psychoactive Drugs 35(2):253–259, 2003 12924748

White WL: Addiction recovery: its definition and conceptual boundaries. J Subst Abuse Treat 33(3):229–241, 2007 17889295

White WL: Recovery: old wine, flavor of the month or new organizing paradigm? Subst Use Misuse 43(12–13):1987–2000, 2008 19016175

Worley J: Recovery in substance use disorders: what to know to inform practice. Issues Ment Health Nurs 38(1):80–91, 2017 27901625

Yudko E, Lozhkina O, Fouts A: A comprehensive review of the psychometric properties of the Drug Abuse Screening Test. J Subst Abuse Treat 32(2):189–198, 2007 17306727

Zedler B, Xie L, Wang L, et al: Risk factors for serious prescription opioid-related toxicity or overdose among Veterans Health Administration patients. Pain Med 15(11):1911–1929, 2014 24931395

9

Opioid Withdrawal Management and Transition to Treatment

Matisyahu Shulman, M.D.
Arthur Robin Williams, M.D., M.B.E.
Adam Bisaga, M.D.

Clinical Vignette: Joe's Intolerable Opioid Withdrawal

Joe is a 45-year-old construction worker who injured his back while picking up a heavy piece of equipment around 1 year ago. His primary care physician prescribed oxycodone 10 mg every 4 hours as needed for pain and spasms. After 3 months, Joe reported, "The original dose doesn't do anything for me anymore." He subsequently began taking extra doses and started running out of his medication earlier than anticipated on a regular basis.

After multiple discussions about his escalating doses of oxycodone, his physician stopped prescribing the medication and Joe used his last pill later that same night. The next morning, he began buying "blue roxies" (a colloquial term for oxycodone 30-mg tablets) from a neighbor and taking 4–6 pills a day, depending on how much he could afford. Over the subsequent months, amid arguments and increasing tension with his wife, he started crushing the pills and using the powder intranasally, noting a faster onset of effect than taking them orally.

Joe soon began missing work frequently in order to continue using the painkillers, and he often felt sick in the morning when he did not use enough. He also became depressed, became uninterested in socializing with his friends, had a poor appetite, and lost his sex drive.

Finally, after 9 months, Joe's brother convinced him to go to the emergency department to seek help for his pill use. He is seen by the emergency room physician. Joe's vital signs are within normal limits, and his basic laboratory studies are unremarkable. Joe is referred for emergency department social work and psychiatric consultation to address his opioid use disorder (OUD).

When speaking with the social worker and psychiatrist, Joe appears dysphoric but calm, and he says he is motivated to stop using opioids because "they have taken over my life." He is concerned about getting off opioids completely, however, because when he stopped taking them in the past he became very sick with nausea, diarrhea, sweats, and insomnia; he is not willing to go through that again. On discussing the case after the interview, the experienced emergency department social worker remarks that Joe is "just not ready for treatment" and should be discharged home.

Several questions arise from this clinical vignette. How can a provider determine whether a patient is "ready for treatment"? What are the pathophysiology, time course, signs, and symptoms of opioid withdrawal? What treatment options exist for someone like Joe? What further assessments are required before recommending a course of treatment? How can someone like Joe be most successfully transitioned to effective treatment for OUD?

Introduction

Opioid detoxification refers to the process in which an individual with a physiological dependence on opioids (someone who is "neuroadapted") is treated with medical supervision to systematically decrease or stop opioid intake while minimizing distressing symptoms of withdrawal. The primary goal of detoxification is to provide for safe cessation of the problematic substance while minimizing withdrawal symptoms. This process is particularly important in many cases to avoid life-threatening medical complications such as severe fluid loss, delirium, or autonomic instability. Equally important, however, is stabilization of the patient's medical and psychological health to allow him or her to benefit from treatment for the underlying substance use disorder (SUD).

Detoxification itself is not a treatment for OUD, and greater emphasis is now placed on "withdrawal management" to help initiate treatment with a U.S. Food and Drug Administration (FDA)–approved medication for OUD (Friedmann and Suzuki 2017). There is no evidence that detoxification programs alone effectively decrease the likelihood that a patient will meet diagnostic criteria for OUD in the subsequent months. Rather, successful detoxification can be measured by whether an individual with OUD enters and remains in a treatment or rehabilitation program facilitated by detoxification, such as starting one of the three medication-assisted treatments (MATs) currently available for OUD: methadone, buprenorphine, or long-acting injectable extended-release naltrexone (XR-naltrexone [Vivitrol]).

In considering how to approach a person seeking treatment for OUD, practitioners must first consider the long-term-care plan for the individual in question. The process of detoxification commonly used in substance use treatment has no clinical utility in the absence of a plan for maintenance treatment and has no evidence for improving outcomes unless serving as a bridge to long-term follow-up options. "Detoxing" a person from opioids also eliminates opioid tolerance, which otherwise serves to protect against the toxic effects of opioids, such as respiratory depression. Without clear motivation by the individual to maintain abstinence or without a follow-up plan that is likely to maintain sustained abstinence through the use of maintenance medications, detoxification increases patients' risk for overdose and death in the case of any return to use (Bird and Hutchinson 2003; Broers et al. 2000; Caplehorn 1998; del Campo et al. 1977; Smyth et al. 2010; Strang et al. 2003). The goal of treatment interactions with any individual experiencing OUD must be to maximize the probability of long-term treatment engagement and to minimize the impact of the OUD on the patient's health and functioning.

In this chapter, we review background information regarding the pathophysiology, time course, and signs and symptoms of opioid withdrawal, followed by clinical approaches to treating individuals requiring or requesting opioid detoxification.

Pathophysiology of Tolerance and Withdrawal

Opioids act at μ, κ, or δ opioid receptors, exerting agonist effects and producing a wide range of physiological effects in the nervous, digestive, and other systems. Opioid receptors are G protein–coupled receptors and respond to endogenous opioids (endorphins), first scientifically characterized in the 1970s (Filizola and Devi 2012). These receptors are widely distributed throughout the body and are especially concentrated in the central nervous system (brain and spinal cord) and the digestive tract (Minami and Satoh 1995). The molecular mechanisms mediating the development of tolerance to exogenous opioids are still not completely clear. One theory posits that opioid receptors are downregulated following chronic agonist exposure, which produces tolerance to some of the opioid agonist effects, such as euphoria or respiratory depression. More recent studies have shown that downregulation does not occur consistently with each agonist, and additional evidence implies desensitization and uncoupling of downstream signaling pathways with chronic exposure. Uncoupling of downstream pathways is mediated by changing levels of intracellular second messengers, such as cyclic adenosine monophosphate (cAMP) and adenylyl cyclase. As a result, there can be variation between individuals in neural adaptations and related physiological effects, such as tolerance and withdrawal severity, depending on the pharmacology and patterns of opioid use (Kreek 2002).

Tolerance and withdrawal often involve multiple organ systems and physiological effects. Some individuals are at greater risk than others of overdose with return to use following detoxification. Additionally, individuals may have different tolerance and withdrawal dose-response curves related to euphoria versus respiratory depression. Following detoxification, individuals typically regain tolerance to the euphoric effects of opioids more quickly than they regain tolerance to the respiratory depression effect, which may be one of the reasons that risk for overdose rises after detoxification (White and Irvine 1999).

There is a critical distinction between symptoms of physical neuroadaptive changes occurring with chronic opioid exposure (i.e., tolerance and withdrawal) and diagnostic criteria for OUD. Although tolerance and withdrawal may help substantiate a diagnosis of OUD, they are insufficient on their own. Physical dependence and tolerance are predictable physiological effects of opioid use. Addiction (i.e., OUD) is additionally characterized by loss of control over opioid use with persistent craving and ongoing, compulsive drug-taking behaviors despite worsening consequences.

Time Course and Signs and Symptoms of Withdrawal

Individuals with chronic opioid exposure experience a well-characterized clinical syndrome of tolerance and opioid withdrawal. Brief periods of exogenous opioid use (4–7 days) generate a sufficient level of neuroadaptations for a spontaneous withdrawal syndrome (following abrupt cessation of opioid use) to be clinically significant, often manifesting with cold- or flu-like symptoms, including malaise, nausea, and runny nose/eyes. The *Diagnostic and Statistical Manual of Mental Disorders*, Fifth Edition (DSM-5; American Psychiatric Association 2013), criteria for opioid withdrawal are listed in Box 9–1. Withdrawal symptoms generally occur spontaneously upon stopping regular use of opioids, but withdrawal can also be precipitated with the administration of an opioid antagonist or partial agonist.

BOX 9–1. Diagnostic Criteria, Opioid Withdrawal

A. Presence of either of the following:

   1. Cessation of (or reduction in) opioid use that has been heavy and prolonged (i.e., several weeks or longer).

   2. Administration of an opioid antagonist after a period of opioid use.

B. Three (or more) of the following developing within minutes to several days after Criterion A:

   1. Dysphoric mood.

   2. Nausea or vomiting.

   3. Muscle aches.

   4. Lacrimation or rhinorrhea.

   5. Pupillary dilation, piloerection, or sweating.

   6. Diarrhea.

   7. Yawning.

8. Fever.

9. Insomnia.

C. The signs or symptoms in Criterion B cause clinically significant distress or impairment in social, occupational, or other important areas of functioning.

D. The signs or symptoms are not attributable to another medical condition and are not better explained by another mental disorder, including intoxication or withdrawal from another substance.

Note. For specific coding and coding notes for opioid withdrawal in DSM-5, visit www.PsychiatryOnline.org for the free DSM-5 Update.

Source. Reprinted from American Psychiatric Association: *Diagnostic and Statistical Manual of Mental Disorders*, 5th Edition. Arlington, VA, American Psychiatric Association, 2013. Copyright © 2013 American Psychiatric Association. Used with permission.

In spontaneous withdrawal, symptoms generally begin 6–8 hours after the last use of short-acting opioids, such as heroin, morphine, oxycodone, or hydrocodone, although symptoms may not occur for up to 12–25 hours after the last use of a longer-acting opioid such as methadone or buprenorphine (Figure 9–1). Severity of symptoms of withdrawal from short-acting opioids peaks around 36–48 hours, and acute symptoms usually resolve after 5–7 days. With longer-acting opioids, symptoms may peak more than a week after cessation and may last 2 or more weeks. Drug effects from larger doses of buprenorphine (16–32 mg or more sublingually) can persist for several days due to the long half-life, and withdrawal symptoms can appear 4 or more days after the last dose of buprenorphine is taken, which can lead to confusion about the etiology of these symptoms.

Most patients in acute opioid withdrawal complain of anxiety and/or irritability, restlessness, an "achy feeling" in the legs and back, abdominal cramps, nausea, diarrhea, and increased sensitivity to pain and stress. It is likely that many individuals with OUD develop a conditioned psychological sensitization to withdrawal, heightening their sense of anxiety and discomfort. Fewer objective signs are present in milder withdrawal although moderate cases may present with vomiting, diarrhea, severe muscle aches, lacrimation and rhinorrhea, yawning, and pupillary dilation, along with increased sweating and chills. In severe withdrawal, these symptoms plus fever, persistent insomnia, confusion, and delirium can occur.

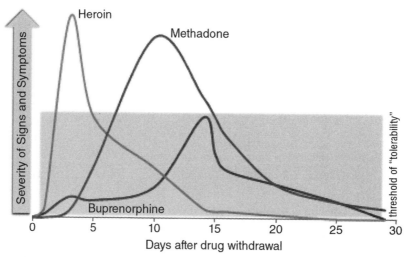

FIGURE 9–1. Progress of the acute phase of opioid withdrawal.

Following the resolution of a well-characterized acute opioid withdrawal syndrome, a lesser-known protracted period of physiological abnormality can last for months. This extended period of withdrawal symptoms is called protracted or post-acute-withdrawal syndrome. It can persist for weeks or months and is characterized by depressed, dysphoric, or labile mood; anhedonia; irritability; stress intolerance; insomnia; and recurrent urges to use opioids. This protracted syndrome is postulated to result from alterations and remodeling of the neural circuitry associated with chronic opioid exposure, such as changes in both the serotonergic and dopaminergic systems. Protracted or post-acute-withdrawal syndrome, although not formally included in DSM-5, is likely a significant contributor to relapse to opioid use. Symptomatic treatment with medications targeting stress intolerance (e.g., clonidine), anxiety and insomnia (e.g., long-acting benzodiazepines such as clonazepam, other γ-aminobutyric acid (GABA)ergic agents, mirtazapine), and diarrhea (e.g., loperamide) during the first few weeks or months of abstinence can help improve patient comfort, minimize triggers, and prevent relapse.

A precipitated withdrawal occurs after administration of an antagonist to an individual who is physically dependent on opioids and begins within minutes of parenteral or intramuscular administration of naloxone or within 1–2 hours after oral administration of naltrexone. Withdrawal precipitated by naloxone and naltrexone is usually more severe than spontaneous withdrawal, but it resolves faster, generally within 2–3 days, and administering small increasing doses of naltrexone is being investigated as a possible therapeutic target for expediting detoxification protocols for initiating XR-naltrexone. Precipitated withdrawal can also occur following the administration of a partial agonist such as buprenorphine to individuals taking regular doses of an agonist (e.g., heroin). In this case, buprenorphine can "antagonize" the effect of a full agonist because it abruptly decreases the activation of the receptor (from a full to a partial effect) and also has high receptor affinity, displacing many full agonists, both of which precipitate withdrawal.

There is considerable variation between individuals in withdrawal in terms of time course, severity, and the specific constellations of symptoms experienced. Symptoms depend on individual biological differences (e.g., genetics, comorbidities) but also on the various properties of the opioid the individual has become accustomed to using—that is, degree of agonism (full vs. partial agonism), potency, dose, duration of use, and rate of opioid discontinuation (e.g., slow taper vs. abrupt cessation). In general, a more severe withdrawal syndrome results with any of the following: higher potency, full agonists, higher doses, longer duration of use and greater addiction severity, co-occurring medical and psychiatric disorders, and abrupt discontinuation. For example, withdrawal symptoms may occur after discontinuation of maintenance treatment with buprenorphine, a partial opioid receptor agonist, but symptoms may be less severe in comparison with those seen with abrupt cessation of a short-acting full agonist such as heroin.

Rating Instruments

Several standardized instruments are available to quantify the severity of opioid withdrawal symptoms in clinical practice. The Clinical Opiate Withdrawal Scale (COWS; Wesson and Ling 2003) is most commonly used and includes ratings of resting pulse rate, restlessness, sweating, pupil dilation, rhinorrhea, pain, gastrointestinal symptoms, tremor, anxiety, yawning, and piloerection. Wesson and colleagues developed the scale to be administered quickly, and it was intended to improve upon existing measurement tools. It was first published in a training manual for buprenorphine treatment (Wesson et al. 1999). The

COWS is available online for clinical use on the National Institute on Drug Abuse website via the following link: www.drugabuse.gov/sites/default/files/files/ClinicalOpiateWithdrawalScale.pdf. The Subjective Opiate Withdrawal Scale (SOWS; Handelsman et al. 1987) is a 16-item self-report scale to quantify withdrawal symptoms. Other rating instruments include the Objective Opiate Withdrawal Scale (OOWS; Handelsman et al. 1987), which rates 13 objective signs as being either present or absent, and the 11-item Clinical Institute Narcotic Assessment (CINA; Peachey and Lei 1988).

Clinical Approaches to Withdrawal Management

OUD is a chronic disorder with severe health and social consequences and an elevated mortality rate (Hser et al. 2017). In light of OUD's chronic nature, individuals with OUD commonly interact with the medical system multiple times when seeking treatment to address substance use and medical complications related to substance use (Substance Abuse and Mental Health Services Administration 2016). In certain situations, individuals may remain in medical settings for an extended time and not use illicit substances. Likewise, if an individual presents to a treatment setting requesting treatment for OUD, the clinician must provide interventions that allow for transition of the individual from active opioid use to treatment with a MAT pharmacotherapy such as methadone, buprenorphine, or XR-naltrexone (Center for Substance Abuse Treatment 2005).

Approaches to detoxification depend on which of the three medications is best suited to a given patient. It should be noted that the most common treatment approach, which was accepted for many years as the standard of care, assumes that the optimal treatment approach for OUD involves detoxification followed by treatment without the use of medication under a 12-step model of recovery for an OUD. This approach was adapted from support groups for alcoholism, such as Alcoholics Anonymous, and insurance reimbursement restrictions stemming from health maintenance organizations (HMOs) in the 1990s (Galanter et al. 2000). Through the early twenty-first century, treatment for OUD was often initiated with a period of detoxification following abrupt opioid cessation, with medications used solely for the management of acute symptoms of opioid withdrawal. This process was frequently followed by residential or outpatient relapse-prevention psychosocial therapy and with encouragement to participate in 12-step self-help groups such as Alcoholics Anonymous or Narcotics Anonymous. Unfortunately, evidence has repeatedly shown that this approach is associated with high rates of treatment dropout, relapse, and complications including fatal overdose (Bird and Hutchinson 2003; Broers et al. 2000; Caplehorn 1998; del Campo et al. 1977; Smyth et al. 2010; Strang et al. 2003). The evidence base for effective treatment now rejects this approach and considers such treatment as inadequate and ineffective (Gowing et al. 2014; Kampman and Jarvis 2015; Lingford-Hughes et al. 2012; World Health Organization 2009). Instead, individuals should be maintained on medication with an effective evidence base, such as methadone or buprenorphine, which have both repeatedly been shown to reduce mortality; they have been promoted by the World Health Organization (2009) as "essential medicines" given their great importance for treating OUD in populations worldwide.

Initial Assessment

Initial assessments of individuals with OUD should build from a motivational interviewing (MI) stance as standard care. Taking an MI stance may increase the likelihood of long-term treatment engagement and appropriate discussions of evidence-based treatment options for opioid maintenance treatment (Smedslund et al. 2011). This stance includes treating all patients with respect and dignity in a nonjudgmental and supportive manner and giving consideration to individual background, ethnicity, religion, disabilities, and strengths. All professionals involved in the care of the patient should be supportive, promote rehabilitation, and encourage remaining in treatment. Active involvement of family and social supports when feasible is often helpful. Additionally, it is important early on to anticipate challenges to treatment retention among patients with OUD and incorporate motivational techniques to improve duration of treatment, starting in the initial assessment (e.g., MI, anticipatory guidance).

The initial assessment of a patient presenting for treatment should include an examination of the patient's medical and psychological status that includes identifying conditions that need to be addressed at treatment outset (Center for Substance Abuse Treatment 2005). Substance use and its sequelae can cause significant medical issues, which should be addressed immediately. Some examples of conditions that need urgent medical care include confusion, disorientation, excessive somnolence or unconsciousness, slow breathing, blue or pale skin color, hallucinations, seizures, fever, significant increases and/or decreases in blood pressure and pulse, upper and lower gastrointestinal bleeding, and heightened deep tendon reflexes indicating an increased risk for seizures.

Further assessment of other drug and alcohol use and for physiological dependence on these substances is crucial because some patients with OUD may also be physically dependent on alcohol or benzodiazepines, which could complicate their withdrawal course and thus may require a concomitant treatment. If an individual is dependent on sedative-hypnotics and/or alcohol as well as opioids, the standard of care involves sequential treatment of alcohol or sedative-hypnotic withdrawal and opioid withdrawal. This is often accomplished by maintaining the patient on an opioid agonist while he or she is being tapered from the sedative-hypnotic, and once the patient is stable, usually after 5–7 days of treatment, the OUD is addressed as described in the next section of this chapter.

For patients not in need of urgent medical care, the assessment should continue with a full medical, psychiatric, social, and substance use history, with a focus on previous treatment episodes and prior complications from withdrawal episodes. With regard to drug use, this assessment should include identifying the primary drug used and patterns of use, including quantity and duration of use as well as the route of administration and other substances used in combination (e.g., among patients with OUD, comorbid cocaine use disorder is often associated with worse outcomes). Important for detoxification treatment planning is determining the time the drug was last used (in relation to half-life), the severity of the dependence, and prior withdrawal symptoms and treatment response. Evaluation should also include the age at first use and periods of abstinence. The assessment should confirm the presence of drug in the body (i.e., through urine toxicology) and physical dependence on the substance. Finally, the clinician should assess the patient's readiness to enter treatment after completion of detoxification (Center for Substance Abuse Treatment 2005).

On the basis of a comprehensive assessment, recommendations should be given for the appropriate level of care, such as inpatient or residential treatment, an intensive outpatient program, or general outpatient treatment. One framework for selecting a level of care is the placement criteria of the American Society of Addiction Medicine (2001). Depending on the level of care needed, withdrawal management can proceed in a variety of inpatient or outpatient settings. For patients with a high disorder severity or with complicating co-occurring disorders and for those with complicated withdrawal episodes in the past inpatient medically managed detoxification is often necessary.

Choosing the Pharmacological Approach

Once it is clear that an individual meets criteria for OUD and is seeking treatment beyond the detoxification phase, the clinician should raise the issue of maintenance treatment with either methadone, buprenorphine, or XR-naltrexone (Lee et al. 2015). Individuals are often unaware of these options, or they or their families harbor misinformation about them. At present, no treatment-matching studies have successfully shown which medication best suits a specific patient population. In general, some patients with more severe burdens of psychiatric comorbidity, such as anxiety, mood, and personality disorders, may respond best to treatment with methadone or buprenorphine provided in the structure of an opioid treatment program (OTP), whereas those with less severe addiction and treatment histories may be better candidates for less frequent monitoring and at-home use of buprenorphine or XR-naltrexone, both of which are available outside OTPs. However, treatment placement should always be individualized to the needs and preferences of each patient and based on the locally available array of services and resources. For instance, certain patients with serious mental illness may do better in a more flexible but still intensive mental health program that offers integrated dual diagnosis treatment (McGovern et al. 2014) in addition to buprenorphine and/or XR-naltrexone, whereas other patients with complex medical comorbidities may do better in an OTP that happens to offer robust integrated medical services. See Chapters 6, "Opioid Use Disorder and Medical Comorbidity," and 7, "Opioid Use Disorder and Psychiatric Comorbidity," for further discussion of considerations for patients with psychiatric and/or medical comorbidities.

Although treatment availability, cost, and patient preferences often determine the treatment approach, it is important to engage the patient in the process of shared decision making to craft an appropriate and individualized treatment plan. This involves a review of available treatment settings by level of care, including residential programs, office-based pharmacological options, and specialized outpatient OTPs. This discussion should also include a review of the following: the differences between methadone, buprenorphine, and XR-naltrexone, including the mechanisms of therapeutic effect; requirements for treatment initiation; comparative risks, benefits, and side effects of each medication; duration of treatment and treatment dropout or termination issues; and the feasibility of each of the potential treatments (e.g., daily visits to an OTP to receive methadone vs. a monthly visit for XR-naltrexone injections). When appropriate, the final discussion should involve an available family member or significant other. The provider should assess the patient's motivation for treatment and preferences for any particular medication before offering a final recommendation for a first-line treatment with a specific medication. In some cases, if the provider lacks familiarity or certification in one of the available treatment options, it may be necessary to assure the patient that a referral for his or her preferred treatment will be arranged (Center for Substance Abuse Treatment 2004).

Transition From Opioid Use to Agonist Maintenance Medication

Once the patient agrees to a treatment plan, the patient can transition from active opioid use to a maintenance medication. Agonist maintenance with methadone (first approved in the early 1960s) and buprenorphine (FDA approved in 2002) are the most studied and utilized approaches to improving treatment retention and reducing problematic substance use, as well as lowering risk of relapse, overdose, and death (Bart 2012).

Methadone, a long-acting agonist at the μ opioid receptor, and buprenorphine, a long-acting partial agonist, are both approved for OUD maintenance treatment. However, methadone can only be administered as a treatment for OUD through federally regulated and state-regulated OTPs (rather than an independent doctor's office), which limits access for many patients. A major advantage of treatment with methadone or buprenorphine is that either can be more easily started than XR-naltrexone, without the requirement of a wait period (beyond the 12–24 hours to avoid toxicity in the case of methadone or the precipitated withdrawal in the case of buprenorphine) and without the need to undergo complete opioid withdrawal (as are both necessary before use of XR-naltrexone). For an individual who is open to maintenance treatment with an opioid agonist, it is possible to use either buprenorphine or methadone in the initial treatment setting to mitigate withdrawal symptoms and also to bridge to long-term maintenance therapy.

Transition to Methadone Maintenance

The major advantage for the use of methadone to prevent withdrawal symptoms is ease of initiation. Methadone can be started readily because it is a full agonist and will not precipitate withdrawal, as buprenorphine, a partial agonist, might (Stotts et al. 2009). However, clinicians must take care when initiating and increasing the dose of methadone because of its long half-life. The first dose is usually given in the morning, when the patient is in a state of mild withdrawal after an overnight abstinence. Administering methadone to a person who just used heroin or a sedative drug may result in excessive sedation or toxicity. Afterward, the dose of methadone has to be increased very slowly, with at least 3- to 4-day intervals between increases, to allow for the development of tolerance and a steady-state blood level to avoid the possibility of sedation or respiratory depression. Even with once-daily dosing, blood levels increase after each subsequent dose because of the slow elimination, which can lead to an excessive buildup of blood levels and to toxicity or death in patients with low opioid tolerance. Risk of toxicity is greatest in the first 2–3 weeks of treatment, and toxic manifestations might be delayed for up to 12 hours after the last dose. It is generally recommended to begin individuals on doses of 20–40 mg/day and to increase weekly by no more than 10–15 mg/day. It is possible that an individual with high daily opioid use will develop withdrawal symptoms during the first 2 weeks while taking comparatively lower doses of methadone, in which case the clinician should manage these symptoms with additional medications as described below. Methadone-treated individuals commonly continue to intermittently use heroin or other opioids when their doses are too low; patients have better outcomes with higher doses of methadone (80–120 mg/day), which can be achieved within 3–4 weeks of starting treatment. Clinicians should continue to increase the methadone dose as long as the individual continues to report cravings or ongoing opioid use and does not exhibit evidence of toxicity.

Transition to Buprenorphine Maintenance

Since 2002, buprenorphine has had FDA approval for the treatment of OUD by physicians authorized under the Drug Addiction Treatment

Act of 2000 (DATA 2000; PL 106-310) with a waiver from the Drug Enforcement Administration (DEA) to prescribe it outside OTPs. In 2017, prescribing access was extended to nurse practitioners and physician assistants who completed required training and obtained a DEA waiver.

Initiating buprenorphine treatment in a patient who is actively using opioid agonists (e.g., heroin, hydrocodone, methadone) and is physically dependent on opioids will often lead to precipitated withdrawal because buprenorphine is a partial agonist with greater receptor affinity than commonly used full agonists. Because its effects at the opioid receptor are only partial in relation to full agonists and because of its strong binding at the receptor, buprenorphine will displace full agonist opioids from the opioid receptor, abruptly diminishing receptor activation and leading to withdrawal symptoms. These symptoms are generally mild to moderate and can be treated with supportive symptomatic management or escalating doses of buprenorphine to restabilize opioid receptors (Bart 2012).

To minimize the risk of precipitating withdrawal, clinicians should give individuals their first dose of buprenorphine during an initial withdrawal state, when fewer receptors are occupied by a full agonist. At that point, receptor activation provided by buprenorphine is unlikely to precipitate withdrawal; rather, the level of activation is likely sufficient to alleviate and prevent further withdrawal. The higher the severity of predose withdrawal is, the better the tolerability of the first dose. Usually, a mild to moderate symptom severity is adequate, corresponding to a minimum score of 10–12 on the COWS, preferably with clear objective signs of withdrawal (e.g., yawning, tremors/shivers, tachycardia).

Once an individual has tolerated the first dose of buprenorphine, further doses can be safely given, with the goal of providing a sufficient dose to alleviate withdrawal and provide consistent relief from both cravings and further withdrawal symptoms. Several schedules have been proposed for titration of buprenorphine, but generally individuals are started with a dose of 1–2 mg, which is repeated as needed every 2–3 hours up to 8–12 mg on the first day. Daily dosing is increased as needed over the next few days. After the initial titration using divided doses, it is preferred that the full daily dose be given once daily in the morning, although some individuals may initially require an additional smaller dose in the evening to counteract residual withdrawal.

The usual maintenance dose is in the range of 8–24 mg/day, with higher doses offering additional benefits (i.e., lower opioid craving and use, improved treatment retention). Higher doses, occasionally up to 32 mg/day, may be necessary to sustain full clinical response early during treatment, but over time in stable patients the maintenance dose may be in the range of 8–16 mg/day.

Once successfully stabilized on buprenorphine, patients should be encouraged to continue this maintenance treatment for a minimum of 1–2 years (World Health Organization 2009), preferably as long as it is clinically indicated with the patient continuing to benefit from treatment and tolerating medication. Many patients will require an indefinite duration of treatment because the risk of relapse and related overdose death remains high after treatment discontinuation, despite years of successful treatment. Although many patients request long-term opioid agonist treatment (Ling 2016; Uebelacker et al. 2016), some do not accept this approach because of ideological or logistical barriers and instead seek to be medication-free (Friedmann and Suzuki 2017; Winstock et al. 2011).

Often, patients entering treatment for OUD will only agree to the short-term use of an agonist to alleviate the most severe opioid withdrawal symptoms, as a temporary detoxification rather than long-term maintenance. Indeed, the majority of patients who receive buprenorphine are thought to receive less than 30–60 days of medication (Timko et al. 2016). However, this brief, limited treatment approach has a high failure rate, with a large proportion of patients unable to remain in sustained abstinence following opioid withdrawal (Bentzley et al. 2015). Individuals who wish to discontinue agonist treatment should be counseled on the risks of discontinuing medications, including the elevated risk of relapse and overdose death (Sordo et al. 2017; Strang et al. 2003). For those patients who wish to discontinue buprenorphine, current evidence has consistently shown superiority for slow tapers, extending over weeks or months, rather than a rapid taper (Dunn et al. 2011). Some patients successfully treated with buprenorphine over the long term will not be able to complete tapers without destabilizing cravings, discomfort, and relapse, and they may need to continue agonist maintenance for a longer duration. For these patients, transition to XR-naltrexone may represent a viable treatment alternative.

Detoxification and Naltrexone Maintenance

Another approach for patients with OUD who are undergoing opioid withdrawal is to follow its management with a relapse-prevention treatment that includes XR-naltrexone. If during treatment planning the individual wishes to be maintained without agonist treatment or cannot access such treatment (i.e., due to a lack of OTPs or buprenorphine-waivered prescribers), naltrexone, an opiate antagonist, may be used successfully as a maintenance treatment for motivated patients.

Oral naltrexone has been available for clinical use in the United States since the 1970s. It is effective in preventing acute opioid intoxication and relapse due to μ opioid receptor antagonist properties. Naltrexone used in an oral dose of 50 mg/day provides blockade of average doses of opioids for 24–48 hours. Effectiveness of oral naltrexone requires daily adherence, which can be a challenge for some patients. Multiple studies have shown low rates of adherence among patients in community settings, which can increase risk of overdose death upon return to active opioid use by a person whose opioid receptors are not blocked with naltrexone and who is no longer tolerant to opioids. Oral naltrexone is recognized in the World Health Organization opioid dependence treatment guidelines for preventing relapse in patients who have withdrawn from opioids (World Health Organization 2009), and it is also approved by the FDA for blockade of exogenously administered opioids. XR-naltrexone received FDA approval in 2010 for prevention of relapse following opioid detoxification. XR-naltrexone administered monthly circumvents some of the naltrexone nonadherence problems. Blood levels of naltrexone are detected for up to 6 weeks after the injection, which reduces the risk of overdose in case of treatment dropout, making it a safer preparation of naltrexone, especially in early phases of treatment. In clinical trials, XR-naltrexone appears to be significantly more effective than the oral preparation. Owing to its efficacy and safety advantage, XR-naltrexone is a much preferred formulation for treatment of patients with OUD.

A patient should not begin naltrexone induction until full detoxification from opioids and the resolution of opioid withdrawal, typically 7–10 days after last opioid use. If XR-naltrexone is administered before the completion of withdrawal, it may precipitate severe opioid withdrawal requiring hospitalization. Because most patients presenting for

OUD treatment are actively using opioids at the time of initial evaluation, they must undergo opioid withdrawal before XR-naltrexone can be initiated. For this reason for populations in institutionalized residential treatment or criminal justice settings that are already fully detoxified, it is typically easier to begin XR-naltrexone treatment (Lee et al. 2016).

A commonly used procedure for naltrexone induction involves a short-term (e.g., 7- to 14-day) taper of buprenorphine followed by a washout period of 7–10 days. This procedure requires that the patient wait at least 2 weeks—and possibly almost 4 weeks—after cessation of active drug use before receiving XR-naltrexone. Importantly, every day that the patient waits to start XR-naltrexone, his or her opioid receptors remain unblocked, with decreasing tolerance and a growing risk of premature treatment dropout and relapse to opioid use. A shorter induction period is preferable but involves the risk of a precipitated withdrawal. Although pharmacological management of opioid withdrawal under medical supervision in the inpatient setting is optimal, such treatment may be unavailable for many patients, in which case the withdrawal and initiation of XR-naltrexone can be done on an outpatient basis (Sullivan et al. 2017).

To shorten the induction period following abrupt discontinuation of an opioid agonist (e.g., heroin), several approaches have been proposed which may be used on an inpatient or outpatient basis. First, buprenorphine can be given for a single day, because it replaces the full agonist at the receptor while providing some (partial) agonist activity to prevent significant withdrawal while reducing activity at the μ opioid receptor. Buprenorphine is followed by 1–2 days of washout and a gradual ascending titration of oral naltrexone over the subsequent 3–5 days, beginning with a low dose of 1–4 mg (Table 9–1). This dose is sufficient to modulate activity at the μ receptor but is not high enough to precipitate a significant withdrawal. Subsequent doses of naltrexone can be higher, escalated to a full blocking dose of 25 mg/day, without the risk of significant withdrawal. Throughout this procedure, patients receive frequent standing doses of adjunctive medications aimed at preventing the emergence of withdrawal (see Table 9–1) (Bisaga et al. 2011, 2014; Sullivan et al. 2017).

The second procedure employs a buprenorphine taper in combination with very low doses of oral naltrexone (< 1 mg/day), beginning after a day of abstinence to allow for buprenorphine induction. On the sub-

TABLE 9–1. Initiating treatment with naltrexone (inpatient and outpatient)

Day	Inpatient procedure
1	Induct and administer buprenorphine 8 mg
2–3	Washout days
4–6	Increase daily doses of oral naltrexone: 3.125 mg, 6.25 mg, 25 mg
7	Administer XR-naltrexone 380-mg injection
Standing dosage with additional doses as necessary	Adjuvant medications: clonidine, clonazepam, prochlorperazine, trazodone, zolpidem
Day	**Outpatient procedure (Sullivan et al. 2017)**
1	Patient comes to clinic in mild to moderate withdrawal. Give buprenorphine starting at 2 mg, titrate up to 8 mg as tolerated
2	Washout day
3–6	Initiate titration of oral naltrexone (total daily doses): 1 mg, 3 mg, 12 mg, 25 mg
7	Administer XR-naltrexone 380-mg injection
Standing dosage with additional doses as necessary	Adjuvant medications: clonidine, clonazepam, prochlorperazine, trazodone or zolpidem (for sleep)

Source. Adapted from Bisaga et al. 2014; Sullivan et al. 2017.

sequent 2–3 days, buprenorphine is initiated and tapered off, while at the same time very low doses of naltrexone are initiated and slowly increased. This is followed by a gradual titration of naltrexone alone to full blocking doses (>25 mg/day), usually accomplished with 7–9 days followed by a gradual titration of naltrexone to full blocking doses, usually accomplished within 7–9 days (Mannelli et al. 2014); see Table 9–2 for more details.

In studies, these procedures allowed 50%–80% of outpatients to successfully initiate treatment with XR-naltrexone (Mannelli et al. 2014; Sullivan et al. 2017) with favorable tolerability and no serious adverse events due to precipitated withdrawal (Bisaga et al. 2011, 2014; Mannelli et al. 2014; Sullivan et al. 2017). Methadone is not recommended as a

TABLE 9–2. Using very low doses of naltrexone to initiate treatment

Day	Outpatient procedure
1	Instruct patient to remain abstinent for 24 hours
2–3	Increase daily dose of oral naltrexone (0.25–1 mg) as tolerated, and decrease daily dose of buprenorphine (4–2 mg)
4–7	Increase daily dose of naltrexone to 30–50 mg by day 7 if possible
8	Administer XR-naltrexone 380-mg injection
As necessary	Adjuvant medications: trazodone, cyclobenzaprine, lorazepam, hydroxyzine

Source. Adapted from Mannelli et al. 2014.

detoxification agent to facilitate XR-naltrexone induction because methadone persists for a long time postcessation, further delaying the first dose of XR-naltrexone.

Stabilizing Patients on XR-Naltrexone

Rapid induction onto XR-naltrexone (approximately 1 week after the last day of agonist use such as heroin or oxycodone) may result in withdrawal-like symptoms during the first few weeks of maintenance therapy and has been attributed to a protracted opioid withdrawal syndrome (Kleber and Kosten 1984; Kosten 1990; Mariani et al. 2009). Symptoms can include disturbances of sleep, low energy, anxiety, irritability, and diarrhea that persist for weeks (or longer in the case of insomnia) (Bisaga et al. 2014; Sullivan et al. 2017). In the majority of patients, these symptoms fully resolve within 3–4 weeks of the first XR-naltrexone injection. Table 9–3 lists adjunctive medication options that can help to symptomatically manage protracted opioid withdrawal. Most of these symptoms can be avoided if naltrexone is started after a longer period of abstinence from opioids, such as 3–4 weeks, which may be an option available to patients treated in residential settings. However, clinicians must weigh the decision to delay the administration of XR-naltrexone (to decrease the risk of precipitated and protracted withdrawal) against

TABLE 9–3. Withdrawal symptoms and pharmacological treatment

Withdrawal symptoms	Drug class
Autonomic arousal (sympathetic)	α_2-Adrenergic agonists (e.g., clonidine 0.1–0.2 mg every 6 hours, lofexidine 0.54–0.72 mg every 6 hours)
Anxiety	Benzodiazepines (e.g., clonazepam 1 mg every 8 hours)
Restlessness	Benzodiazepines (e.g., clonazepam 1 mg every 8 hours)
	α_2-Adrenergic agonists (e.g., clonidine 0.1–0.2 mg every 6 hours, lofexidine 0.54–0.72 mg every 6 hours)
Insomnia	Sedative-hypnotics (e.g., zolpidem 10 mg, clonazepam 1 mg) at bedtime
	Sedating antidepressants (e.g., trazodone 100 mg, mirtazapine 7.5 mg) at bedtime
	Sedating atypical neuroleptics (e.g., quetiapine 50 mg) at bedtime
Musculoskeletal pain	Nonsteroidal anti-inflammatory drugs (e.g., ibuprofen 600 mg every 8 hours)
Gastrointestinal distress (nausea, vomiting, diarrhea)	Oral hydration (e.g., water, Pedialyte) and supportive care
	Antiemetics (e.g., chlorpromazine 10 mg every 8–12 hours)
	Antidiarrheals (e.g., loperamide 2 mg every 6 hours)

the risk of treatment dropout among patients whose opioid receptors are not blocked—that is, giving the XR-naltrexone injection earlier may cause more severe withdrawal, but giving it later may increase the risk of relapse and overdose.

Because of the difficulty many patients with severe OUD experience when attempting a full detoxification before initiating XR-naltrexone, there is growing interest in strategies to facilitate success. Intermittent use of marijuana may alleviate withdrawal symptoms and improve induction and adherence with XR-naltrexone (Bisaga et al. 2014; Church et al. 2001; Raby et al. 2009), likely because of reduced anxiety and improved sleep. Additionally, experimental use of dopaminergic medications such as stimulants, the use of ketamine, and devices such as the NSS-2 Bridge (an over-the-ear device that modulates cranial nerve activity) are being investigated.

Although it involves some consideration and treatment planning to perform properly, the transition of patients from active opioid use to maintenance treatment can be a rewarding experience for clinicians. In light of the current opioid crisis in the United States, a successful command of such procedures can help save countless lives.

Key Chapter Points

▶ Individuals who are chronically exposed to opioids develop physical dependence and experience withdrawal symptoms if the daily dose of opioids is reduced or stopped abruptly. Detoxification is a process of removing physiological dependence while managing the severity of opioid withdrawal symptoms.

▶ Detoxification alone is not a treatment for OUD and increases an individual's risk for relapse, overdose, and death when not followed with medication-assisted treatment.

▶ Several medications help to reduce the symptoms of opioid withdrawal during the detoxification process. Determining the approach to managing opioid withdrawal for individual patients depends on their plans for treatment. Therefore, prior to initiating the detoxification process, it is important to discuss with patients their individual motivations for treatment as well as long-term plans for sustaining gains made in treatment.

▶ If the medication-assisted treatment choice is methadone, this option allows for initiation immediately upon entering treatment, with minimal need to manage opioid withdrawal. However, doses must be raised slowly because of methadone's long half-life and related toxicity risks.

▶ If the treatment choice is buprenorphine, the individual needs to be in moderate withdrawal at the start of treatment to avoid causing precipitated withdrawal. Once treatment has been established, the dosage can be rapidly titrated upward to reduce discomfort associated with withdrawal.

▶ If the treatment choice is XR-naltrexone, treatment is initiated after full detoxification and the resolution of opioid withdrawal, at the risk of precipitating severe opioid withdrawal requiring hospitalization if extended-release naltrexone (XR-naltrexone) is initiated too soon.

▶ Clinicians should use a motivational and nonjudgmental stance in supporting patients through treatment and present them with all available treatment options to develop an individualized and most suitable approach.

▶ Although it involves some consideration and treatment planning to perform properly, transitioning patients from active opioid use to maintenance treatment can be a rewarding experience for clinicians. In light of the current opioid crisis in the United States, a successful command of such procedures can help save countless lives.

References

American Psychiatric Association: Diagnostic and Statistical Manual of Mental Disorders, 5th Edition. Arlington, VA, American Psychiatric Association, 2013

American Society of Addiction Medicine: Patient Placement Criteria for the Treatment of Substance-Related Disorders, 2nd Edition. Chevy Chase, MD, American Society of Addiction Medicine, 2001

Bart G: Maintenance medication for opiate addiction: the foundation of recovery. J Addict Dis 31(3):207–225, 2012 22873183

Bentzley BS, Barth KS, Back SE, et al: Discontinuation of buprenorphine maintenance therapy: perspectives and outcomes. J Subst Abuse Treat 52:48–57, 2015 25601365

Bird SM, Hutchinson SJ: Male drugs-related deaths in the fortnight after release from prison: Scotland, 1996–99. Addiction 98(2):185–190, 2003 12534423

Bisaga A, Sullivan MA, Cheng WY, et al: A placebo controlled trial of memantine as an adjunct to oral naltrexone for opioid dependence. Drug Alcohol Depend 119(1–2):e23–e29, 2011 21715107

Bisaga A, Sullivan MA, Glass A, et al: A placebo-controlled trial of memantine as an adjunct to injectable extended-release naltrexone for opioid dependence. J Subst Abuse Treat 46(5):546–552, 2014 24560438

Broers B, Giner F, Dumont P, et al: Inpatient opiate detoxification in Geneva: follow-up at 1 and 6 months. Drug Alcohol Depend 58(1–2):85–92, 2000 10669058

Caplehorn JR: Deaths in the first two weeks of maintenance treatment in NSW in 1994: identifying cases of iatrogenic methadone toxicity. Drug Alcohol Rev 17(1):9–17, 1998 16203464

Center for Substance Abuse Treatment: Substance abuse treatment and family therapy, in Substance Abuse Treatment and Family Therapy (Treatment Improvement Protocol [TIP] Series, No 39, SMA-04-3957). Rockville, MD, Substance Abuse and Mental Health Services Administration, 2004. Available at: https://www.ncbi.nlm.nih.gov/books/NBK64269/. Accessed April 3, 2018.

Center for Substance Abuse Treatment: Clinical pharmacotherapy, in Medication-Assisted Treatment for Opioid Addiction in Opioid Treatment Programs (Treatment Improvement Protocol [TIP] Series, No 43, SMA-12-4214). Rockville, MD, Substance Abuse and Mental Health Services Administration, 2005. Available at: https://www.ncbi.nlm.nih.gov/books/NBK64152/. Accessed April 3, 2018.

Church SH, Rothenberg JL, Sullivan MA, et al: Concurrent substance use and outcome in combined behavioral and naltrexone therapy for opiate dependence. Am J Drug Alcohol Abuse 27(3):441–452, 2001 11506261

del Campo EJ, John DS, Kauffman CC: Evaluation of the 21-day outpatient heroin detoxification. Int J Addict 12(7):923–935, 1977 591146

Dunn KE, Sigmon SC, Strain EC, et al: The association between outpatient buprenorphine detoxification duration and clinical treatment outcomes: a review. Drug Alcohol Depend 119(1–2):1–9, 2011 21741781

Filizola M, Devi LA: Structural biology: how opioid drugs bind to receptors. Nature 485(7398):314–317, 2012 22596150

Friedmann PD, Suzuki J: More beds are not the answer: transforming detoxification units into medication induction centers to address the opioid epidemic. Addict Sci Clin Pract 12(1):29, 2017 29141667

Galanter M, Keller DS, Dermatis H, et al: The impact of managed care on substance abuse treatment: a report of the American Society of Addiction Medicine. J Addict Dis 19(3):13–34, 2000 11076117

Gowing L, Ali R, Dunlop A, et al: National Guidelines for Medication-Assisted Treatment of Opioid Dependence. Canberra, ACT, Commonwealth of Australia, 2014, pp 38–39

Handelsman L, Cochrane KJ, Aronson MJ, et al: Two new rating scales for opiate withdrawal. Am J Drug Alcohol Abuse 13(3):293–308, 1987 3687892

Hser YI, Mooney LJ, Saxon AJ, et al: High mortality among patients with opioid use disorder in a large healthcare system. J Addict Med 11(4):315–319, 2017 28426439

Kampman K, Jarvis M: American Society of Addiction Medicine (ASAM) national practice guideline for the use of medications in the treatment of addiction involving opioid use. J Addict Med 9(5):358–367, 2015 26406300

Kleber HD, Kosten TR: Naltrexone induction: psychologic and pharmacologic strategies. J Clin Psychiatry 45(9 Pt 2):29–38, 1984 6469934

Kosten TR: Current pharmacotherapies for opioid dependence. Psychopharmacol Bull 26(1):69–74, 1990 2196628

Kreek MJ: Molecular and cellular neurobiology and pathophysiology of opiate addiction, in Neuropsychopharmacology: The Fifth Generation of Progress. Edited by Davis KL, Charney D, Coyle JT, et al. Philadelphia, PA, Lippincott Williams & Wilkins, 2002, pp 1491–1506

Lee J, Kresina TF, Campopiano M, et al: Use of pharmacotherapies in the treatment of alcohol use disorders and opioid dependence in primary care. Biomed Res Int 2015:137020, 2015 25629034

Lee JD, Friedmann PD, Kinlock TW, et al: Extended-release naltrexone to prevent opioid relapse in criminal justice offenders. N Engl J Med 374(13):1232–1242, 2016 27028913

Ling W: A perspective on opioid pharmacotherapy: where we are and how we got here. J Neuroimmune Pharmacol 11(3):394–400, 2016 27008037

Lingford-Hughes AR, Welch S, Peters L, et al; British Association for Psychopharmacology, Expert Reviewers Group: BAP updated guidelines: evidence-based guidelines for the pharmacological management of substance abuse, harmful use, addiction and comorbidity: recommendations from BAP. J Psychopharmacol 26(7):899–952, 2012 22628390

Mannelli P, Wu LT, Peindl KS, et al: Extended release naltrexone injection is performed in the majority of opioid dependent patients receiving outpatient induction: a very low dose naltrexone and buprenorphine open label trial. Drug Alcohol Depend 138:83–88, 2014 24602363

Mariani JJ, Sullivan MA, Bisaga A, et al: Naltrexone-induced protracted opioid withdrawal symptoms. Presented at the College on Problems of Drug Dependence 71st Annual Scientific Meeting, Reno/Sparks, NV, June 20–25, 2009

McGovern MP, Lambert-Harris C, Gotham HJ, et al: Dual diagnosis capability in mental health and addiction treatment services: an assessment of programs across multiple state systems. Adm Policy Ment Health 41(2):205–214, 2014 23183873

Minami M, Satoh M: Molecular biology of the opioid receptors: structures, functions and distributions. Neurosci Res 23(2):121–145, 1995 8532211

Peachey JE, Lei H: Assessment of opioid dependence with naloxone. Br J Addict 83(2):193–201, 1988 3345396

Raby WN, Carpenter KM, Rothenberg J, et al: Intermittent marijuana use is associated with improved retention in naltrexone treatment for opiate-dependence. Am J Addict 18(4):301–308, 2009 19444734

Smedslund G, Berg RC, Hammerstrøm KT, et al: Motivational interviewing for substance abuse. Cochrane Database Syst Rev (5):CD008063, 2011 21563163

Smyth BP, Barry J, Keenan E, et al: Lapse and relapse following inpatient treatment of opiate dependence. Ir Med J 103(6):176–179, 2010 20669601

Sordo L, Barrio G, Bravo MJ, et al: Mortality risk during and after opioid substitution treatment: systematic review and meta-analysis of cohort studies. BMJ 357:j1550, 2017 28446428

Stotts AL, Dodrill CL, Kosten TR: Opioid dependence treatment: options in pharmacotherapy. Expert Opin Pharmacother 10(11):1727–1740, 2009 19538000

Strang J, McCambridge J, Best D, et al: Loss of tolerance and overdose mortality after inpatient opiate detoxification: follow up study. BMJ 326(7396):959–960, 2003 12727768

Substance Abuse and Mental Health Services Administration: Health care systems and substance use disorders, in Facing Addiction in America: The Surgeon General's Report on Alcohol, Drugs, and Health. U.S. Department of Health and Human Services, 2016. Available at: https:// www.ncbi.nlm.nih.gov/books/NBK424848/. Accessed April 3, 2018.

Sullivan MA, Bisaga A, Pavlicova M, et al: Long-acting injectable naltrexone induction: a randomized trial of outpatient opioid detoxification with naltrexone versus buprenorphine. Am J Psychiatry 174:459–467, 2017 28068780

Timko C, Schultz NR, Cucciare MA, et al: Retention in medication-assisted treatment for opiate dependence: a systematic review. J Addict Dis 35(1):22–35, 2016 26467975

Uebelacker LA, Bailey G, Herman D, et al: Patients' beliefs about medications are associated with stated preference for methadone, buprenorphine, naltrexone, or no medication-assisted therapy following inpatient opioid detoxification. J Subst Abuse Treat 66:48–53, 2016 27211996

Wesson DR, Ling W: The Clinical Opiate Withdrawal Scale (COWS). J Psychoactive Drugs 35(2):253–259, 2003 12924748

Wesson DR, Ling W, Jara G: Buprenorphine in pharmacotherapy of opioid addiction: Implementation in office-based medical practice, in Translating the Experience of Clinical Trials Into Clinical Practice, Edited by Committee on Treatment of Opioid Dependence. San Francisco, CA, California Society of Addiction Medicine, 1999

White JM, Irvine RJ: Mechanisms of fatal opioid overdose. Addiction 94(7):961–972, 1999 10707430

Winstock AR, Lintzeris N, Lea T: "Should I stay or should I go?" Coming off methadone and buprenorphine treatment. Int J Drug Policy 22(1):77–81, 2011 20956077

World Health Organization: Guidelines for the Psychosocially Assisted Pharmacological Treatment of Opioid Dependence. Geneva, World Health Organization, 2009. Available at: http://www.who.int/substance_abuse/publications/opioid_dependence_guidelines.pdf. Accessed April 3, 2018.

10

Medication-Assisted Treatment for Opioid Use Disorder

Leslie Marino, M.D., M.P.H.
Sarah Oreck, M.D., M.S.
Samuel Kolander, M.D.

Clinical Vignette: Jonathan's Use of Medication-Assisted Treatment to Support His Recovery

Jonathan is a 29-year-old man who is presenting to a general adult psychiatrist for the first time to explore options for medication-assisted treatment (MAT) for opioid use disorder (OUD). At age 13, he began smoking marijuana with his friends, "to be cool." Around age 17, he started hanging out in clubs in New York City, experimenting with many different drugs, including ketamine, ecstasy, cocaine and other stimulants, Xanax (alprazolam), and Klonopin (clonazepam). He also tried opioids for the first time, both OxyContin (oxycodone extended-release tablets) and Vicodin (hydrocodone and acetaminophen). He states that although he always found the other drugs "fun," the first time he took an opioid he felt a sense of "calm euphoria" that he had never experienced before. His use quickly escalated to upward of 20–30 pills per day. He was struggling in school, skipping classes, lying to his parents, stealing money, and engaging in other illegal activity to get more pills.

In his early 20s, he was in and out of various detoxification and re-habilitation programs, including one long-term residential program for 3 months. His longest period of abstinence after completing a rehab program was 3 months. When he turned 23, he decided to move to California, hoping to "start over." He maintained abstinence from opi-oids for nearly 2 years before relapsing to pills and eventually trying in-travenous hydromorphone. He returned home to New York to live with his family and found easy access to heroin. He started using 10–15 bags of heroin intravenously daily until he experienced an accidental over-dose and was sent to a detox program for 5 days. He refused rehab after that, saying, "I've been through it many times." In detox, he was given buprenorphine for withdrawal symptoms and then tapered off, but he found that he felt good when taking the buprenorphine and wanted to explore options for maintenance treatment. His family is very support-ive, but they are also worried about his recent overdose and the risk of overdose and death on "another drug" (buprenorphine).

The psychiatrist completes a full psychiatric evaluation, including a thorough review of substance use history, current substance use, and medical history and a risk assessment. She asks about Jonathan's social support, housing, and employment status, and explores what his motiva-tion for treatment is and whether he is engaged in other psychosocial treatments for his OUD. The psychiatrist conducts a urine toxicology test in the office and also performs a Clinical Opiate Withdrawal Scale (COWS; Wesson and Ling 2003) assessment to determine whether or not Jonathan is in active withdrawal. After discussing the options for MAT, including buprenorphine, methadone, and naltrexne, and risks and benefits of each, the psychiatrist and Jonathan agree to a trial of buprenorphine/naloxone sublingual film with a plan to complete a home induction given that he is not currently in withdrawal and still has opioids in his system.

This vignette demonstrates how clinicians should approach and eval-uate patients for MAT in an office-based setting. Psychiatrists treating patients with OUD may have the following specific questions, which will be answered in this chapter: How does an individual's (past and current) experience with substance use affect MAT decision making and manage-ment? How does an individual's motivation for treatment and engage-ment in psychosocial treatments for substance use disorders (SUDs) affect MAT decision making and management? What are the different options for MAT? How do they work, and which options are best suited to which individuals? What are the risks for patients? What are the chal-lenges associated with MAT? Are there any special considerations?

Introduction

Medication-assisted treatment, the use of U.S. Food and Drug Administration (FDA)–approved medications for the treatment of OUD in combination with psychosocial therapies, is an effective yet underutilized approach for the treatment of opioid addiction. Medication options include full opioid receptor agonists (methadone), partial opioid receptor agonists (buprenorphine with or without naloxone), and opioid receptor antagonists (oral and extended-release naltrexone) (Table 10–1). In numerous studies, MAT has been demonstrated to be effective in reducing illicit opioid use, reducing transmission of human immunodeficiency virus (HIV) and hepatitis C virus (HCV), reducing criminality, and decreasing opioid overdose deaths (Center for Substance Abuse Treatment 2005). Despite MAT's effectiveness, the rates of adoption by providers and rates of use by individuals with OUD remain low. Among Substance Abuse and Mental Health Services Administration (SAMHSA)–certified addiction treatment centers and opioid treatment programs, the proportion providing any buprenorphine services increased from 11% in 2006 to 27% in 2016, while the proportion providing injectable extended-release naltrexone (XR-naltrexone) rose from 10% in 2012 to 21% in 2016 (Substance Abuse and Mental Health Services Administration 2017). Of clients with OUD in all treatment settings (inpatient, outpatient, hospital, residential, etc.), the proportion receiving methadone was 30% in 2016, but only 5% of clients received buprenorphine and 1% received XR-naltrexone (Substance Abuse and Mental Health Services Administration 2018) (Figure 10–1). Challenges to expanding access include federal and state regulations, funding for MAT, and stigma toward MAT from policy makers, providers, families, and patients (Jones et al. 2015).

The decision to begin MAT with a patient is based on many factors and should be based on shared decision making between medical providers and patients. Initial steps include screening and assessment of the patient for OUD and clarifying the scope of the problem and the resources in the patient's life to manage it. When considering treatment, providers must also give consideration to the treatment setting and level of intensity, based on the patient's preferences; history; medical or psychiatric comorbidities, if any; and readiness to change. A thorough discussion of the various options for MAT should occur, including the risks, benefits, and alternatives of each. Once patients are stabilized and in a maintenance

TABLE 10–1. U.S. Food and Drug Administration–approved medications for opioid addiction treatment

Product	Formulations	Receptor pharmacology	DEA schedule	Treatment settings
Methadone	Oral solution	Full μ opioid agonist	II	OTP
	Liquid concentrate			
	Tablet/diskette powder			
Buprenorphine				
Subutex	Sublingual tablet	Partial μ opioid agonist	III	Physician's office, OTP, or other health care setting
Probuphine	Subdermal implant			
Sublocade	Extended-release subcutaneous injection			
Buprenorphine-naloxone				
Suboxone	Sublingual film	Partial μ opioid agonist– μ opioid antagonist	III	Physician's office, OTP, or other health care setting
Zubsolv	Sublingual tablet			
Naltrexone				
ReVia	Oral tablet	μ Opioid antagonist	Not scheduled	Physician's office, OTP, or other health care setting
Vivitrol	Extended-release intramuscular injection			

Note.   DEA=U.S. Drug Enforcement Administration; OTP=opioid treatment program.

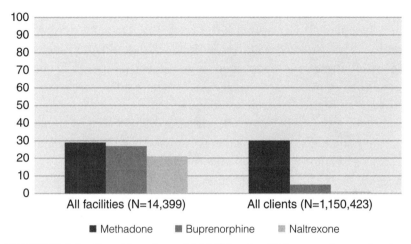

FIGURE 10–1. Uptake of MAT by facilities and uptake by clients in various addiction treatment settings, 2016.

MAT=medication-assisted treatment.

phase of MAT, providers need to continue to assist the patients with other areas of life—including psychiatric, medical, family, employment, financial, and legal issues—to help them achieve full recovery. These practices highlight the importance of ongoing psychosocial treatments in combination with MAT to help patients achieve treatment goals and maintain abstinence (Center for Substance Abuse Treatment 2004).

In this chapter, we review the pharmacology of the most commonly prescribed medications for OUD, as well as the effectiveness of these medications and the challenges faced in increasing access. In the final section, we give an overview of the use of MAT in special populations, with a focus on those in the criminal justice system, women, and adolescents and young adults.

Methadone

History of Methadone and Federal Regulations Regarding Its Use

Methadone was first discovered in Germany in the late 1930s by scientists looking to develop a synthetic opioid to address the country's opium shortage. After World War II, the novel compound, its patent, and research were seized by the United States, and it was eventually brought to market in the United States in 1947 as an analgesic under the brand name Dolphine. It was not until the 1960s that Drs. Dole, Nyswander, and Kreek at Rockefeller University in New York City began studying the use of long-acting opioid agonists as a treatment for OUD and suggested that opioid addiction, specifically heroin addiction, was a brain disease with behavioral manifestations and not a result of a personality disorder or criminal behavior. Despite decades of studies documenting the safety and efficacy of methadone pharmacotherapy, strict federal regulations and stigma prevented widespread implementation of maintenance treatment for opioid addiction (Kreek 2000).

The FDA approved methadone for use in opioid addiction in 1972 with unprecedented regulations under the categories of Investigational New Drug Application and New Drug Application. The regulations specified which patients would be eligible for methadone treatment depending on duration of drug dependence and outlined strict record-keeping practices, the maximum initial dosages that could be used, the minimum amount of counseling required, and limitations on take-home medications (Jaffe and O'Keeffe 2003). The distribution of methadone for opioid addiction was further restricted to hospital pharmacies and to physicians approved by the FDA and Drug Enforcement Administration (DEA), with annual registration required to dispense medication only within federally approved opioid treatment programs (OTPs) and not in individual outpatient practices. It was not until the Institute of Medicine published its study titled "Federal Regulations of Methadone Treatment" in 1995 and the National Institutes of Health conference on effective medical treatment of opiate addiction in 1997 that significant changes were made to the original FDA regulations on methadone prescribing (Center for Substance Abuse Treatment 2005).

In 2001, SAMHSA issued final regulations governing the use of methadone for opioid addiction (Center for Substance Abuse Treatment 2005). These regulations repealed the FDA regulations of 1972 and created a new accreditation-based regulatory system overseen by SAMHSA. The new regulations replaced the FDA's proscriptive rules with best practice guidelines that allowed for more individualized, patient-centered treatment that could also be updated based on expert consensus and medical research (Center for Substance Abuse Treatment 2005). To limit its illicit use and diversion, the DEA continues to subject methadone to increased regulation and monitoring as a Schedule II controlled substance with high potential for abuse and dependence. Further complicating this regulatory system is the fact that the federal regulations in 2001 preserved states' authority to regulate methadone treatment programs (Center for Substance Abuse Treatment 2005). This means that states can establish their own requirements and regulations that do not necessarily parallel the federal recommendations. Therefore, state and local governments can disallow dispensing of any take-home doses of methadone, and they have the ability to determine significant elements of clinical care in methadone programs, as well as the number, size, and location of methadone treatment programs.

Pharmacology of Methadone

Methadone is a synthetic, long-acting μ opioid receptor agonist. It was initially created as an analgesic and can be administered orally, rectally, or intravenously. Oral methadone is available in a variety of formulations, including tablets, oral solution, diskettes, powder, and liquid concentrate (Center for Substance Abuse Treatment 2005). It has an oral bioavailability of 70%–80% and a half-life that varies significantly between individuals but, on average, is approximately 24 hours. This long half-life allows for daily dosing in patients with OUD. It should be noted that the analgesic effects of methadone last only 4–6 hours, and methadone for pain control requires dosing 2–4 times per day (Galanter et al. 2015).

Methadone is mostly metabolized in the liver by the cytochrome P450 (CYP) system into inactive metabolites, and about 10% is excreted unchanged in the urine. Several liver enzymes—predominantly CYP3A4, as well as CYP2B6 and CYP2D6—are involved in the metabolism of methadone. Some of these enzymes play a role in metabolizing other medications, including benzodiazepines, antidepressants, anticonvulsants, and antiviral medications, which if coadministered with methadone could impact the level of methadone in a patient's blood. At therapeutic daily doses, methadone can suppress withdrawal, decrease cravings for opioids, and create a cross-tolerance for short-acting opioids, such as morphine or heroin. This cross-tolerance means that while taking methadone, the patient is unable to experience a high or euphoric effect from shorter-acting opioids. Methadone is a medium-potency opioid, which has a lower affinity than fentanyl and buprenorphine at the μ opioid receptor and roughly equivalent affinity to morphine, but it has a higher intrinsic activity at the receptor than morphine. As such, methadone's sustained activity at the μ opioid receptor allows for normalization of many of the physiological disturbances resulting from repeated intoxication and withdrawal cycles with short-acting opioids, including profound disruption of the stress-responsive hypothalamic-pituitary-adrenal (HPA) axis (Center for Substance Abuse Treatment 2005).

In addition to producing analgesia, methadone can produce sedation, respiratory depression, miosis or constriction of the pupils, nausea, vomiting, constipation, itching, flushing, and sweating, effects that can be more pronounced in individuals who are not dependent on opioids (Galanter et al. 2015). Some other common side effects include insomnia, early morning awakening, and decreased libido and sexual performance (Center for Substance Abuse Treatment 2005). There is some evidence that methadone, especially at high doses, can prolong the QT interval on the electrocardiogram and increase the risk of a fatal cardiac arrhythmia called torsades de pointes. QT prolongation can be influenced by a patient's age, heart rate, gender, cardiovascular history, and use of other medications; clinicians should closely consider these factors and the need for electrocardiographic monitoring when making clinical decisions about the safety of methadone for a particular patient.

Clinical Guidelines for Methadone

In the United States, methadone treatment for OUD is restricted to OTPs that are federally and locally regulated. In addition to dispensing methadone, these clinics provide a variety of services, including counseling, urine testing, primary medical and psychiatric care, and even vocational training. Liquid methadone diluted with flavored juice or water is commonly dispensed at these facilities because it is less subject to diversion and provides dosing flexibility through a computer-assisted dispensing pump system (Center for Substance Abuse Treatment 2005). Patients attend the clinic on a daily basis to receive their dose of methadone and are supervised by clinic staff while taking the medication to further deter diversion.

Admission criteria for OTPs became more inclusive with the revision of the regulations by SAMHSA in 2001. According to the most recent federal regulation criteria for admission to methadone maintenance programs, it must be determined "using accepted medical criteria such as those listed in the *Diagnostic and Statistical Manual for Mental Disorders* (DSM-IV) that the person is addicted to an opioid drug, and that the person became addicted at least one year before admission for treatment" (Substance Abuse and Mental Health Services Administration 2018). Further, the patient must be voluntarily entering treatment and must sign a written consent to treatment. Maintenance treatment for persons under age 18 years requires two documented unsuccessful attempts at short-term medical detoxification or drug-free treatment within a 12-month period, and a parent or legal guardian must sign consent to treatment. Exceptions to these admission criteria include patients released from a penal institution within the past 6 months with a documented history of OUD, pregnant patients, and previously treated patients within 2 years of discharge from a methadone maintenance program. A physician may waive the requirement for a 1-year history of addiction to opioids if clinically appropriate (Substance Abuse and Mental Health Services Administration 2018).

Phases of treatment include induction, stabilization, and maintenance. The induction phase is the 24- to 48-hour period after the initial dose of methadone is administered. The typical starting dose of methadone is 20–30 mg, with a possible addition of 5–10 mg depending on symptoms of withdrawal in the first 2–3 hours after the initial dose is given (Galanter et al. 2015). Federal regulations stipulate that the total first-day dose should be limited to 40 mg unless a physician clearly documents that this dose was insufficient to suppress opioid withdrawal symptoms (Center for Substance Abuse Treatment 2005). During stabilization, the second phase of treatment, the patient's optimal methadone dose is determined. Dosing increases should be limited to 5–10 mg every 3–4 days and should never occur more frequently than every 2 days (Galanter et al. 2015). Serum levels of methadone can accumulate over several days, putting the patient at risk for sedation and, in rare cases, overdose if the dose is increased too rapidly. Some illicit opioid use may occur during this time, but the trend should be toward reduction in use and engagement in treatment. The final phase is the maintenance period, in which a stable dose of methadone is administered, there is no concurrent illicit opioid use, and other drug use or psychosocial stressors are being adequately addressed (Galanter et al. 2015). Maintenance doses are generally between 80 and 120 mg/day, although some patients respond to smaller or larger doses. Methadone dosing should be personalized to the individual patient and meet several important criteria: prevention of opioid withdrawal for 24 hours, elimination of drug craving, blockade of euphoric effects of self-administered opioids, tolerance for the side effects of the medication so that patients can function normally, and tolerance for most of the medication's analgesic effects.

Initially, the patient is required to attend the clinic 6 or 7 days per week. On days when the OTP is closed, the patient is allowed one take-home or unsupervised dose. Patients also can earn increasing privileges for take-home doses, beyond those permitted when the clinic is closed, through regular attendance, negative urine toxicology screens, absence of recent criminal activity, greater length of time in the program, and assurance of safe storage space of take-home doses. After 2 years of continuous treatment and evidence of stability, it is possible for patients to receive a 1-month's supply of take-home medications and visit the OTP monthly.

Effectiveness of Methadone

Many studies have demonstrated the efficacy of methadone treatment measured through treatment retention rates and toxicology screening for illicit opioids. Mattick and colleagues (2009) performed a systematic review of randomized controlled clinical trials of methadone maintenance treatment compared with either placebo maintenance or other nonpharmacological therapy for opioid dependence. Eleven studies met inclusion criteria for the review; all were randomized and two were double-blind, with a total of 1,969 participants. The researchers found that methadone was significantly more effective than nonpharmacological methods in retaining patients in treatment and in decreased heroin use both by self-report and by urine/hair analysis. Another large review found evidence for decreased HIV risk behaviors, mortality, and criminality in patients on methadone maintenance treatment compared with placebo or nonpharmacological interventions (Fullerton et al. 2014).

The California Department of Alcohol and Drug Programs published a large-scale study in 1994 on the effectiveness, benefits, and costs of substance abuse treatment in California (Gerstein et al. 1994). In that report, patients on methadone maintenance showed significant reductions in criminal activity (down 84%) and drug selling (down 86%), as well as decreased health care utilization, with the greatest reduction in number of days of hospitalization (down 58%). Moreover, methadone treatment was found to be one of the most cost-effective substance abuse treatments in California, providing savings of $3–$4 for every dollar spent.

Regulatory Challenges in Increasing Access to Methadone in the Community

The uniquely stringent federal, state, and local regulations on methadone exacerbate the already existing stigma around drug use and harm reduction models for SUDs in the United States. The requirement for methadone to be dispensed in specialized OTPs or inpatient hospitals restricts its potential use to specific geographic locations and populations. In fact, while rural areas are currently seeing the greatest increases in individuals with OUD, a large proportion of methadone programs are in urban settings (Center for Substance Abuse Treatment 2005). Further, treatment at OTPs may not be acceptable for patients who work full time, are primary caretakers, or desire a greater level of privacy in their treatment. An additional challenge is the limited availability of slots within the OTPs, which have been unable to meet the growing demand. Federal restrictions limit methadone prescribing to physicians who are registered annually with the DEA and who work in specific settings, which limits methadone prescribing to specialized addiction psychiatry or addiction medicine practitioners. These restrictions keep the prescribing of methadone for OUD outside mainstream medical practice and out of most medical school curricula. The lack of education early in medical training contributes to misperceptions and stigma around methadone use even within the medical community.

To combat stigma and discrimination, methadone patients and advocates formed the National Alliance for Methadone Advocates (Joseph et al. 2000), now known as the National Alliance for Medication Assisted Recovery (www.methadone.org). To harness the potential life-saving benefits of this MAT option, methadone must become more acceptable to patients with OUD. Moreover, education and advocacy within the medical field and in the general public are still needed to decrease the stigma around methadone maintenance treatment and to increase its use.

Buprenorphine

History of Buprenorphine and the Federal Regulations Guiding its Use in Office-Based Settings

Buprenorphine was developed in 1966 by researchers at Reckitt & Colman (later known as Reckitt Benckiser) who were looking for safer opioid compounds for analgesia. Buprenorphine's efficacy for treatment of addiction was tested in the 1970s at the Addiction Research Center in Lexington, Kentucky, among federal inmates at a prison. In 1978, Don Jasinski, a researcher at the Addiction Research Center, published a landmark paper delineating the potential use of buprenorphine as a treatment for opioid addiction (Jasinski et al. 1978); despite these findings, it took nearly three decades for buprenorphine to receive FDA approval for the treatment of OUD. The medication faced many challenges, including scheduling issues, reluctance of pharmaceutical companies to take on addiction medicine, concerns about diversion and abuse, and restrictive addiction treatment systems (Campbell and Lovell 2012). Subutex (buprenorphine) and Suboxone (a combination of buprenorphine and naloxone in a 4:1 ratio in a sublingual film) were approved by the FDA in 2002, 2 years after passage of the Drug Addiction Treatment Act of 2000 (DATA 2000; P.L. 106-310), which allowed physicians to prescribe FDA-approved, DEA Schedule III, IV, and V narcotics to treat patients with opioid dependence in an office-based setting, despite there not being any approved medications available when the act was passed (Center for Substance Abuse Treatment 2004).

DATA 2000 allowed for physicians to complete an 8-hour training course and request a waiver from the DEA to prescribe buprenorphine for OUD in office-based settings. The initial cap of 30 patients was extended to 100 after 1 year of practice. The Comprehensive Addiction and Recovery Act of 2016 (P.L. 114-198) was intended to increase access to MAT in response to the opioid epidemic by further increasing the patient cap for physicians to 275 and allowing nurse practitioners and physician assistants to prescribe buprenorphine for up to 30 patients (temporarily through 2021) after completing 24 hours of training and similarly applying for a waiver from the DEA (Substance Abuse and Mental Health Services Administration 2018).

Pharmacology of Buprenorphine

Buprenorphine is a thebaine (opioid alkaloid derived from the poppy plant) derivative that has been used for decades as an analgesic in many countries. It is a partial agonist that has a very high affinity at the μ opioid receptor. It is more potent than morphine at low doses and displaces morphine, methadone, and other full opioid agonists from opioid receptors. Owing to its high affinity, it also blocks the receptors from binding to other opioid agonists and antagonists, with a dose-related blocking effect against heroin (Comer et al. 2001). As a partial agonist, buprenorphine is described as having a "ceiling effect," in that its maximal opioid effects are less than those of full agonists, and at a certain point, no further effect can be obtained despite continued increase in dose. Generally, this makes buprenorphine alone less likely than full agonists to cause respiratory depression, but its mild subjective opioid effects can aid in patient adherence to treatment, in contrast to antagonists such as naltrexone (Center for Substance Abuse Treatment 2004). In addition to having a high affinity at the μ opioid receptors, buprenorphine has a slow rate of dissociation, which allows it to be effectively dosed at a minimum of 3 times per week (Center for Substance Abuse Treatment 2004).

Buprenorphine is metabolized in the liver by the CYP3A4 enzyme system into norbuprenorphine, and this first-pass effect accounts for the medication's low bioavailability. Given the poor gastrointestinal absorption of buprenorphine, FDA-approved oral formulations come in the form of sublingual tablets or soluble film. Buprenorphine can be abused, although the abuse potential is much lower than that for methadone or other full opioid agonists. Injection of buprenorphine as a method of abuse has been reported internationally (Center for Substance Abuse Treatment 2004). As a way of limiting the abuse potential, sublingual naloxone, a μ opioid receptor antagonist, was added to buprenorphine and marketed under the trade name Suboxone. Sublingual naloxone has poor bioavailability but is highly bioavailable when injected. Essentially, when taken in combination with sublingual buprenorphine, the naloxone component has no effect, but if the combination were to be injected, the naloxone would block opioid receptors from exerting buprenorphine's effect.

An injectable buprenorphine implant was approved by the FDA in 2016 for the treatment of OUD under the brand name Probuphine. It is composed of a polymeric matrix of ethylene vinyl acetate and buprenorphine in the form of four implantable rods that are placed subdermally and deliver approximately 80 mg at a measured rate over 6 months. The implants have demonstrated observed steady-state blood levels of buprenorphine in patients after 21 days (Barnwal et al. 2017). Candidates for Probuphine must be stably maintained on 8 mg or less of sublingual buprenorphine for consideration. Sublocade, an extended-release monthly subcutaneous injection of buprenorphine, received FDA approval in November 2017 and is also indicated for individuals who have been on a stable dose of sublingual buprenorphine for at least 7 days. The monthly 300-mg dose results in steady-state plasma levels of around 2 ng/mL of buprenorphine for up to 1 month and has been shown to fully block the drug-liking effects of hydromorphone in clinical studies (Nasser et al. 2016).

Side effects of buprenorphine are similar to those of other opioid medications; they include headache, drowsiness, nausea, constipation, sleep problems, depression, anxiety, and dizziness. Buprenorphine in combination with other respiratory depressants, such as alcohol or benzodiazepines, can result in life-threatening respiratory depression (Center for Substance Abuse Treatment 2004), although recent FDA guidance suggests that neither comorbid alcohol use disorder nor benzodiazepine use is a contraindication to buprenorphine treatment or reason to withhold it, but careful medication management is key (U.S. Food and Drug Administration 2017). In addition, other medications that affect the CYP system, specifically CYP3A4, may increase or decrease metabolism of buprenorphine.

Clinical Guidelines for Buprenorphine

Because buprenorphine can be prescribed in office-based settings, the criteria for inclusion are much less stringent than those for methadone in OTPs. Some conditions or circumstances that may preclude individuals from buprenorphine treatment include acute psychiatric risk, significant medical complications, poor response to prior well-conducted attempts at buprenorphine treatment, and multiple previous treatments for drug abuse with frequent relapses (although arguably multiple prior detox episodes with relapses are a strong indication for buprenorphine) (Center for Substance Abuse Treatment 2004).

The three treatment stages for buprenorphine—induction, stabilization, and maintenance—are similar to those for methadone. In the induction phase, the goals of treatment are to successfully cross-titrate the patient from the opioid of abuse to buprenorphine, while decreasing overall illicit opioid use, controlling withdrawal symptoms, and reducing craving. The initial starting dose of buprenorphine generally ranges from 2 to 8 mg, with follow-up doses every 2–3 hours as needed, depending on symptoms. The dose is titrated over the next few days to meet the goals of this phase. The maximum dose on the first day should not exceed 8–12 mg; the second day, 16 mg; and for the overall induction phase, 32 mg (Center for Substance Abuse Treatment 2004). Although it is recommended to give the initial dose in the office and observe the patient for a few hours afterward, home induction protocols have been developed and demonstrated to be feasible and safe (Lee et al. 2014). Unlike with methadone, treatment with buprenorphine can cause a precipitated opioid withdrawal syndrome in individuals who are opioid dependent when opioids are still present at the receptors (Center for Substance Abuse Treatment 2004). Adequate assessment of objective signs of opioid withdrawal symptoms prior to initiation of the first dose can help to reduce this risk. Use of validated tools such as the Clinical Opiate Withdrawal Scale (COWS; Wesson and Ling 2003) can assist providers in making the assessment. The main goals of the stabilization phase are to eliminate use of illicit opioids and reduce craving. This may require 1–2 months and doses up to 32 mg/day. As with any treatment, the ideal dose is the lowest dose that results in good effect with minimal side effects. There may be many dose adjustments during this phase, and it is recommended that patients be seen at least weekly. In the maintenance phase, just as with methadone, there are no formal scientific guidelines for the length of time that patients should maintain treatment with buprenorphine, and continuation depends on treatment effectiveness and patient preference.

Effectiveness of Buprenorphine

Many studies have established the effectiveness of buprenorphine in comparison with placebo and methadone. A Cochrane Review from 2014 summarized findings from 31 clinical trials to evaluate buprenorphine maintenance compared with placebo and methadone maintenance for OUD (Mattick et al. 2014). Overall, the review found buprenorphine to be an effective treatment for OUD, especially at medium and higher doses, and generally safe with few adverse events. Buprenorphine improved treatment retention compared with placebo but had mixed results when compared with methadone. At fixed medium or high doses, buprenorphine performs similarly to methadone on outcomes related to treatment retention and use of illicit opioids. In addition, treatment with buprenorphine has also been shown to be effective in reducing risks for both HIV and HCV infection among injection drug users, similar to methadone (Kraus et al. 2011). Several studies have examined the public health impact of buprenorphine on overdose deaths. In Baltimore,

Maryland, researchers demonstrated a significant association between treatment with buprenorphine and reduction in heroin overdose deaths from 2003 to 2009 after controlling for heroin purity and number of patients receiving methadone (Schwartz et al. 2013).

Research has also explored the effectiveness of induction of buprenorphine in various medical settings with linkage to outpatient treatment. At Yale University in New Haven, Connecticut, researchers conducted a randomized controlled trial with three arms: 1) emergency department (ED) initiation of buprenorphine including a brief motivational intervention and linkage to outpatient treatment, 2) only a referral to treatment (usual care), and 3) brief intervention plus referral to treatment. The main outcome measure was engagement in addiction treatment at 30 days. Those who received buprenorphine in the ED were more likely to be engaged in treatment at 30 days (78%) compared with those who received only a referral to treatment (37%) or a brief intervention plus referral to treatment (45%) (D'Onofrio et al. 2015). In the STOP (Suboxone Transition to Opiate Program) trial, Liebschutz et al. (2014) randomly assigned opioid-dependent patients to one of two groups: 1) in-hospital buprenorphine induction, stabilization, and linkage to outpatient care or 2) hospital detoxification without linkage. Patients in the linkage group were more likely to enter outpatient treatment (72%) than were those who did not receive linkage (11.9%), and linkage decreased patients' odds of illicit opioid use during the subsequent 6 months.

Challenges and Innovations in Enhancing Access to Buprenorphine in Office-Based Settings

Despite the effectiveness of buprenorphine in various settings, adoption by providers and OTPs remains low. It is estimated that on average, only 50% of waivered providers prescribe buprenorphine, and most others do so below capacity (Jones et al. 2015). In 2016, only 37% of OTPs and 27% of all addiction treatment programs provided buprenorphine (Substance Abuse and Mental Health Services Administration 2018). Systems-level barriers include limited geographic availability, cost, and provider willingness to prescribe buprenorphine (Jones et al. 2015). In addition, providers cite lack of time, concerns about diversion, low reimbursement rates, patients with addiction being too complex, and lack of access to psychosocial supports as reasons for not prescribing buprenorphine in the office (Jones et al. 2015). Among OTPs there has been greater adoption of buprenorphine for opioid detox compared with maintenance, and it has been hypothesized that market factors and financial incentives may play a role in these differential rates of adoption (Andrews et al. 2014).

Several implementation models have been developed to enhance adoption of buprenorphine in outpatient settings. Project ECHO (Extension for Community Healthcare Outcomes) has employed a telemedicine clinic model to support primary care providers in New Mexico in treating SUDs. The project has greatly increased the number of buprenorphine-waivered providers in the state, particularly in underserved areas, since 2005 (Komaromy et al. 2016). Massachusetts implemented a collaborative care model in community health centers, using nurse care managers initially funded by the state to evaluate for OUD and monitor patients taking buprenorphine. This model has greatly increased access to buprenorphine in community health settings (LaBelle et al. 2016). The Collaborative Opioid Prescribing (CoOP) model developed at Johns Hopkins University in Baltimore, Maryland, links primary care sites with addiction treatment centers (Stoller 2015). The Vermont hub-and-spoke model utilizes OTPs as "hubs" for more complex care and a network of office-based providers as "spokes" when patients have been stabilized on buprenorphine. It has greatly increased the state's capacity to provide buprenorphine treatment (Brooklyn and Sigmon 2017). In addition, a SAMHSA-funded online initiative, the Providers Clinical Support System for MAT (https://pcssnow.org), provides free training and support for physicians, including online and in-person training, webinars, and clinical consultation services.

Naltrexone

History and Development of Naltrexone

Naltrexone is a direct opioid receptor antagonist used in the treatment of OUD. It was originally created by Endo Products (now Endo), a small New York–based pharmaceutical company, in 1963, and then patented in 1967. Shortly thereafter, in 1969, DuPont bought Endo Laboratories, thereby acquiring the rights to naltrexone. In 1972, the Nixon administration–created Special Action Office for Drug Abuse Prevention, which encompassed all federal agencies involved in substance abuse research, asked DuPont for permission to use naltrexone for clinical purposes. The first clinical trials using naltrexone as a treatment for heroin addiction began in 1973, and in 1984 the New Drug Application for naltrexone for the treatment of heroin addiction was approved. Du-Pont marketed the drug under the name Trexan, and it was the first opioid antagonist tested and developed for treatment of heroin addiction.

Studies on oral naltrexone from the 1980s showed that about one-quarter of participants dropped out after a few days and up to one-half of participants dropped out after a few weeks (Mannelli et al. 2011). This high rate of nonadherence was anticipated as early as the 1970s, and during that time, the National Institute on Drug Abuse (NIDA) is-sued six different contracts to begin development of a long-acting in-jectable formulation (Gastfriend 2011). Development stalled over the next 30 years, as the available technology could not produce an effective injectable agent free of the residual solvents needed for manufacturing of the drug. In the early 2000s, in response to the 1994 approval of oral naltrexone for treatment of alcohol use disorder, the National Institute on Alcohol Abuse and Alcoholism joined forces with NIDA to create two grant mechanisms to spur innovation on an injectable naltrexone. Finally, XR-naltrexone, marketed under the trade name Vivitrol by the pharmaceutical company Alkermes, was approved by the FDA in 2006 for alcohol dependence and in 2010 for the treatment of opioid depen-dence (Gastfriend 2011).

Pharmacology of Naltrexone

Naltrexone is a derivative of the opiate noroxymorphone and is a com-petitive opioid antagonist at the μ, κ, and δ opioid receptors. It has no, or insignificantly little, agonist activity. XR-naltrexone is a microsphere formulation that is typically administered as a 380-mg injection in the gluteal muscle once every 4 weeks. There is a brief initial peak con-centration 2 hours after injection, with a second peak occurring about 2–3 days after injection. The serum concentrations of naltrexone then slowly decrease after day 14. A steady-state plasma concentration is reached at around the time the second dose is due.

Oral naltrexone undergoes extensive first-pass metabolism in the liver, with a resulting bioavailability of 5%–40%, and is converted to the active metabolite 6β-naltrexol, an opioid antagonist that likely adds to the therapeutic effect of the drug. The injectable formulation generates significantly less 6β-naltrexol than its oral counterpart due to decreased first-pass metabolism. Half-lives for oral naltrexone and 6β-naltrexol are 4 hours and 13 hours, respectively. The elimination half-life after XR-naltrexone administration for both the drug and its active metabolite is 5–10 days. Naltrexone is predominantly renally cleared, and due to its extensive metabolism, the amount of unchanged naltrexone in the urine is less than 2% of the original oral dose. For both oral and intramuscular formulations, naltrexone is 21% protein bound.

Naltrexone is typically well tolerated by patients and, aside from opioids, does not usually interact with other medications (American Society of Addiction Medicine 2015). Common side effects include nausea and vomiting, myalgias, headache, anxiety, insomnia, fatigue, and, in the intramuscular formulation, reactions at the injection site. There is risk of hepatotoxicity (described in a black box warning in the drug's labeling) if naltrexone is given in excess doses, and caution should be used in patients with liver disease. It is contraindicated in patients with liver failure or acute hepatitis.

Clinical Guidelines for Naltrexone

Before starting treatment with naltrexone, patients must refrain from using opioids and must no longer be physically dependent (American Society of Addiction Medicine 2015). This is because naltrexone can cause severe withdrawal symptoms in patients who have not had adequate detoxification. It is recommended that prior to starting naltrexone, patients stop using short-acting opioids for a minimum of 6 days and long-acting opioids for at least 7–10 days. If it is unclear whether a patient has been adequately detoxified from opioids prior to initiation of treatment, the patient can be given the short-acting opioid antagonist naloxone and then monitored for withdrawal symptoms. Induction procedures for XR-naltrexone are discussed more extensively in Chapter 9, "Opioid Withdrawal Management and Transition to Treatment." When dosing oral naltrexone, clinicians have the option of giving either a daily dose of 50 mg or three doses a week in which the first two doses are 100 mg and the third dose is 150 mg (American Society of Addiction Medicine 2015). The XR-naltrexone formulation is dosed as a standard 380-mg gluteal injection once every 4 weeks. As with all MAT, it is important for psychosocial treatment to be used in conjunction with naltrexone therapy. It is crucial for clinicians to remember that during treatment with naltrexone, patients will have decreased opioid tolerance (American Society of Addiction Medicine 2015). Therefore, if patients discontinue treatment and resume using opioids in pretreatment amounts, they are at an increased risk of overdose, particularly if they are receiving oral naltrexone, which has very low rates of adherence (discussed below). Patients must be informed of this risk, and clinicians should use the intramuscular formulation for maintenance treatment whenever possible.

Effectiveness of Naltrexone

In a Cochrane Review and meta-analysis examining the efficacy of oral naltrexone for opioid dependence, when oral naltrexone was compared with placebo or no drug, there was no statistically significant difference in terms of abstinence, but two studies showed a decreased risk of reincarceration (relative risk=0.47; 95% confidence interval, 0.26–0.84) (Minozzi et al. 2011). Only in subgroup analyses in participants who were mandated to treatment were there statistically significant differences in favor of naltrexone for both abstinence and retention in treatment over a range of 6–9 months of follow-up. The results of this meta-analysis were limited by a 28% retention rate in the included studies, and therefore the authors do not recommend oral naltrexone as a maintenance therapy for the treatment of OUD.

The FDA approved XR-naltrexone for opioid dependence in 2010 based on the results of an Alkermes-funded, multicenter randomized controlled trial. This 24-week study involved 250 participants from 13 different sites in Russia who were assigned to receive XR-naltrexone or placebo. The XR-naltrexone group had significantly more weeks free of opioids relative to the placebo group and had a significantly greater proportion of participants achieving abstinence (35.7%) relative to the placebo group (22.6%) (Krupitsky et al. 2011). Although this study informed the FDA's decision to approve XR-naltrexone, it had several limitations. The study population was quite narrow, with participants being mostly white males; it did not include people with external mandates for treatment; and participants in the study had daily monitoring, which is not typical for many patients in clinical practice. The study also compared XR-naltrexone with placebo, not methadone or buprenorphine.

Two recent trials of XR-naltrexone addressed this latter point and compared XR-naltrexone with buprenorphine; outcomes were reported to be generally equivalent between the two drugs. One 24-week randomized controlled trial investigated differences in opioid relapse among opioid-dependent participants assigned to receive either buprenorphine or XR-naltrexone (Lee et al. 2018). Fewer patients were able to initiate treatment with XR-naltrexone relative to buprenorphine, and when data were analyzed using the intention-to-treat principle, the XR-naltrexone group was more likely to have relapses (65%) compared to those receiving buprenorphine (57%). However, among those who were able to adhere to the study protocols, there were no significant differences in relapse rates between the two groups (Lee et al. 2018). Another study, funded by the National Institutes of Health with medication provided by Alkermes, examined the difference between opioid detoxification, using either oral buprenorphine or oral naltrexone, prior to initiation of XR-naltrexone therapy. The trial found that those participants who underwent naltrexone-assisted detoxification were more likely both to be induced with XR-naltrexone and to receive a second injection of XR-naltrexone 1 month later than were those who received buprenorphine-assisted detoxification (Sullivan et al. 2017). The study authors speculate that this difference may be because those who received the buprenorphine taper had to wait an additional 7 days before receiving their injection of XR-naltrexone, whereas those who underwent naltrexone-assisted detoxification did not have this additional waiting time.

Relatively limited data are available on long-term outcomes of naltrexone for opioid dependence. In 2013, Krupitsky and colleagues published the results from a 52-week extension of the original Russian study (Krupitsky et al. 2011); in the extension, participants in the original placebo group received the XR-naltrexone for 52 weeks, and participants who had received XR-naltrexone for 24 weeks received the injection for an additional 52 weeks. At the end of the 52-week extension, after a total of 18 months, 50.9% of participants had urine samples negative for opioids at all of the monthly assessments (49.3% of the original XR-naltrexone group and 53.2% of the original placebo group). Of the original 126 participants who initially started in the XR-naltrexone group, only 39 (31%) continued XR-naltrexone for the entire 18-month period (Krupitsky et al. 2013). An additional open-label XR-naltrexone study investigating opioid-dependent health care professionals in the United States for 2 years found that only 36.8% of participants received all of the monthly XR-naltrexone injections for the entire 2-year period, but only 4 of the study's 38 participants tested positive for opioids on monthly urine drug screens (Earley et al. 2017). Both studies suggest that XR-naltrexone is safe and well tolerated and that it is effective when used consistently. However, they both show relatively low adherence, likely due to the lack of opioid agonist activity.

Challenges and Limitations of Using and Prescribing Naltrexone

One of the major challenges in using XR-naltrexone for OUD in clinical practice, as demonstrated in most studies, is the large number of patients who stop using the medication. Because naltrexone is an antagonist therapy, it does not have the reinforcing effects of agonist therapies such as buprenorphine and methadone, which may assist with patient adherence. Many clinicians feel that naltrexone is most appropriate for patients who are either highly motivated or who are supervised in adhering to the medication regimen, although the decision about whether to use it should be based on the physician's assessment and patient's preference.

XR-naltrexone is also far more expensive than methadone and buprenorphine. Each XR-naltrexone injection costs about $1,000, whereas methadone typically costs about $150 a month and buprenorphine costs approximately $300–$450 each month (Tabachnik 2015). Also, because there is less evidence for the efficacy of naltrexone relative to methadone and buprenorphine, many prescribers are reluctant to offer naltrexone, which can make it difficult for patients to access it in the community.

There are also select populations and circumstances for which naltrexone poses particular challenges. The medication can only be given to patients who are not presently physiologically dependent on opioids, and this initial detoxification can be difficult for some patients. Because naltrexone is hepatotoxic in excess doses, it cannot be given to patients with acute hepatitis or liver failure. Patients who discontinue naltrexone are at increased risk of opioid overdose, as tolerance decreases during naltrexone treatment. Finally, when patients using naltrexone have acute and severe pain requiring opioid analgesia, they need close monitoring for respiratory depression from high-dose opioids.

Advantages and Disadvantages of Medication-Assisted Treatment

The various forms of MAT have advantages and disadvantages that are important to consider in the evaluation and treatments of patients with

OUD (Table 10–2). Methadone is relatively inexpensive and provides patients with a structured setting and treatment program, but because of federal regulations, it is limited to prescribing only in OTPs, which have limited geographic availability in many states and challenges with capacity and funding. Buprenorphine is much more accessible because of its availability in office-based settings and may be less stigmatizing than methadone, but it requires substantial provider training and can also be diverted. XR-naltrexone is an opioid antagonist without any subjective opioid effects, which may be preferable for some patients. It also allows for monthly dosing, but it is challenging to begin treatment in the community because patients must be abstinent and discontinuation rates are high.

Medication-Assisted Treatment and Special Populations

Medication-Assisted Treatment in the Criminal Justice System

Use of opioids and other recreational drugs is pervasive in the U.S. criminal justice system. Still, many U.S. jails and prisons fail to provide MAT for individuals with OUD despite the fact that when inmates receive MAT while incarcerated, they are more likely to continue their treatment after release (National Institute on Drug Abuse 2017). A study on former prisoners found that 68.6% of inmates who were treated with methadone while incarcerated subsequently sought treatment at methadone clinics in the community. However, only 50% of those who were treated with counseling and referred to a methadone clinic actually received treatment at the community clinic (Kinlock et al. 2007). Treating inmates with buprenorphine while they are incarcerated increases the average amount of time that patients stay in treatment after release (20.3 weeks) relative to those who are only referred for treatment (13.2 weeks) (Zaller et al. 2013). In addition, inmates treated with naltrexone while incarcerated have significantly lower relapse rates while incarcerated compared with inmates treated with counseling alone (National Institute on Drug Abuse 2017).

Pretrial diversion and drug courts are additional ways of getting individuals in the criminal justice system access to MAT, although use of these alternatives varies from state to state. In the diversion model, drug

TABLE 10–2. Pros and cons of medications for opioid addiction treatment

Product	Pros	Cons
Methadone	Daily administration	Can only be dispensed at OTPs, which are limited geographically and have fixed hours of operation
	Additional supports and resources, including counseling and primary care services, available for patients at OTPs	Increased risk of respiratory depression when combined with benzodiazepines or alcohol; can overdose on drug
	Found to be safe in pregnant women	Risk of prolonging QT interval, which can lead to fatal cardiac arrhythmia
	Not necessary for patients to undergo complete withdrawal prior to induction	Significant stigma around methadone use and attending OTPs
	Inexpensive	Diversion and potential for abuse
Buprenorphine	Ease of prescribing in an office-based health care setting	Requires significant provider training, initially and ongoing
	Not necessary for patients to undergo complete withdrawal prior to induction	Prescriber caseload caps (majority of prescribers limited to 30 patients and higher limits often not applied for)
	Can dose less than daily (i.e., every other day)	Diversion and potential for abuse (although less than with methadone)
	Less stigmatizing than methadone	Increased risk of respiratory depression when combined with benzodiazepines or alcohol; can overdose on drug (although less than with methadone)
	Provides moderate subjective effect, which helps with adherence	
	Moderate cost	

TABLE 10–2. Pros and cons of medications for opioid addiction treatment *(continued)*

Product	Pros	Cons
Naltrexone	Blocks opioid receptors for up to 4 weeks while reducing craving	Difficult to start given that patients must be abstinent from opioids
	Monthly dosing easier for patient adherence	High rates of discontinuation
	Preferred in criminal justice settings or after inpatient residential drug treatment	Increased risk of overdose with relapse immediately after discontinuation
		Management of opioid analgesia for severe pain difficult
		Few providers familiar with prescribing and performing injection
		Expensive

Note. OTP=opioid treatment program.

charges are dismissed and guilty pleas are withdrawn for arrestees who complete a drug treatment program. Diversion programs are typically run by the district attorney. A prospective evaluation found that individuals who went to diversion programs had lower rates of reincarceration, and an average of nearly $90,000 was saved over the 6-year study period per participant compared with those who went to state prisons for drug offenses (Belenko et al. 2004). A meta-analysis examining the effectiveness of drug courts found that the rate of recidivism among drug court participants was 38%, compared with 50% for those not in drug courts (Mitchell et al. 2012).

Unfortunately, negative attitudes toward MAT in the criminal justice system play a large role in limiting its use. One study surveyed employees from 50 different criminal justice agencies to determine how their beliefs affected the treatment, or lack thereof, of individuals with OUD (Friedmann et al. 2012). The top three factors cited by employees as influencing their agency's use of MAT were concerns about security, the availability of MAT via community treatment programs, and the agency's preference for treatment without using drugs. Moreover, agencies in the criminal justice system that did not provide MAT rated lack of adequate information, not having qualified staff, concerns over liability, and objections from staff as more important factors than did those agencies that did provide MAT. Agencies that did not provide MAT were also more likely to ascribe to the notion that MAT is replacing one drug with another (Friedmann et al. 2012). It therefore seems prudent to address negative attitudes among criminal justice agencies through education and outreach to expand existing infrastructure that is currently serving only limited populations.

Women and Pregnancy

Women who are pregnant or have young children can potentially face more difficulties seeking treatment both because of lack of child care and because of the fear that they might have their children removed if they are discovered to be using drugs. Attending an OTP 6–7 times per week can become untenable and overwhelming for a woman with young children who is working and taking care of family responsibilities. Office-based opioid treatments, to which a mother can feel comfortable taking her children, provide more flexibility for women in these circumstances.

Pregnancy also presents challenges for women with OUD. The use of short-acting opioids during pregnancy subjects the fetus to dangerous fluctuations between intoxication and withdrawal, which can result in a number of deleterious outcomes, including but not limited to premature birth, stillbirth, and low birth weight. Although there are no approved medications to treat OUD in pregnant women, a comprehensive drug treatment program in which women receive either methadone or buprenorphine maintenance has been found to significantly improve outcomes for such women and their children (Jones et al. 2010). Federal law gives priority to pregnant women for admission into publicly funded substance use treatment programs (Center for Substance Abuse Treatment 2009).

Newborns whose mothers used opioids during pregnancy are at a high risk of a postnatal opioid withdrawal syndrome, called neonatal abstinence syndrome (NAS). NAS has been described as a complex disorder involving the central and autonomic nervous systems and gastrointestinal system, with symptoms that range from mild tremors and irritability to fever, excessive weight loss, and seizures (McQueen and Murphy-Oikonen 2016). It usually occurs within the first few days after birth, but clinical signs may manifest later for infants exposed to opioids with a longer half-life, such as methadone or buprenorphine. Reported cases of NAS alarmingly increased by 300% in the United States between 2000 and 2009 (Centers for Disease Control and Prevention 2017). Methadone treatment during pregnancy has been studied since the 1960s and is considered the standard of care. There is evidence that buprenorphine is comparable to methadone in terms of safety and could result in a shorter NAS (Jones et al. 2010). Recent studies indicate better outcomes with buprenorphine than with methadone, as evaluated by Apgar score, birth length, respiratory distress, and preterm labor (Brogly et al. 2014). Suboxone, the combination of buprenorphine and naloxone, is contraindicated in pregnancy because of the presence of naloxone, an opioid antagonist. Similarly, naltrexone, another opioid antagonist, is contraindicated in pregnancy because it can precipitate opioid withdrawal and result in placental abruption, spontaneous abortion, premature labor, or stillbirth (Galanter et al. 2015). Although there is a small transmission of methadone and buprenorphine to breast milk, breast-feeding is not contraindicated during MAT and should be encouraged, with close monitoring of the infant for any signs of drowsiness, difficulty breathing, or difficulty feeding. Naltrexone and opioid antagonists are contraindicated in women who are breast-feeding.

Adolescents and Young Adults

Despite increasing rates of opioid use among adolescents, few receive treatment with MAT. In a recent study, Hadland and colleagues (2017) found that roughly one-quarter of adolescents diagnosed with OUD were given medication, with the vast majority (almost 90%) receiving buprenorphine over naltrexone. There are numerous barriers to accessing MAT for adolescents, including limited research regarding efficacy, limited training of pediatricians in providing MAT, stigma and misinformation about MAT, and cost/financing (Saloner et al. 2017).

Use of methadone in adolescents is very limited, because federal restrictions require two documented unsuccessful attempts at short-term medical detoxification or drug-free treatment within a 12-month period, as well as parental consent. Naltrexone has FDA approval only for adults age 18 years and older, and although providers, patients, and families may prefer naltrexone in youth as an antagonist therapy instead of an agonist therapy, no research has been published on the use of naltrexone in adolescents; use therefore remains very low. Buprenorphine has FDA approval for use in adolescents age 16 and over, and several studies have demonstrated efficacy in this population, with outcomes including less opioid use and better treatment retention (Marsch et al. 2016; Woody et al. 2008). The American Academy of Pediatrics recently released a policy statement recommending MAT for the treatment of OUD in adolescents (Saloner et al. 2017).

Additional research on the effectiveness of MAT in adolescents is needed, but other, more quickly realized interventions may help enhance uptake of MAT for this age group. More training of pediatricians around screening and assessment for OUD is necessary, in addition to training on the use of MAT. Psychoeducation of families and adolescents regarding MAT may also be helpful to reduce some of the stigma surrounding it. Finally, policy and systems-level interventions may be helpful in reducing cost and ensuring health insurance coverage of MAT for adolescents.

Key Chapter Points

▶ Methadone is a synthetic, long-acting μ opioid receptor agonist that suppresses withdrawal, decreases cravings for opioids, and has cross-tolerance for short-acting opioids. Methadone administration is highly regulated by federal and local authorities, and the medication can only be dispensed at opioid treatment programs, which limits its use to particular geographic areas and populations.

▶ Buprenorphine is a partial agonist at the opioid receptor and an effective treatment for OUD. Federal legislation through the Drug Addiction Treatment Act of 2000 and subsequent laws allows for buprenorphine to be prescribed by doctors, nurse practitioners, and physician assistants in office-based settings after they complete training and receive a waiver from the Drug Enforcement Administration; however, uptake remains low due to many systems- and provider-level barriers.

▶ When used as directed after a period of opioid detoxification, extended-release naltrexone is an effective and well-tolerated medication for OUD that increases the likelihood of opioid abstinence; however, only about one-third of patients adhere to naltrexone for an extended period of time.

▶ Negative attitudes toward medication-assisted treatment (MAT) in the criminal justice system contribute to its relatively low level of utilization in such settings. When MAT is used, patients are generally more likely to engage in treatment upon reentry to the community and have lower rates of recidivism.

▶ Women using short-acting opioids during pregnancy expose the newborn to intoxication and withdrawal cycles and should be encouraged to begin maintenance treatment with buprenorphine or methadone.

▶ There is limited research on the use of MAT in adolescents with OUD, but based on the available knowledge, MAT is recommended as a treatment for adolescents, including by the American Academy of Pediatrics.

References

American Society of Addiction Medicine: National practice guideline for the use of medications in the treatment of addiction involving opioid use. 2015. Available at: www.asam.org/docs/default-source/practice-support/guidelines-and-consensus-docs/asam-national-practice-guideline-supplement.pdf. Accessed November 4, 2017.

Andrews CM, D'Aunno TA, Pollack HA, et al: Adoption of evidence-based clinical innovations: the case of buprenorphine use by opioid treatment programs. Med Care Res Rev 71(1):43–60, 2014 24051897

Barnwal P, Das S, Mondal S, et al: Probuphine (buprenorphine implant): a promising candidate in opioid dependence. Ther Adv Psychopharmacol 7(3):119–134, 2017 28348732

Belenko S, Foltz C, Lang MA, et al: Recidivism among high-risk drug felons: a longitudinal analysis following residential treatment. J Offender Rehabil 40:105–132, 2004

Brogly SB, Saia KA, Walley AY, et al: Prenatal buprenorphine versus methadone exposure and neonatal outcomes: systematic review and meta-analysis. Am J Epidemiol 180(7):673–686, 2014 25150272

Brooklyn JR, Sigmon SC: Vermont hub-and-spoke model of care for opioid use disorder: development, implementation, and impact. J Addict Med 11(4):286–292, 2017 28379862

Campbell ND, Lovell AM: The history of the development of buprenorphine as an addiction therapeutic. Ann NY Acad Sci 1248:124–139, 2012 22256949

Center for Substance Abuse Treatment: Clinical guidelines for the use of buprenorphine in the treatment of opioid addiction (Treatment Improvement Protocol [TIP] Series 40, DHHS Publ No SMA-04-3939). Rockville, MD, Substance Abuse and Mental Health Services Administration, 2004. Available at: https://www.naabt.org/documents/TIP40.pdf. Accessed April 4, 2018.

Center for Substance Abuse Treatment: Medication-assisted treatment for opioid addiction in opioid treatment programs (Treatment Improvement Protocol [TIP] Series 43, HHS Publ No SMA-09-4314). Rockville, MD, Substance Abuse and Mental Health Services Administration. 2005. Available at: https://www.ohsu.edu/xd/health/for-healthcare-professionals/telemedicine-network/for-healthcare-providers/ohsu-echo/addiction-medicine/upload/Medication-Assisted-Treatment-for-Opioid-Addiction.pdf. Accessed April 4, 2018.

Center for Substance Abuse Treatment: Substance abuse treatment: addressing the special needs of women (Treatment Improvement Protocol [TIP] Series 51, HHS Publ No SMA-14- 4426). Rockville, MD, Substance

Abuse and Mental Health Services Administration. 2009. Available at: https://store.samhsa.gov/shin/content/SMA13-4426/SMA13-4426.pdf. Accessed April 4, 2018.

Centers for Disease Control and Prevention: Prescription painkiller overdoses: a growing epidemic, especially among women. CDC Vital Signs, March 23, 2017. Available at: https://www.cdc.gov/vitalsigns/Prescription PainkillerOverdoses/index.html. Accessed November 4, 2017.

Comer SD, Collins ED, Fischman MW: Buprenorphine sublingual tablets: effects on IV heroin self-administration by humans. Psychopharmacology (Berl) 154(1):28–37, 2001 11292003

D'Onofrio G, O'Connor PG, Pantalon MV, et al: Emergency department-initiated buprenorphine/naloxone treatment for opioid dependence: a randomized clinical trial. JAMA 313(16):1636–1644, 2015 25919527

Earley PH, Zummo J, Memisoglu A, et al: Open-label study of injectable extended-release naltrexone (XR-NTX) in healthcare professionals with opioid dependence. J Addict Med 11(3):224–230, 2017 28358754

Friedmann PD, Hoskinson R, Gordon M, et al; MAT Working Group of CJ-DATS: Medication-assisted treatment in criminal justice agencies affiliated with the Criminal Justice-Drug Abuse Treatment Studies (CJ-DATS): availability, barriers, and intentions. Subst Abus 33(1):9–18, 2012 22263709

Fullerton CA, Kim M, Thomas CP, et al: Medication-assisted treatment with methadone: assessing the evidence. Psychiatr Serv 65(2):146–157, 2014 24248468

Galanter M, Kleber HD, Brady KT: The American Psychiatric Publishing Textbook of Substance Abuse Treatment, 5th Edition. Arlington, VA, American Psychiatric Publishing, 2015

Gastfriend DR: Intramuscular extended-release naltrexone: current evidence. Ann NY Acad Sci 1216:144–166, 2011 21272018

Gerstein DR, Johnson RA, Harwood HJ, et al: Evaluating recovery services: the California Drug and Alcohol Treatment Assessment (CALDATA), 1994. Available at: https://www.ncjrs.gov/pdffiles1/Photocopy/157812NCJRS.pdf. Accessed October 15, 2017.

Hadland SE, Wharam JF, Schuster MA, et al: Trends in receipt of buprenorphine and naltrexone for opioid use disorder among adolescents and young adults, 2001–2014. JAMA Pediatr 171(8):747–755, 2017 28628701

Jaffe JH, O'Keeffe C: From morphine clinics to buprenorphine: regulating opioid agonist treatment of addiction in the United States. Drug Alcohol Depend 70(2)(suppl):S3–S11, 2003 12738346

Jasinski DR, Pevnick JS, Griffith JD: Human pharmacology and abuse potential of the analgesic buprenorphine: a potential agent for treating narcotic addiction. Arch Gen Psychiatry 35(4):501–516, 1978 215096

Jones CM, Campopiano M, Baldwin G, et al: National and state treatment need and capacity for opioid agonist medication-assisted treatment. Am J Public Health 105(8):e55–e63, 2015 26066931

Jones HE, Kaltenbach K, Heil SH, et al: Neonatal abstinence syndrome after methadone or buprenorphine exposure. N Engl J Med 363(24):2320–2331, 2010 21142534

Joseph H, Stancliff S, Langrod J: Methadone maintenance treatment (MMT): a review of historical and clinical issues. Mt Sinai J Med 67(5–6):347–364, 2000 11064485

Kinlock TW, Gordon MS, Schwartz RP, et al: A randomized clinical trial of methadone maintenance for prisoners: results at 1-month post-release. Drug Alcohol Depend 91(2–3):220–227, 2007 17628351

Komaromy M, Duhigg D, Metcalf A, et al: Project ECHO (Extension for Community Healthcare Outcomes): a new model for educating primary care providers about treatment of substance use disorders. Subst Abus 37(1):20–24, 2016 26848803

Kraus ML, Alford DP, Kotz MM, et al; American Society of Addiction Medicine: Statement of the American Society of Addiction Medicine Consensus Panel on the use of buprenorphine in office-based treatment of opioid addiction. J Addict Med 5(4):254–263, 2011 22042215

Kreek MJ: Methadone-related opioid agonist pharmacotherapy for heroin addiction: history, recent molecular and neurochemical research and future in mainstream medicine. Ann NY Acad Sci 909:186–216, 2000 10911931

Krupitsky E, Nunes EV, Ling W, et al: Injectable extended-release naltrexone for opioid dependence: a double-blind, placebo-controlled, multicentre randomised trial. Lancet 377(9776):1506–1513, 2011 21529928

Krupitsky E, Nunes EV, Ling W, et al: Injectable extended-release naltrexone (XR-NTX) for opioid dependence: long-term safety and effectiveness. Addiction 108(9):1628–1637, 2013 23701526

LaBelle CT, Han SC, Bergeron A, et al: Office-based opioid treatment with buprenorphine (OBOT-B): statewide implementation of the Massachusetts collaborative care model in community health centers. J Subst Abuse Treat 60:6–13, 2016 26233698

Lee JD, Vocci F, Fiellin DA: Unobserved "home" induction onto buprenorphine. J Addict Med 8(5):299–308, 2014 25254667

Lee JD, Nunes EV Jr, Novo P, et al: Comparative effectiveness of extended-release naltrexone versus buprenorphine-naloxone for opioid relapse prevention (X:BOT): a multicentre, open-label, randomised controlled trial. Lancet 391(10118):309–318, 2018 29150198

Liebschutz JM, Crooks D, Herman D, et al: Buprenorphine treatment for hospitalized, opioid-dependent patients: a randomized clinical trial. JAMA Intern Med 174(8):1369–1376, 2014 25090173

Mannelli P, Peindl KS, Wu LT: Pharmacological enhancement of naltrexone treatment for opioid dependence: a review. Subst Abuse Rehabil 2011(2):113–123, 2011 21731898

Marsch LA, Moore SK, Borodovsky JT, et al: A randomized controlled trial of buprenorphine taper duration among opioid-dependent adolescents and young adults. Addiction 111(8):1406–1415, 2016 26918564

Mattick RP, Breen C, Kimber J, et al: Methadone maintenance therapy versus no opioid replacement therapy for opioid dependence. Cochrane Database Syst Rev (3):CD002209, 2009 19588333

Mattick RP, Breen C, Kimber J, et al: Buprenorphine maintenance versus placebo or methadone maintenance for opioid dependence. Cochrane Database Syst Rev (2):CD002207, 2014 24500948

McQueen K, Murphy-Oikonen J: Neonatal abstinence syndrome. N Engl J Med 375(25):2468–2479, 2016 28002715

Minozzi S, Amato L, Vecchi S, et al: Oral naltrexone maintenance treatment for opioid dependence. Cochrane Database Syst Rev (4):CD001333, 2011 21491383

Mitchell O, Wilson D, Eggers A, et al: Drug courts' effects on criminal offending for juveniles and adults. Campbell Systematic Reviews, 2012. Available at: https://www.campbellcollaboration.org/media/k2/attachments/Mitchell_DrugCourts_Review.pdf. Accessed April 4, 2018.

Nasser AF, Greenwald MK, Vince B, et al: Sustained-release buprenorphine (RBP-6000) blocks the effects of opioid challenge with hydromorphone in subjects with opioid use disorder. J Clin Psychopharmacol 36(1):18–26, 2016 26650971

National Institute on Drug Abuse: Treatment of opioid use disorder in the criminal justice system. May 2017. Available at: www.drugabuse.gov/publications/research-reports/medications-to-treat-opioid-addiction/treatment-opioid-use-disorder-in-criminal-justice-system. Accessed October 28, 2017.

Saloner B, Feder KA, Krawczyk N: Closing the medication-assisted treatment gap for youth with opioid use disorder. JAMA Pediatr 171(8):729–731, 2017 28628699

Schwartz RP, Gryczynski J, O'Grady KE, et al: Opioid agonist treatments and heroin overdose deaths in Baltimore, Maryland, 1995–2009. Am J Public Health 103(5):917–922, 2013 23488511

Stoller KB: A collaborative opioid prescribing (CoOP) model linking opioid treatment programs with office-based buprenorphine providers. Addict Sci Clin Pract 10:A63, 2015

Substance Abuse and Mental Health Services Administration, National Survey of Substance Abuse Treatment Services (N-SSATS): 2016, Data on Substance Abuse Treatment Facilities (BHSIS Series S-93, HHS Publ No SMA-17-5039), Rockville, MD, Substance Abuse and Mental Health Services Administration, 2017. Available at: https://www.samhsa.gov/data/sites/default/files/2016_NSSATS.pdf. Accessed April 4, 2018.

Substance Abuse and Mental Health Services Administration: Buprenorphine waiver management. January 18, 2018. Available at: https://www.samhsa.gov/programs-campaigns/medication-assisted-treatment/training-materials-resources/buprenorphine-waiver. Accessed November 1, 2017.

Sullivan M, Bisaga A, Pavlicova M, et al: Long-acting injectable naltrexone induction: a randomized trial of outpatient opioid detoxification with naltrexone versus buprenorphine. Am J Psychiatry 174(5):459–467, 2017 28068780

Tabachnik C: Breaking good: Vivitrol, a new drug given as a monthly shot, is helping addicts stay clean. The Washington Post, March 13, 2015

U.S. Food and Drug Administration: FDA urges caution about withholding opioid addiction medications from patients taking benzodiazepines or CNS depressants: careful medication management can reduce risks. September 20, 2017. Available at: https://www.fda.gov/downloads/Drugs/DrugSafety/UCM576377.pdf. Accessed January 10, 2018.

Wesson DR, Ling W: The Clinical Opiate Withdrawal Scale (COWS). J Psychoactive Drugs 35:253–259, 2003

Woody GE, Poole SA, Subramaniam G, et al: Extended vs short-term buprenorphine-naloxone for treatment of opioid-addicted youth: a randomized trial. JAMA 300(17):2003–2011, 2008 18984887

Zaller N, McKenzie M, Friedmann PD, et al: Initiation of buprenorphine during incarceration and retention in treatment upon release. J Subst Abuse Treat 45(2):222–226, 2013 23541303

Psychosocial Approaches to the Treatment of Opioid Use Disorder

Karen L. Dugosh, Ph.D.
David S. Festinger, Ph.D.
S. Brook Burkley, M.S.W.

Clinical Vignette: Tim's "Doubling Up" on His Dosage

Tim is a 24-year-old man who recently completed college and is currently living at home with his parents, with plans of finding his own place. He works in the information technology department at a local retail chain and likes to play football with his college friends on the weekends. He sustained a knee injury during one of these games. He put off going to the doctor for a few weeks but eventually sought treatment when the pain did not subside. His family doctor prescribed 1 month's supply of Vicodin (hydrocodone 5 mg combined with acetaminophen 500 mg), with instructions to take one or two every 4–6 hours as needed for his pain, and referred him for X-rays. Tim found that the medication significantly reduced his discomfort. Within 2 weeks, Tim began "doubling up" on his dosage to obtain the same relief that he had ini-

311

tially. After refilling the medication twice, Tim's doctor informed him that she would not provide any more refills, suggested that he begin to use ibuprofen as needed for the pain, and recommended an appointment with an orthopedist. When Tim stopped using the Vicodin, he began to experience symptoms of withdrawal, including anxiety, trouble sleeping, chills, sweating, dizziness, and irritability, because he had developed physical dependence on the opioid medication. To alleviate these withdrawal symptoms, he first took his mother's unused Percocet tablets (oxycodone combined with acetaminophen) and then began buying it on the street. Eventually, the cost of these pills became prohibitive, and Tim moved on to heroin.

During this time period, Tim's functioning in many areas of life began to deteriorate. He stopped engaging in social activities that he once greatly enjoyed and became isolated. His performance and attendance at work began to slip, and he was in jeopardy of losing his job. Tim's parents began to notice this dramatic change in his behavior and knew that something was wrong. After finding a pile of empty bags and syringes in his room, his mother and father confronted him, and Tim admitted that he had developed a heroin addiction. After he initially refused detoxification and treatment, his parents were able to convince him to seek care. He completed a 7-day inpatient detoxification and a course of intensive outpatient psychosocial treatment that included a family-based component. In addition, he regularly attended self-help groups. After achieving a 6-month period of abstinence, he relapsed. This led to some brief periods of treatment and abstinence followed by relapses, and eventually to more sustained abstinence.

Tim's story brings up a number of questions. How can health care professionals address individuals' different levels of ambivalence about and motivation toward changing their lives and entering treatment for opioid use disorder (OUD)? What treatments can help patients correct maladaptive thinking related to drug use, engage in adaptive behaviors, develop effective coping mechanisms, and understand and manage cravings and triggers? What types of effective psychosocial treatments are available for OUD? What can family members and significant others do to engage patients in treatment and improve outcomes? What role can mutual-help groups play in the recovery process? What does the overall course of treatment for OUD look like, and how is it determined?

Introduction

Medication-assisted treatment (MAT) is a first-line treatment for patients with OUD. Regardless of the type of MAT that an individual receives (e.g., methadone, buprenorphine, long-acting injectable extended-release naltrexone [XR-naltrexone]), it is generally recommended that individuals receive an adjunctive psychosocial treatment with the pharmacotherapy (Kampman and Jarvis 2015). The sections that follow provide a review of different types of psychosocial approaches to the treatment of substance use disorders (SUDs) and present evidence for their effectiveness for OUD in particular.

Motivational Approaches

Two of the primary barriers that prevent individuals with SUDs from obtaining and engaging in treatment are a lack of understanding of the need for treatment and poor awareness of the benefits of therapeutic intervention. Poor access to and limited availability of services are additional roadblocks. These factors, combined with the highly rewarding effects of psychoactive substances, prevent individuals in need of treatment from initiating it. Research indicates that a very small percentage of individuals with SUDs engage in treatment. Only about 11% of the 21.7 million people who need SUD treatment actually receive it (Lipari et al. 2016), and only about half of individuals who schedule an initial treatment appointment attend it (Fehr et al. 1990; Festinger et al. 1995; Stark et al. 1990). Furthermore, another 40% of those who attend the initial appointment drop out before their second appointment, and roughly another half drop out before completing what might be considered a therapeutically meaningful dosage of treatment (e.g., 30–90 days) (Festinger et al. 2002; Loveland and Driscoll 2014). These statistics underscore the importance of exploring each individual's readiness for change and gaining an understanding of what can be done to more effectively and efficiently engage and motivate those individuals in SUD treatment.

Readiness for Change

According to the transtheoretical model (TTM) (Prochaska and DiClemente 2005; Prochaska et al. 1992), individuals vary along a continuum in the degree to which they acknowledge that they have a substance use problem and are ready to change their behavior. Individuals in the first stage in this continuum, *precontemplation*, are not even considering changing their substance use–related behaviors. Individuals in the second stage, *contemplation*, have begun to acknowledge that they have a problem and consider the possibility of changing their behavior. Those in the third stage, *preparation* (also called *determination*), have accepted that they have a problem and have begun working toward change. Individuals who are in the process of changing their behavior are in the fourth stage, *action*. Finally, individuals in the *maintenance* stage have achieved, and are working to sustain, healthier substance use–related behaviors, including abstinence. This model has been quite useful in helping therapists and other treatment providers to identify where clients are in terms of their treatment motivation and to develop strategies to move clients along the continuum.

Motivational Interviewing

One of the most widely known approaches to enhancing treatment motivation is motivational interviewing (MI; Rollnick and Miller 1995). MI is a brief, structured strategy designed to help people recognize the potential benefits of behavioral change. Motivational enhancement therapy (Miller et al. 1995) is a manualized variant of MI. According to Miller and Rollnick (2012), the spirit of MI encompasses collaboration between the client and the provider, the provider's acceptance of the client, evocation of the client's own thoughts, and demonstration of compassion toward the client. The core communication skills utilized in MI can be summarized by the acronym OARS: open-ended questions, affirmations, reflections, and summaries. Each of these skills, along with examples, is described in Table 11–1. The four processes or strategies involved in MI are *engaging* or establishing a connection and working relationship between the client and provider, *focusing* or maintaining a particular agenda throughout a conversation, *evoking* or eliciting the client's own motivation for change, and *planning* or developing commitment to change and formulating a plan of action.

Rather than confronting a client with the dangers of drug use or the ways in which the client's behaviors are maladaptive, the therapist using the MI approach seeks to guide the client toward identifying how changing harmful behaviors can help the client achieve what he or she wants in life and, conversely, how current actions prevent him or her from achieving those goals. Therapists using an MI approach can work with the client to discover discrepancies between current behaviors and proximal and distal goals.

MI is typically provided in one to four sessions, with each session addressing a specific behavior for which the client is experiencing some

TABLE 11–1. OARS: core communication skills in motivational interviewing

O	Open-ended questioning	Ask open-ended questions that invite the client to reflect before responding and that provide latitude in how the client may respond.
		How have you been since we last spoke?
		Where do you see this path leading you?
A	Affirming	Recognize and acknowledge the positive, such as the client's self-worth, strengths, intentions, and efforts. Provide support and encouragement.
		You really have been working hard!
		It's so great that you came in today despite the setback that you had this week!
R	Reflecting	Reflect what the client has said.
		It sounds like you are saying...
		You feel like...
S	Summarizing	Pull together and highlight the different pieces of information that the client has provided during the interview and reflect this summary back to the client.
		So, you said that you hope to have a regular job in the next year that will allow you to support yourself. You also indicated that it is important to work on improving your relationship with your wife and children. What else can you think of that you would like to change in the coming year?

Source. Adapted from Miller and Rollnick 2012.

level of ambivalence or reluctance to change. Although MI provides a different conceptual framework from TTM described above, the two are "complementary and compatible" (Miller and Rollnick 2012, p. 35). Unlike TTM, MI is not intended to be a comprehensive theory of change, but it can serve as a practical therapeutic style to assist individuals in the earlier stages of change (i.e., precontemplation, contemplation, and preparation) in resolving their ambivalence about change and moving toward action and maintenance.

MI may be viewed as a form of cognitive-behavioral therapy (CBT, described in the next section) in that it assists the client in 1) resolving ambivalence by identifying thoughts and feelings that cause and maintain maladaptive, unhealthy behaviors and 2) engaging in new, more adaptive thoughts and perceptions to facilitate behavior change. As with most therapeutic strategies, this technique is generally more effective after the client and therapist have developed some degree of rapport and established a positive therapeutic relationship.

MI has been demonstrated to have a generally positive impact on SUDs. A meta-analysis of 59 randomized studies of individuals with SUDs found that MI resulted in a significant reduction in substance use shortly after intervention and at 12-month follow-up (Smedslund et al. 2011). Research support for MI within the context of OUD is more limited, but MI has been shown to be efficacious as an adjunct to MAT. Saunders et al. (1995) experimentally compared the efficacy of MI relative to a psychoeducational session among methadone maintenance treatment clients. Findings revealed that individuals receiving the MI intervention had longer periods of abstinence and fewer opioid-related problems at the 6-month follow-up assessment. Another study (Nyamathi et al. 2011) examined the efficacy of two 3-day MI conditions (individual and group) and a non-MI attention control condition for reducing drug use among methadone maintenance clients. Although no during-treatment effects were found, participants in the two MI conditions reported significantly less past-month drug use at the 6-month follow-up than those in the attention control condition.

In a recent clinical trial, Coffin et al. (2017) investigated the comparative efficacy of a repeated-dose brief MI-based intervention (called REBOOT) versus treatment as usual (i.e., educational information and referrals) in reducing opioid overdoses. Participants ranged in age from 18 to 65 years, met DSM-5 criteria (American Psychiatric Association 2013) for OUD, had experienced an opioid overdose within the past 5 years, and had previously received naloxone kits. Findings indicated that participants assigned to REBOOT were less likely to experience any overdose than participants assigned to treatment as usual.

Chang et al. (2015) examined the utility of an office-based MI intervention to reduce prescription opioid misuse among older adults with chronic pain. In the pre-post study, 30 chronic pain patients who had been prescribed opioids for their pain participated in weekly manualized MI sessions that were delivered over the course of 4 weeks. Findings demonstrated a significantly reduced risk of prescription opioid misuse, decreased substance use, increased self-efficacy, increased motivation to change, and decreased depression both at posttest and at 1-month follow-up.

Cognitive-Behavioral Approaches

Cognitive-Behavioral Therapy

CBT is a widely used form of psychotherapy that focuses on the relationships and interplay between thoughts, feelings, and behaviors. Rather than being a single therapeutic approach, CBT refers to a class of interventions that share the basic premise that psychological disorders and distress are maintained by cognitive factors. The core principle of this treatment approach, as pioneered by Beck (1970) and Ellis (1962), is that maladaptive thoughts and beliefs create and maintain emotional distress and behavioral problems. According to Beck's model, these thoughts include generalized beliefs, or schemas, about the world, oneself, and the future. These schemas lead to automatic thoughts that occur in specific situations.

The primary aims of CBT, therefore, include helping individuals to monitor their thoughts, beliefs, and perceptions; to examine and test their veracity and rationality; and to restructure and/or replace them with more rational ones as a means of improving negative feelings and changing problematic behaviors. The client and therapist work collaboratively to develop constructive ways of thinking that will produce healthier and more adaptive beliefs and behaviors. Typically, CBT also includes structured between-session homework designed to help the client learn to monitor his or her thoughts, feelings, and behaviors and to practice skills learned in sessions. For this purpose, CBT typically relies on a number of structured forms, such as the dysfunctional thought record, the activity schedule, and costs-benefits lists, among others.

One common maladaptive thought process (also referred to as a *cognitive distortion*) experienced by individuals with an SUD is "all-or-nothing thinking." This is essentially the expectation that life events and plans will either work out entirely as planned or will be utter failures (e.g., "I used drugs once again, so I will never succeed in treatment"). For example, clients in treatment for OUD often "slip" and use opioids after a period of abstinence. Someone who engages in all-or-nothing thinking may view this as a complete failure and consequently drop out of treatment and begin using regularly. In this case, the job of the CBT clinician is to help the client realize that such events often happen within the course of treatment and that they do not erase all progress that has been made to this point. For this reason, CBT for SUDs often involves teaching the client to differentiate between a "lapse," which is a brief, one-time slip-up, and a "relapse," which is a full return to the pretreatment, baseline level of drug use. Other cognitive distortions include catastrophic thinking, mind reading, fortune-telling, overgeneralization, and discounting the positive, to name a few (Leahy 1996).

Two very essential components of CBT are functional analysis and case formulation. *Functional analysis* helps the therapist identify all of the factors that may contribute to the client's substance use and develop a working hypothesis about what is sustaining the addiction. It also provides important information about high-risk situations that may trigger a client's substance use and when and how the client should engage in coping skills. The *case conceptualization* or *formulation* is essentially a hypothesis about the mechanisms causing and maintaining the patient's problems; this is used to develop and guide the treatment plan and clinical decisions.

Relapse Prevention

Another key cognitive-behavioral approach for SUD treatment is relapse prevention; its primary aim is to educate clients about ways to reduce the risk of relapse (Cummings et al. 1980). Relapse prevention is a psychoeducational approach that helps individuals learn to identify, anticipate, and prevent a full relapse following a period of abstinence using a variety of behavioral and cognitive techniques. These techniques focus on 1) learning to avoid high-risk situations; 2) identifying triggers, both internal (e.g., anxiety, boredom, depression) and external (e.g., people, places, things), that precipitate lapses and relapses; 3) developing coping skills to assist in dealing with triggers and cravings; 4) establishing and practicing refusal skills to help deal with interpersonal pressures to use; and 5) understanding the difference between a lapse and a full-blown relapse, as discussed above. A recent variant of relapse prevention, mindfulness-based relapse prevention (Bowen et al. 2011), builds on traditional relapse prevention by incorporating mindfulness training to help clients raise their awareness of triggers, monitor internal reactions, and foster more skillful behavioral choices. These practices are also intended to increase acceptance and tolerance of positive and negative physical, emotional, and cognitive states, such as craving, and decrease the need to alleviate the discomfort by engaging in substance use.

Other Adjunctive Approaches

Although restructuring maladaptive thinking through CBT and relapse prevention represent the core cognitive-behavioral approaches to SUD treatment, a number of other related techniques, including problem solving and training, are also important. Problem solving can be a very useful adjunct to CBT. Although a variety of problem-solving models exist, problem solving generally involves training clients to define problems, generate alternative solutions, evaluate the consequences of each potential solution, implement the solutions, and then examine the results. Training in relaxation techniques, including progressive muscle relaxation and deep breathing, is also frequently used in CBT to help clients manage stress while exploring and reframing maladaptive thoughts and beliefs, resisting cravings, and maintaining sobriety.

Research supports the use of cognitive-behavioral approaches for SUDs more generally (e.g., Dutra et al. 2008; Magill and Ray 2009); however, support for the utility of these approaches in treating OUD specifically is more limited. Researchers have recently begun to examine the efficacy of combining CBT with first-line MAT for OUD. For example, Fiellin et al. (2013) experimentally compared the use of primary care–based buprenorphine treatment with or without adjunctive manualized CBT. Findings indicated that the two conditions were similarly effective in significantly reducing frequency of opioid use, suggesting no incremental benefit of CBT over primary care–based buprenorphine treatment alone. Future research should seek to identify what client factors may moderate the effect of CBT for individuals with OUD and how CBT can be leveraged to improve the efficacy of MAT.

Contingency Management

Contingency management (CM) is a behavioral intervention that has been shown to improve outcomes for individuals with OUD (Dugosh et al. 2016; Lussier et al. 2006; Prendergast et al. 2006). It is most often used in combination with other treatment approaches such as MAT,

CBT, and community reinforcement approaches rather than as a stand-alone treatment. CM is based on principles of operant conditioning in which behaviors that are rewarded are more likely to continue and those that are not rewarded are likely to be eliminated (Skinner 1953). According to operant theory, opioid use is a behavior that is maintained due to the reinforcing effects of the drug. When applying CM to SUDs, specific behaviors are targeted, such as providing a drug-negative urine specimen, attending a treatment session, or taking prescribed medications for the SUD. When an individual displays the targeted behavior, he or she earns a reward that serves to reinforce the behavior and increase the likelihood that it will occur in the future. Because these alternative reinforcers are intended to compete with the reinforcing properties of drug use and related behaviors, it is critical that the reinforcer be meaningful to the individual (Bigelow et al. 1981). Reinforcers that have been examined for use with individuals with OUD include take-home methadone privileges (Stitzer et al. 1982, 1992), increased methadone dosing (Stitzer et al. 1986), employment (Silverman et al. 1996a), food (Gruber et al. 2000), services (Tuten et al. 2012), and cash (Festinger et al. 2014).

Two types of CM that have been extensively studied within the context of SUD treatment are voucher-based reinforcement (Budney and Higgins 1994; Higgins et al. 1994) and intermittent reinforcement (e.g., prize bowl method) (Petry et al. 2000). In voucher-based CM (Budney and Higgins 1994; Festinger et al. 2014; Higgins et al. 1994), individuals earn rewards (historically, rewards were vouchers that could be exchanged for goods or services) each time they perform a targeted behavior. The reward or voucher is withheld when the individual fails to perform the behavior. Typically, the value of the voucher escalates with each successive display of the targeted behavior and resets when the behavior is not performed. Often, individuals have the opportunity to earn a bonus when they have performed a prespecified number of consecutive targeted behaviors. Studies of the efficacy of voucher-based CM have generally involved a 12-week reinforcement period.

The intermittent reinforcement or prize bowl method (Petry et al. 2000) was developed to be more cost-effective than voucher-based CM. In the prize bowl method, after individuals perform the targeted behavior, they earn a chance to draw from a prize bowl that contains slips of paper that vary in value. Typically, about half of the slips say "Good job!" and the other half contain varying prize amounts that usually range in value from $1 to $100. Generally, the majority of prize slips are for small prizes (e.g., $1) and a single prize slip is for a jumbo prize (e.g., $100). As in voucher-based methods, the number of draws earned increases with each successive display of the targeted behavior and the number of draws resets when the targeted behavior is not observed.

The efficacy of CM for individuals with OUD has largely been studied within the context of MAT using a range of targeted behaviors, including abstinence from drug use, treatment attendance, and medication adherence (Benishek et al. 2014; Griffith et al. 2000; Lussier et al. 2006; Prendergast et al. 2006). The large majority of this research has been conducted with individuals who are receiving methadone maintenance therapy (Griffith et al. 2000). Findings have demonstrated that CM can be effective in reducing opioid use (Chen et al. 2013; Griffith et al. 2000; Higgins et al. 1986; Hser et al. 2011; Robles et al. 2002). Evidence also points to the effectiveness of CM in reducing concurrent cocaine use among individuals who are receiving methadone maintenance therapy (Festinger et al. 2014; Ghitza et al. 2007; Petry and Martin 2002; Silverman et al. 1996b, 1998). Furthermore, CM has been found to be effective in improving non-drug-use outcomes for methadone maintenance clients, including treatment attendance and medication adherence (Chen et al. 2013; Gerra et al. 2011; Hser et al. 2011). Studies have used a variety of reinforcers, including vouchers, take-home methadone doses, and methadone increases, as well as a number of targeted behaviors, such as urinalysis-confirmed opioid and/or cocaine abstinence and methadone maintenance treatment program attendance.

More recent studies have examined the efficacy of providing CM as an adjunct to other types of MAT. CM has been shown to improve adherence with XR-naltrexone. Two studies (DeFulio et al. 2012; Everly et al. 2011) demonstrated that individuals received more injections and had greater treatment retention when they were granted access to a therapeutic workplace as a reinforcer for receiving an injection than when access was not contingent on behavior. However, no differences in rates of urinalysis-verified opioid use were observed between the two groups in either study.

To summarize, CM is generally delivered not as an isolated intervention for OUD but as an adjunct to other treatment approaches. It has been most extensively studied within the context of MAT for individuals who have OUD. Studies of CM have employed a range of targeted behaviors, including opioid abstinence, cocaine abstinence, medication adherence, and treatment attendance, and a host of reinforcers, such as vouchers for goods and services, access to a therapeutic workplace, and take-home methadone doses. Overall, CM has been shown to reduce drug use, increase treatment retention, and improve medication adherence among individuals with OUD who are receiving MAT.

Family-Based Approaches

Like all SUDs, OUD has a substantial impact not only on the affected individuals, but also on their families and loved ones. Individuals with SUDs often have considerable relationship conflict or distress, which can have a significant impact on recovery and relapse (Emmelkamp and Vedel 2002; Maisto et al. 1995). Similarly, family members often report substantial emotional distress and interpersonal conflict (Kirby et al. 2005). Accordingly, family members can play a critical role in the recovery process by learning how to address relationship issues and motivate behavioral change. Several family-based therapies have been developed to address SUDs, including behavioral couples therapy (BCT) and community reinforcement and family training (CRAFT). Both of these interventions have been shown to be effective in promoting abstinence and improving psychosocial functioning within the context of the family unit. Other family-based interventions, such as multisystemic family therapy (Henggeler 1999) and multidimensional family therapy (Liddle 2015), have been studied extensively within the context of adolescent drug use and are beyond the scope of this chapter.

Behavioral Couples Therapy

BCT (O'Farrell and Fals-Stewart 2000) is a behavioral approach in which the person using substances and his or her partner meet for 15–20 outpatient sessions over the course of approximately 6 months. BCT is based on the premises that 1) partners have the ability to reward one another's abstinence and 2) decreasing relationship distress is a way to reduce the likelihood that a person experiences a relapse to drug use. A goal of BCT is to develop behavioral self-control and coping skills that are necessary to achieve and maintain drug abstinence and improve relationship functioning. In BCT, the couple completes a daily sobriety contract in which the drug user states his or her intentions to not use drugs that day and the partner indicates how he or she will support the partner's efforts. The two record their respective behaviors in a sobriety contract calendar and agree to reserve any discussion surrounding drug use for their therapy sessions. They then review their calendars with the therapist during these sessions, and the therapist verbally rewards the partners for their progress. Through BCT, couples learn to interact with one another in more positive, constructive, and supportive ways that are conducive to achieving and maintaining abstinence.

Research indicates that BCT can be effective in improving outcomes for individuals with OUD (Powers et al. 2008). Several studies examined the efficacy of BCT for men in methadone maintenance treatment who were married or cohabitating with significant others (Fals-Stewart et al. 1996, 2001); in these studies, the men who received BCT had reduced opioid and other drug use, increased relationship happiness, and improved relationship adjustment relative to the men who received individual treatment with no partner involvement.

Community Reinforcement and Family Training

CRAFT (Meyers et al. 1998) is a behavioral approach designed to engage a treatment-resistant individual (called the *identified person*) in SUD treatment by involving a concerned family member (called a *concerned significant other*) in the process. Concerned significant others are typically parents or spouses who reside with or spend a large amount of time with the identified person. The CRAFT intervention is designed to achieve the following aims: 1) engage the identified person in treatment, 2) reduce the identified person's drug use, and 3) improve the concerned significant other's social and emotional functioning. Over the course of approximately 12 sessions, the concerned significant other is trained to interact with the identified person in a way that promotes reduced drug use and increases treatment motivation. Through these sessions, the concerned significant other learns to change the home environment by rewarding behaviors that promote abstinence and withholding rewards when the identified person uses drugs (Meyers et al. 2011). The CRAFT intervention comprises six elements: 1) functional analysis to identify the function of substance use for the identified person; 2) contingency management training in which the concerned significant other learns to reward sobriety; 3) no disruption of the natural negative consequences of drug use; 4) communication skills training to assist the concerned significant other in delivering contingencies (i.e., positive reinforcement for desirable behavior and negative reinforcement for undesirable behavior) and avoiding engaging in confrontational and unproductive interactions; 5) treatment entry training in which the concerned significant other learns when and how to discuss treatment entry with the identified person; and 6) self-care in which the concerned significant other learns to engage in independent positive relationships and activities (Kirby et al. 2017; Meyers et al. 1996).

Studies have demonstrated that CRAFT is efficacious in increasing rates of treatment entry among individuals with SUDs, including those who use opioids (Kirby et al. 1999; Meyers et al. 1998, 2002). Furthermore, these studies found that CRAFT results in improved concerned significant other functioning, including reductions in physical problems, anxiety, depression, and anger. Results from a pilot study (Brigham et al. 2014) suggest that CRAFT can be modified to improve treatment retention for patients who have completed opioid detoxification (i.e., CRAFT for treatment retention [CRAFT-TR]). The CRAFT-TR intervention worked with concerned significant others of identified persons who were in treatment, and concerned significant others were trained to use behavioral principles to increase the identified person's retention in treatment and reduce substance use. The intervention had a moderate effect on treatment retention, significantly reduced the identified person's opioid and other drug use, and was more effective when the concerned significant other was a parent, rather than a romantic partner.

Mutual-Help Approaches

Mutual-help groups, sometimes referred to as self-help groups, are voluntary peer groups that emphasize sobriety and recovery from addiction through in-person or online meetings. These groups include Alcoholics Anonymous (AA) and Narcotics Anonymous (NA); they offer support, fellowship, recovery activities, and one-on-one support to members (Kelly and Yeterian 2008). A mutual-help approach can serve as an easily accessible ancillary service to most SUD treatment modalities. It connects people with others who are in the process of recovery and with sobriety-based activities. Mutual-help groups can serve as a valuable bridge between formal treatment sessions.

In the mutual-help approach, members are encouraged to attend meetings on a regular basis and share personal experiences related to their addiction and recovery experiences. Mutual-help groups typically follow the "12 steps to recovery" model, a set of guidelines to overcome addiction, to achieve sobriety, and to remain abstinent. These steps begin with a person admitting that he or she has a problem that needs to be overcome. Subsequent steps for the individual include, but are not limited to, admitting wrongdoing, asking a higher power to remove personal shortcomings, making amends with those who have been wronged as a result of the addiction, admitting when he or she is wrong, and continuing to work to improve himself or herself. With recovery viewed as a lifelong journey, members may revisit some steps or "work" more than one step at a time.

Despite the widespread use of mutual-help approaches, clinical trials focused on their efficacy for individuals with OUD are virtually nonexistent. Given the assurance of anonymity in these groups, it is difficult to enroll individuals in a clinical trial. For this reason, much of the research is observational and/or correlational in nature and has focused on the relationships between frequency of mutual-help group attendance and outcomes, including perceived helpfulness and rates of opioid and/or alcohol abstinence (Gossop et al. 2008; Kaskutas 2009; Kelly et al. 2013; Tonigan et al. 2003; White et al. 2013). For example, Gossop et al. (2008) found that mutual-help group attendance was associated with increased posttreatment abstinence in residential SUD treatment clients. Similarly, Kelly et al. (2013) found that active mutual-help group involvement resulted in an increase in the percentage of days abstinent for young adults in residential treatment. In a survey study, White et al. (2013) reported that more than 75% of those with OUD who participated in mutual-help groups found the groups to be "very" or "extremely" helpful.

Because of the drug-free nature of the model, individuals who are receiving some forms of MAT are often precluded from attending mutual-help groups. Studies have demonstrated that the use of MAT is often stigmatized within these groups (Ginter 2012; Olsen and Sharfstein 2014). For this reason, it is important that clinicians who are treating individuals with MAT are aware of alternative options, including existing mutual-help groups that are more accepting of these patients, as well as Internet-based support groups.

Determining the Optimal Level of Care

As with any chronic, relapsing medical condition, a one-size-fits-all approach to OUD treatment is inefficient and ineffective and may produce iatrogenic effects. For this reason, it is critical to ascertain the severity of an individual's SUD and identify any other issues that need to be addressed through treatment, including but not limited to psychiatric comorbidity, homelessness and other adverse social factors, acute and chronic medical conditions, and family and/or relationship problems. Following identification of problematic substance use, a comprehensive assessment—such as the Addiction Severity Index (ASI) (Cacciola et al. 2011) or the Global Appraisal of Individual Needs (GAIN) (Dennis et al. 2003)—can be used to identify the optimal level of care for the individual. Table 11–2 describes the different levels of treatment for individuals with OUD at varying levels of severity and at different points within the treatment continuum.

A person who has just begun experimenting with opioids but has not developed physical dependence may be best suited for a prevention-based psychosocial intervention to address drug use and avoid further escalation. Conversely, an individual who has been diagnosed with a severe OUD is likely to be referred to medically managed inpatient services that provide detoxification, followed by MAT initiation in less intensive inpatient treatment and eventually outpatient treatment. Optimally, individuals who are misusing opioids are placed in the level of care indicated by a comprehensive and valid assessment (e.g., ASI, GAIN) and sequentially stepped down as their symptoms and functioning improve. Regular progress monitoring should ensure that individuals continue to receive the most appropriate level of treatment services given their current needs and level of functioning.

Monitoring and Continuing Care

As is the case for treatment of individuals with other chronic conditions, it is critical to monitor the status and progress of individuals engaged in OUD treatment on a regular basis (Goodman et al. 2013; Institute of Medicine 2006). These monitoring activities may pertain to urine drug screens, treatment attendance, and medication adherence. Regular monitoring of progress will alert the treatment provider when an individual is responding to treatment or when the intensity and/or

TABLE 11–2.   Levels of care for opioid use disorder treatment

Level of care	Description
Early intervention	Psychoeducational services designed for individuals at risk of developing opioid use disorder
Outpatient services	Less than 9 hours per week of multimodal treatment including pharmacotherapy; appropriate for individuals living in a supportive environment who are medically and psychiatrically stable and in the action stage of change
Intensive outpatient or partial hospitalization services	Intensive outpatient: 9 or more hours per week of multimodal treatment; appropriate for individuals requiring close monitoring and frequent contact who may lack awareness of their opioid use disorder or be ambivalent about treatment
	Partial hospitalization: 20 or more hours per week of multimodal treatment including direct access to medical and psychiatric care; appropriate for individuals who are at high risk of relapse and have a history of failing intensive outpatient treatment; often serves as a step down from residential treatment
Residential services	Around-the-clock, drug-free environment with professional and/or peer support and multimodal services; appropriate for individuals who have severe functional deficits and require a stable living environment; ranges from clinically managed, low-intensity services to medically monitored, high-intensity services depending on the needs of the patient
Medically monitored/ managed inpatient services	Around-the-clock nursing care, 16 hours per day of counselor availability, and physician services for medical and psychiatric problems; appropriate for individuals with severe functional deficits, cognitive difficulties, and the potential need for care under a physician

Source.   Adapted from Mee-Lee et al. 2013.

type of treatment being provided needs to be adjusted (Brooner and Kidorf 2002; Marlowe et al. 2012).

In addition to tracking these clinical indicators, the provider can administer any of a number of validated instruments at regular intervals to monitor an individual's progress in OUD treatment. Such instruments may be brief (e.g., Brief Addiction Monitor [Cacciola et al. 2013], Treatment Outcomes Profile [Marsden et al. 2008]) or more extensive (e.g., ASI, GAIN). Although they vary in comprehensiveness, these instruments provide an assessment of current functioning across multiple life domains (e.g., emotional status, legal involvement, family and social functioning). Information gleaned from this measurement-based monitoring approach may be used in indicating when treatment and/or services need to be adjusted.

Given the chronic, relapsing nature of addiction (McLellan 2002), it is critical to continue to monitor the patient following the initial episode of intensive treatment and provide aftercare or continuing care (McKay et al. 2005). Continuing care may take many forms, including group counseling, telephonic counseling, brief check-ins, and self-help groups. In a systematic review of the effectiveness of continuing care interventions, McKay (2009) drew three important conclusions regarding effective continuing care approaches: 1) interventions with a longer duration of therapeutic contact were more effective than those with shorter durations; 2) interventions with more active and direct attempts to connect with the individual (e.g., aggressive outreach, telephonic counseling) were more effective; and 3) a significant proportion of individuals do not engage in continuing care, which highlights the need to develop new engagement approaches (e.g., using new technologies, incorporating greater patient choice, ensuring minimal patient burden).

Key Chapter Points

▶ Identifying the extent to which a person acknowledges that he or she has a substance use problem and is motivated to change behavior is essential to making a determination about the best treatment approach.

▶ Motivational interviewing, a nonjudgmental communication style in which the therapist guides the patient to understand the importance of changing behaviors, has been shown to be effective in reducing overall substance use. Within the context of OUD, evidence for the effectiveness of motivational interviewing is less robust. However, when combined with medication-assisted treatment (MAT), it has been shown to reduce drug use, reduce the rate of opioid overdoses, and prevent prescription opioid misuse.

▶ Cognitive-behavioral approaches such as cognitive-behavioral therapy (CBT) and relapse prevention are based on the premise that maladaptive thoughts and beliefs create emotional distress and behavioral problems. These approaches seek to help individuals to monitor their thoughts and beliefs, evaluate veracity and rationality of those thoughts and beliefs, and restructure or replace them as a means to change problematic behaviors. Evidence supporting CBT's effectiveness for the treatment of OUD is limited, but more recent studies suggest that it may be effective when used in combination with MAT.

▶ Contingency management (both voucher- and prize bowl–based methods) is an adjunctive intervention that targets a particular behavior (e.g., urinalysis-validated opioid and other drug abstinence, treatment attendance, and medication adherence). This approach delivers rewards (e.g., vouchers that can be exchanged for goods and services, take-home methadone privileges, access to a therapeutic workplace, cash) when targeted behaviors are displayed. The combination of contingency management and MAT has been shown to reduce opioid and other drug use, increase treatment retention, and improve medication adherence.

▶ Family members can play a key role in the treatment process. Family-based interventions include behavioral couples therapy that involves the individual using substances and his or her romantic partner and the community reinforcement and family training approach for concerned significant others. These interventions have been found to be effective in improving outcomes for individuals with OUD, as well as their partners and loved ones.

▶ Mutual-help groups are recovery-oriented groups in which members share their personal experiences related to addiction and recovery, often following the "12 steps to recovery" model. Mutual-help group attendance has been shown to be positively related to abstinence for individuals with substance use disorders; however, because many mutual-help groups are drug-free, individuals who are receiving MAT may not be accepted into all such groups.

▶ OUD is a chronic, often relapsing, condition. In making initial treatment placement decisions, the clinician needs to conduct a comprehensive assessment to determine the appropriate level of care. Furthermore, regular progress monitoring can help to ensure that individuals are receiving the optimal level and type of services for their current needs and functioning.

References

American Psychiatric Association: Diagnostic and Statistical Manual of Mental Disorders, 5th Edition. Arlington, VA, American Psychiatric Association, 2013

Beck AT: Cognitive therapy: nature and relation to behavior therapy. Behav Ther 1(2):184–200, 1970 27993332

Benishek LA, Dugosh KL, Kirby KC, et al: Prize-based contingency management for the treatment of substance abusers: a meta-analysis. Addiction 109(9):1426–1436, 2014 24750232

Bigelow GE, Stitzer ML, Griffiths RR, et al: Contingency management approaches to drug self-administration and drug abuse: efficacy and limitations. Addict Behav 6(3):241–252, 1981 7293847

Bowen S, Chawla N, Marlatt GA: Mindfulness-Based Relapse Prevention for Addictive Behaviors: A Clinician's Guide. New York, Guilford, 2011

Brigham GS, Slesnick N, Winhusen TM, et al: A randomized pilot clinical trial to evaluate the efficacy of Community Reinforcement and Family Training for Treatment Retention (CRAFT-T) for improving outcomes for patients completing opioid detoxification. Drug Alcohol Depend 138:240–243, 2014 24656054

Brooner RK, Kidorf M: Using behavioral reinforcement to improve methadone treatment participation. Sci Pract Perspect 1(1):38–47, 2002 18567965

Budney A, Higgins ST: A Community Reinforcement Plus Vouchers Approach: Treating Cocaine Addiction (NIDA Publ No 98-4309). Rockville, MD, National Institute on Drug Abuse, 1994

Cacciola JS, Alterman AI, Habing B, et al: Recent status scores for version 6 of the Addiction Severity Index (ASI-6). Addiction 106(9):1588–1602, 2011 21545666

Cacciola JS, Alterman AI, Dephilippis D, et al: Development and initial evaluation of the Brief Addiction Monitor (BAM). J Subst Abuse Treat 44(3):256–263, 2013 22898042

Chang YP, Compton P, Almeter P, et al: The effect of motivational interviewing on prescription opioid adherence among older adults with chronic pain. Perspect Psychiatr Care 51(3):211–219, 2015 25159493

Chen W, Hong Y, Zou X, et al: Effectiveness of prize-based contingency management in a methadone maintenance program in China. Drug Alcohol Depend 133(1):270–274, 2013 23831409

Coffin PO, Santos GM, Matheson T, et al: Behavioral intervention to reduce opioid overdose among high-risk persons with opioid use disorder: a pilot randomized controlled trial. PLoS One 12(10):e0183354, 2017 29049282

Cummings C, Gordon JR, Marlatt GA: Relapse: prevention and prediction, in The Addictive Behaviors: Treatment of Alcoholism, Drug Abuse, Smoking, and Obesity. Edited by Miller RW. New York, Pergamon, 1980, pp 291–321

DeFulio A, Everly JJ, Leoutsakos JM, et al: Employment-based reinforcement of adherence to an FDA approved extended release formulation of naltrexone in opioid-dependent adults: a randomized controlled trial. Drug Alcohol Depend 120(1–3):48–54, 2012 21782353

Dennis ML, Titus JC, White MK, et al: Global Appraisal of Individual Needs: Administration Guide for the GAIN and Related Measures. Bloomington, IL, Chestnut Health Systems, 2003

Dugosh K, Abraham A, Seymour B, et al: A systematic review on the use of psychosocial interventions in conjunction with medications for the treatment of opioid addiction. J Addict Med 10(2):93–103, 2016 26808307

Dutra L, Stathopoulou G, Basden SL, et al: A meta-analytic review of psychosocial interventions for substance use disorders. Am J Psychiatry 165(2):179–187, 2008 18198270

Ellis A: Reason and Emotion in Psychotherapy. New York, Lyle-Stuart, 1962

Emmelkamp PM, Vedel E: Spouse-aided therapy, in The Encyclopedia of Psychotherapy. Edited by Hersen M, Sledge W. New York, Academic Press, 2002, pp 693–698

Everly JJ, DeFulio A, Koffarnus MN, et al: Employment-based reinforcement of adherence to depot naltrexone in unemployed opioid-dependent adults: a randomized controlled trial. Addiction 106(7):1309–1318, 2011 21320227

Fals-Stewart W, O'Farrell TJ, Finneran S, et al: The use of behavioral couples therapy with methadone maintenance patients: effects on drug use and dyadic adjustment. Paper presented at the 30th annual meeting of the Association for the Advancement of Behavior Therapy, New York, November 1996

Fals-Stewart W, O'Farrell TJ, Birchler GR: Behavioral couples therapy for male methadone maintenance patients: effects on drug-using behavior and relationship adjustment. Behav Ther 32(2):391–411, 2001

Fehr BJ, Weinstein SP, Sterling S, et al: "As soon as possible": an initial treatment engagement strategy. Subst Abus 3:180–183, 1990

Festinger DS, Lamb RJ, Kountz MR, et al: Pretreatment dropout as a function of treatment delay and client variables. Addict Behav 20(1):111–115, 1995 7785476

Festinger DS, Lamb RJ, Marlowe DB, et al: From telephone to office: intake attendance as a function of appointment delay. Addict Behav 27(1):131–137, 2002 11800219

Festinger DS, Dugosh KL, Kirby KC, et al: Contingency management for cocaine treatment: cash vs. vouchers. J Subst Abuse Treat 47(2):168–174, 2014 24746956

Fiellin DA, Barry DT, Sullivan LE, et al: A randomized trial of cognitive behavioral therapy in primary care-based buprenorphine. Am J Med 126(1):74.e11–74.e17, 2013 23260506

Gerra G, Saenz E, Busse A, et al: Supervised daily consumption, contingent take-home incentive and non-contingent take-home in methadone maintenance. Prog Neuropsychopharmacol Biol Psychiatry 35(2):483–489, 2011 21147192

Ghitza UE, Epstein DH, Schmittner J, et al: Randomized trial of prize-based reinforcement density for simultaneous abstinence from cocaine and heroin. J Consult Clin Psychol 75(5):765–774, 2007 17907858

Ginter W: Methadone Anonymous and mutual support for medication-assisted recovery. J Groups Addict Recover 7(2–4):189–201, 2012

Goodman JD, McKay JR, DePhilippis D: Progress monitoring in mental health and addiction treatment: a means of improving care. Prof Psychol Res Pr 44(4):231–246, 2013

Gossop M, Stewart D, Marsden J: Attendance at Narcotics Anonymous and Alcoholics Anonymous meetings, frequency of attendance and substance use outcomes after residential treatment for drug dependence: a 5-year follow-up study. Addiction 103(1):119–125, 2008 18028521

Griffith JD, Rowan-Szal GA, Roark RR, et al: Contingency management in outpatient methadone treatment: a meta-analysis. Drug Alcohol Depend 58(1–2):55–66, 2000 10669055

Gruber K, Chutuape MA, Stitzer ML: Reinforcement-based intensive outpatient treatment for inner city opiate abusers: a short-term evaluation. Drug Alcohol Depend 57(3):211–223, 2000 10661672

Henggeler SW: Multisystemic therapy: an overview of clinical procedures, outcomes, and policy implications. Child Psychology and Psychiatry Review 4(1):2–10, 1999

Higgins ST, Stitzer ML, Bigelow GE, et al: Contingent methadone delivery: effects on illicit-opiate use. Drug Alcohol Depend 17(4):311–322, 1986 3757767

Higgins ST, Budney AJ, Bickel WK, et al: Incentives improve outcome in outpatient behavioral treatment of cocaine dependence. Arch Gen Psychiatry 51(7):568–576, 1994 8031230

Hser YI, Li J, Jiang H, et al: Effects of a randomized contingency management intervention on opiate abstinence and retention in methadone maintenance treatment in China. Addiction 106(10):1801–1809, 2011 21793958

Institute of Medicine: Improving the Quality of Health Care for Mental and Substance-Use Conditions. Washington, DC, The National Academies Press 2006

Kampman K, Jarvis M: American Society of Addiction Medicine (ASAM) national practice guideline for the use of medications in the treatment of addiction involving opioid use. J Addict Med 9(5):358–367, 2015 26406300

Kaskutas LA: Alcoholics anonymous effectiveness: faith meets science. J Addict Dis 28(2):145–157, 2009 19340677

Kelly JF, Yeterian JD: Mutual-help groups, in Evidence-Based Adjunctive Treatments. Edited by O'Donohue W, Cunningham JA. New York, Elsevier, 2008, pp 61–105

Kelly JF, Stout RL, Slaymaker V: Emerging adults' treatment outcomes in relation to 12-step mutual-help attendance and active involvement. Drug Alcohol Depend 129(1–2):151–157, 2013 23122600

Kirby KC, Marlowe DB, Festinger DS, et al: Community reinforcement training for family and significant others of drug abusers: a unilateral intervention to increase treatment entry of drug users. Drug Alcohol Depend 56(1):85–96, 1999 10462097

Kirby KC, Dugosh KL, Benishek LA, et al: The Significant Other Checklist: measuring the problems experienced by family members of drug users. Addict Behav 30(1):29–47, 2005 15561447

Kirby KC, Benishek LA, Kerwin ME, et al: Analyzing components of Community Reinforcement and Family Training (CRAFT): is treatment entry training sufficient? Psychof Addict Behav 31(7):818–827, 2017 28836796

Leahy RL: Cognitive Therapy: Basic Principles and Applications. Lanham, MD, Rowman & Littlefield, 1996

Liddle HA: Multidimensional family therapy, in Handbook of Family Therapy. Edited by Sexton T, Lebow J. New York, Routledge, 2015, pp 231–249

Lipari RN, Park-Lee E, Van Horn S: America's need for and receipt of substance use treatment in 2015. Center for Behavioral Health Statistics and Quality, Substance Abuse and Mental Health Services Administration, September 29, 2016. Available at: https://www.samhsa.gov/data/sites/default/files/report_2716/ShortReport-2716.pdf. Accessed April 4, 2018.

Loveland D, Driscoll H: Examining attrition rates at one specialty addiction treatment provider in the United States: a case study using a retrospective chart review. Subst Abuse Treat Prev Policy 9(1):41, 2014 25255797

Lussier JP, Heil SH, Mongeon JA, et al: A meta-analysis of voucher-based reinforcement therapy for substance use disorders. Addiction 101(2):192–203, 2006 16445548

Magill M, Ray LA: Cognitive-behavioral treatment with adult alcohol and illicit drug users: a meta-analysis of randomized controlled trials. J Stud Alcohol Drugs 70(4):516–527, 2009 19515291

Maisto SA, McKay JR, O'Farrell TJ: Relapse precipitants and behavioral marital therapy. Addict Behav 20(3):383–393, 1995 7653319

Marlowe DB, Festinger DS, Dugosh KL, et al: Adaptive programming improves outcomes in drug court: an experimental trial. Crim Justice Behav 39(4):514–532, 2012 22923854

Marsden J, Farrell M, Bradbury C, et al: Development of the Treatment Outcomes Profile. Addiction 103(9):1450–1460, 2008 18783500

McKay JR: Continuing care research: what we have learned and where we are going. J Subst Abuse Treat 36(2):131–145, 2009 19161894

McKay JR, Lynch KG, Shepard DS, et al: The effectiveness of telephone-based continuing care for alcohol and cocaine dependence: 24-month outcomes. Arch Gen Psychiatry 62(2):199–207, 2005 15699297

McLellan AT: Have we evaluated addiction treatment correctly? Implications from a chronic care perspective. Addiction 97(3):249–252, 2002 11964098

Mee-Lee D, Shulman GD, Fishman MJ, et al: The ASAM Criteria: Treatment Criteria for Addictive, Substance-Related, and Co-occurring Conditions, 5th Edition. Carson City, NV, The Change Companies, 2013

Meyers RJ, Dominguez TP, Smith JE: Community reinforcement training with concerned others, in Sourcebook of Psychological Treatment Manuals for Adult Disorders. Edited by Van Hasselt VB, Hersen M. New York, Plenum, 1996, pp 257–294

Meyers RJ, Miller WR, Hill DE, et al: Community reinforcement and family training (CRAFT): engaging unmotivated drug users in treatment. J Subst Abuse 10(3):291–308, 1998 10689661

Meyers RJ, Miller WR, Smith JE, et al: A randomized trial of two methods for engaging treatment-refusing drug users through concerned significant others. J Consult Clin Psychol 70(5):1182–1185, 2002 12362968

Meyers RJ, Roozen HG, Smith JE: The community reinforcement approach: an update of the evidence. Alcohol Res Health 33(4):380–388, 2011 23580022

Miller WR, Rollnick S: Applications of Motivational Interviewing: Helping People Change, 3rd Edition (Applications of Motivational Interviewing Series). New York, Guilford, 2012

Miller WR, Zweben A, DiClemente CC, et al: Motivational enhancement therapy manual: a clinical research guide for therapists treating individuals with alcohol abuse and dependence. National Institute on Alcohol Abuse and Alcoholism (Project MATCH Monograph Series, Vol 2; Mattson ME, series ed). 1995. Available at: https://casaa.unm.edu/download/met.pdf. Accessed April 4, 2018.

Nyamathi AM, Sinha K, Greengold B, et al: Effectiveness of intervention on improvement of drug use among methadone maintained adults. J Addict Dis 30(1):6–16, 2011 21218306

O'Farrell TJ, Fals-Stewart W: Behavioral couples therapy for alcoholism and drug abuse. J Subst Abuse Treat 18(1):51–54, 2000 10636606

Olsen Y, Sharfstein JM: Confronting the stigma of opioid use disorder—and its treatment. JAMA 311(14):1393–1394, 2014 24577059

Petry NM, Martin B: Low-cost contingency management for treating cocaine- and opioid-abusing methadone patients. J Consult Clin Psychol 70(2):398–405, 2002 11952198

Petry NM, Martin B, Cooney JL, et al: Give them prizes, and they will come: contingency management for treatment of alcohol dependence. J Consult Clin Psychol 68(2):250–257, 2000 10780125

Powers MB, Vedel E, Emmelkamp PM: Behavioral couples therapy (BCT) for alcohol and drug use disorders: a meta-analysis. Clin Psychol Rev 28(6):952–962, 2008 18374464

Prendergast M, Podus D, Finney J, et al: Contingency management for treatment of substance use disorders: a meta-analysis. Addiction 101(11):1546–1560, 2006 17034434

Prochaska JO, DiClemente CC: The transtheoretical approach, in Handbook of Psychotherapy Integration (Oxford Series in Clinical Psychology). Edited by Norcross JC, Goldfried MR. New York, Oxford University Press, 2005, pp 147–171

Prochaska JO, DiClemente CC, Norcross JC: In search of how people change: applications to addictive behaviors. Am Psychol 47(9):1102–1114, 1992 1329589

Robles E, Stitzer ML, Strain EC, et al: Voucher-based reinforcement of opiate abstinence during methadone detoxification. Drug Alcohol Depend 65(2):179–189, 2002 11772479

Rollnick S, Miller WR: What is motivational interviewing? Behav Cogn Psychother 23(4):325–334, 1995

Saunders B, Wilkinson C, Phillips M: The impact of a brief motivational intervention with opiate users attending a methadone programme. Addiction 90(3):415–424, 1995 7735025

Silverman K, Chutuape MAD, Bigelow GE, et al: Voucher-based reinforcement of attendance by unemployed methadone patients in a job skills training program. Drug Alcohol Depend 41(3):197–207, 1996a 8842632

Silverman K, Higgins ST, Brooner RK, et al: Sustained cocaine abstinence in methadone maintenance patients through voucher-based reinforcement therapy. Arch Gen Psychiatry 53(5):409–415, 1996b 8624184

Silverman K, Wong CJ, Umbricht-Schneiter A, et al: Broad beneficial effects of cocaine abstinence reinforcement among methadone patients. J Consult Clin Psychol 66(5):811–824, 1998 9803700

Skinner BF: Science and Human Behavior. New York, Macmillan, 1953

Smedslund G, Berg RC, Hammerstrøm KT, et al: Motivational interviewing for substance abuse. Cochrane Database Syst Rev (5):CD008063, 2011 21563163

Stark MJ, Campbell BK, Brikerhoff CV: "Hello, may we help you?" A study of attrition prevention at the time of the first phone contact with substance-abusing clients. Am J Drug Alcohol Abuse 16(1–2):67–76, 1990 2330937

Stitzer ML, Bigelow GE, Liebson IA, et al: Contingent reinforcement for benzodiazepine-free urines: evaluation of a drug abuse treatment intervention. J Appl Behav Anal 15(4):493–503, 1982 6130059

Stitzer ML, Bickel WK, Bigelow GE, et al: Effect of methadone dose contingencies on urinalysis test results of polydrug-abusing methadone-maintenance patients. Drug Alcohol Depend 18(4):341–348, 1986 3816530

Stitzer ML, Iguchi MY, Felch LJ: Contingent take-home incentive: effects on drug use of methadone maintenance patients. J Consult Clin Psychol 60(6):927–934, 1992 1460154

Tonigan JS, Connors GJ, Miller WR: Participation and involvement in Alcoholics Anonymous, in Treatment Matching in Alcoholism. Edited by Babor TF, Del Boca FK. New York, Cambridge University Press, 2003, pp 184–204

Tuten M, DeFulio A, Jones HE, et al: Abstinence-contingent recovery housing and reinforcement-based treatment following opioid detoxification. Addiction 107(5):973–982, 2012 22151478

White WL, Campbell MD, Shea C, et al: Coparticipation in 12-step mutual aid groups and methadone maintenance treatment: a survey of 322 patients. J Groups Addict Recovery 8(4):294–308, 2013

Harm Reduction

Caring for People Who Misuse Opioids

Sharon Stancliff, M.D.
Bethany Medley, M.S.W.
William Mathews, R.P.A.-C.

Clinical Vignette: Jackie After Abstinence-Based Treatment

Jackie is a 22-year-old woman who has been using heroin intravenously for the past 3 years. She typically self-injects several times a day and has had repeated skin infections due to her injection drug use. Jackie is unemployed and lives with her boyfriend, who also uses heroin regularly. Jackie and her boyfriend often share their injecting equipment, including syringes, cookers, water, and cotton. When she fails to obtain heroin, Jackie reports that she will often get buprenorphine from a friend to alleviate her opioid withdrawal symptoms. Jackie states that her boyfriend once overdosed while she was with him, but she called 911, the responders administered naloxone, and he survived. Recently, Jackie checked herself into an inpatient drug treatment facility. She stated that she was depressed and hated the lifestyle that daily heroin use entailed.

At the treatment facility where Jackie was admitted, clients participate in individual, group, and family counseling; psychoeducation; 12-step groups; relapse prevention planning; and case management. The treatment facility advertises its services as "abstinence-based," meaning that the facility has a zero-tolerance policy for any form of illicit drug use and does not offer opioid agonist treatment (OAT), such as buprenorphine or methadone, and does not offer overdose prevention training. Most staff members strongly believe that OAT is merely "substituting one drug for another." Although all daytime activities are coeducational, sleeping quarters are separated by sex.

One night Jackie snuck into a male client's room, and the two were caught having sex by an overnight staff member. Because sexual relationships among clients are strictly forbidden, Jackie and the male client were kicked out of the treatment facility. The only resources they were given were the number to a local homeless shelter and a list of 12-step meetings. Jackie became extremely upset when she learned that she had to leave. She stated that she would be unable to return to staying with her boyfriend after cheating on him. In addition, she feared that she would use heroin again outside the protective environment of the treatment facility. At this point, Jackie had been abstinent from using any opioid for 27 days, but she was also technically homeless.

Jackie agreed to move to the local homeless shelter while figuring out her next steps. She did not attend any 12-step groups but managed to avoid an opioid relapse. A few weeks later, she developed fever with chills, night sweats, a throbbing headache, an intensely sore throat, diarrhea, and a generalized rash. She attended an appointment with Dr. Smith, a family practice physician who worked one evening per week at the homeless shelter, who noted swollen lymph nodes. Suspecting acute human immunodeficiency virus (HIV) infection, Dr. Smith sent the appropriate blood work, including an enzyme-linked immunosorbent assay (ELISA) and an HIV RNA level. When Dr. Smith took a history for HIV risk factors, he uncovered Jackie's recent history of injecting heroin, and he gave her a naloxone rescue kit provided by a local harm reduction organization.

A week later, Jackie attended a follow-up appointment with Dr. Smith, who informed her that she had tested positive for HIV on the RNA test and began discussing treatment options with her. Jackie was unsettled and overwhelmed by this news, in combination with all the other stresses in her life. Later that evening, she purchased a bag of heroin and injected it with a friend she had made at the homeless shelter. About 10 minutes after finishing the injection, she lost consciousness. Her friend had received education about using naloxone to prevent overdose death from the local harm reduction organization and noticed Jackie's naloxone kit sitting next to Jackie's other belongings. She quickly used the kit to administer an intranasal dose of naloxone to Jackie and called 911. Emergency medical technicians arrived 8 minutes later, administered more naloxone, and took Jackie to the hospital. She survived.

Jackie's case illustrates several key questions to consider. What is harm reduction, and how can it prevent drug-related health consequences? How can health care providers incorporate harm reduction interventions into their practices? What is naloxone, and what are opioid overdose prevention programs? What does the research say about the harm reduction aspects of OAT? What are the options for sterile syringe access? Last, what other innovative harm reduction approaches are emerging in the United States? These questions are explored in depth in the remainder of this chapter.

Introduction

Harm reduction is a public health approach that aims to reduce the negative consequences associated with drug use on both individuals and communities (Stancliff et al. 2015). The harm reduction approach has evolved from a collection of pragmatic strategies developed within drug-using communities and then gradually combined with professionally based public health interventions and policies with the goal of improving health and quality of life for individuals who use drugs. Specific harm reduction interventions vary depending on the type of drug. Table 12–1 lists common harm reduction interventions for mitigating the health risks of problematic opioid use. In addition to being an approach to care with a variety of specific strategies, harm reduction is also a social justice movement with a philosophy based on the belief that people who use drugs are entitled to the same basic human rights, dignity, and respect as all people (Hawk et al. 2017). The harm reduction approach recognizes abstinence as a valuable and in many cases desirable outcome; the approach also understands drug use along a continuum from safer to potentially harmful. Use of harm reduction interventions can and should be integrated into strategies to prevent drug use, as well as the care and treatment of people who use drugs. Through this integration, the potential harms associated with drug use, which may occur before, after, and/or during treatment, can be proactively addressed and often averted. The harm reduction approach also acknowledges that many of

TABLE 12–1.   Harm reduction approaches for people who use opioids

Syringe access programs (syringe and needle exchange programs)

Overdose prevention education (including naloxone training and dispensing)

Education for safe injecting practices

Facilitating access to opioid agonist treatment

the adverse health consequences associated with drug use are not due directly to the drug itself but rather result from poorly conceived social policies and programs that have failed to address the needs and rights of people who use drugs. Thus, harm reduction emphasizes the importance of positive health-related, social, and economic outcomes over quantification of drug consumption.

Harm reduction interventions can be delivered across diverse settings to promote engagement in and access to health care for people who use drugs, and these interventions frequently extend to social services, which, for example, provide access to food and housing resources. To effectively implement harm reduction, interventions must recognize both the strengths and challenges of individuals who use drugs and must acknowledge that an abstinence-only approach may not be feasible or even desirable. Advocates frequently say that harm reduction seeks to "meet individuals where they are" while working to improve each individual's health and quality of life. Providers must fully collaborate with those who use drugs to guarantee that all aspects of care are designed and delivered with dignity and respect for the individuals the interventions are intended to help. Fundamentally, harm reduction approaches are built for—and by—individuals who use drugs, with an emphasis on their human rights, individualism, and destigmatization.

The history of current harm reduction models as they relate to drug use can be traced back to the first organized drug user group in the Netherlands during the 1970s (Friedman et al. 1992). The group referred to themselves as the Junkiebond ("Junkie League") and advocated for less repressive national policies and proposed strategies to reduce the risks of HIV transmission during drug use. Junkiebond was eventually able to successfully collaborate with public health officials to increase access to methadone treatment and syringe exchange programs (Friedman et al. 1992). Countries across Europe, as well as Australia, have since widely adopted harm reduction strategies to reduce the spread of HIV and prevent other common drug-related harms (Bramson et al. 2015).

In the United States, ideology and political discourse around drug use have severely hindered the development and uptake of harm reduction approaches. Although the first legally sanctioned syringe exchange program in the United States was established in Tacoma, Washington, in 1988, widespread adoption of syringe exchange programs in the United States did not follow. Instead, most interventions for people who used drugs were strongly punitive, consequently reinforcing the stigma around drug use. Largely influenced by the "War on Drugs" movement, mounting evidence that public health approaches such as access to sterile syringes could reduce the spread of HIV was mostly ignored (Bramson et al. 2015). In 1988, Congress instituted a ban on federal funding to support syringe exchange. It was briefly lifted between 2009 and 2011 and then was reinstated. In 2016, the ban was partially lifted, allowing for federal support of staff and supplies but requiring that syringes and needles be paid for by local resources. Moreover, there have been stark divisions over the use of medications to treat opioid dependence that have hindered the acceptance of harm reduction–oriented treatment innovations, such as OAT (Bertram et al. 1996). The commonly held belief that OAT is merely "substituting one drug for another," as exemplified in the vignette, remains one of the most significant stigmatizing barriers to adoption of harm reduction interventions (White 2012).

Despite these barriers, advocates have made steady progress in challenging and overcoming policies and strategies that either intentionally or unintentionally contribute to drug-related harms. For example, state governments have widely enacted Good Samaritan laws, which provide varying degrees of protection against arrest and/or prosecution for drug possession for individuals responding to an emergency, including an overdose. Harm reductionist advocates have also managed to implement innovative approaches without changing any laws, such as educating people about safer injection practices. To date, there are many community-based harm reduction organizations throughout the United States engaging in collaborative advocacy efforts and providing services with and for people who use drugs.

Implementing Harm Reduction as a Health Care Provider

Harm reduction recognizes that drug use should not be a barrier to receiving comprehensive, high-quality health care. Although not extensive, the literature on stigma and drug use within health care settings demonstrates that "negative attitudes of health professionals towards patients with substance use disorders are common and contribute to suboptimal health care for these patients" (van Boekel et al. 2013). To implement harm reduction techniques in medical settings, clinicians can look to several principles to provide health care to people who use drugs (Table 12–2). Some of these principles are not unique to those who use drugs but are basic to high-quality health care in general, particularly for patients facing complicated psychosocial issues.

Often, the language associated with substance use and people who use drugs is stigmatizing. Person-first language, such as "person with a substance use disorder" or "people who use drugs," is preferred to "addict," "drug abuser," or even "drug user." Toxicology tests should be referred to clinically without using judgmental terms about results, such as calling them "clean" or "dirty." Even when patients use stigmatizing language about themselves, professionals should refrain from reinforcing this usage in their conversations with patients (Kelly et al. 2016). In addition to this general approach, clinicians should develop a basic understanding of commonly used substances, including not only the potential dangers of the drug use and treatments for misuse of these substances, but also the reasons why people choose to use them. This will help health care providers to understand their patients' drug use better and to meet them "where they are." In addition to understanding the medical literature about various drugs, clinicians should remain curious about the reasons their patients use drugs and their perceived effects. This will help to develop rapport and establish respectful therapeutic relationships. A harm reduction approach also includes looking attentively for any positive changes, however small, and celebrating them enthusiastically with patients. This concept of incrementalism not only benefits patients but also can be a source of satisfaction for provider teams (Hawk et al. 2017).

The remainder of this chapter will present several harm reduction interventions that can be incorporated into clinical practice and conclude with an outlook for the future.

TABLE 12–2.   Principles for a harm reduction approach when providing care for people who use drugs

---

1. Use a person/patient–centered approach to develop a rapport based on mutual respect.

2. Encourage patients to share about their drug use while reminding them about confidentiality regulations and noncoercive provision of services.

3. Maintain an approach that reflects the aim of enhancing patients' overall well-being, including reducing drug-related harms.

4. Educate patients using nontechnical language about their medical status, proposed treatments, and potential side effects.

5. Include patients in decision making, including about strategies to promote safer drug use (e.g., safe injecting practices, overdose prevention).

6. For patients with multiple comorbidities, coordinate a multidisciplinary team consisting of medical providers, psychiatrists, social workers, and nurses.

7. Eliminate barriers for continued care (e.g., penalties for missed visits, lack of treatment adherence, or positive urine toxicology reports).

8. Work collaboratively with the patient to set realistic, healthier-behavior goals.

9. Acknowledge that abstinence is not always a realistic, feasible, or even desired goal for some patients.

10. Develop partnerships with local harm reduction organizations.

Naloxone

Naloxone is a prescription medication that reverses the effects of an opioid overdose by acting as a pure antagonist at the μ opioid receptor. During an opioid overdose, naloxone will counteract the potentially life-threatening depression of the central nervous system and respiratory drive, restoring respiration in an overdose victim (Sporer 1999). Naloxone has a stronger affinity for opioid receptors than most opioid agonists. Thus, naloxone works by displacing or "blocking" opioid agonists at opioid receptors in the brain. This blocking effect can last for 20–90 minutes after naloxone administration (Sporer 2003). Naloxone has essentially no other effects or mechanisms of action.

Naloxone is a nonscheduled medication, approved by the U.S. Food and Drug Administration (FDA). Naloxone access laws and prescribing regulations vary by state. The most up-to-date naloxone-related state regulations can be viewed at the website for the Prescription Drug Abuse Policy System (www.pdaps.org), which is funded by the National Institute on Drug Abuse. Because naloxone is safe and has no potential for abuse, there are low to no risks for allowing laypersons to administer the medication (Burris et al. 2001). No evidence has been found that training individuals who use heroin in overdose response and giving them a take-home naloxone rescue kit encourages drug use (Lim et al. 2016; McDonald and Strang 2016). Because naloxone simply displaces opioids from opioid receptors, it will not influence the effects of drug testing. Naloxone itself does not invoke adverse reactions; however, in individuals who are opioid dependent, naloxone may induce temporary opioid withdrawal symptoms such as agitation, vomiting, and diarrhea (Enteen et al. 2010; Lim et al. 2016; Maxwell et al. 2006). Tolerance to naloxone does not develop, and the medication can be effectively used for repeated overdoses.

Methods of naloxone administration include injection (intramuscular, subcutaneous, or intravenous) and intranasal administration. Two delivery devices have been approved by the FDA for use outside the medical setting: a nasal device delivering 4 mg in a 0.1-cc dose and an auto-injector delivering 2 mg in a 0.4-cc dose. Each package contains two doses. There is also a generic formulation of naloxone with 0.4 mg/cc for intramuscular use, which is prescribed with an intramuscular needle and syringe. Naloxone has an average shelf life of 12–18 months and should be stored at room temperature, although it loses little potency when exposed to heat or cold (Gammon et al. 2018).

In the early 1990s, a syringe exchange, Chicago Recovery Alliance, began distributing naloxone to clients (Maxwell et al. 2006). Since then, programs to distribute take-home naloxone have become increasingly widespread in the United States and are now a leading response in communities impacted by the opioid overdose crisis (Fairbairn et al. 2017). Notably, evidence from communities with naloxone distribution and training programs for people who use drugs showed significantly lower overdose death rates compared with communities with no such programs (Walley et al. 2013). In one systematic review, nonmedical laypersons who were trained in overdose response programs were able to recognize opioid overdoses and successfully administer naloxone to victims with a nearly 100% survival rate (Clark et al. 2014). On a national level, gathering the collective total number of prevented overdose fatalities with the use of naloxone is difficult because of the various avenues through which naloxone is administered (e.g., emergency medical services, trained laypeople, law enforcement) and the lack of streamlined reporting. However, in a recent survey of 140 naloxone-distributing organizations—including public health departments, pharmacies, health care facilities, substance use treatment facilities, and community-based organizations—109 collected overdose reversal reports were tallied, totaling 26,463 overdose reversals from 1996 to 2014 (Wheeler et al. 2015). It is important to note that epidemiological data are likely significantly underestimated, and there is great need for a streamlined data collection approach.

Opioid overdose prevention programs have been established in many venues, including syringe access programs, HIV prevention outreach programs, methadone maintenance clinics, inpatient detoxification programs, and hospital-based settings. The primary purposes of opioid overdose prevention programs are to educate and train laypersons on overdose prevention and reversal with the use of naloxone and to distribute naloxone rescue kits. Naloxone rescue kits typically contain two doses of naloxone, instructions, gloves, and a rescue breathing face mask. Although using opioids alone is one of the primary risk factors for dying of an overdose, research shows that people who use drugs typically use them in the company of another person (Lim et al. 2016). Thus, providing naloxone kits to people who use drugs as well as anyone else who might be a bystander to an overdose is strongly recommended. Populations with the highest risk for overdose include those who have experienced a previous nonfatal overdose, those who have chronic illness (particularly illness that impacts drug metabolism), and those who have recently experienced any periods of abstinence (e.g., detoxification, staying in abstinence-based residential facilities, incarceration) (Lim et al. 2016). Special attention should be given to these at-risk populations when planning naloxone distribution and identifying training sites.

Clinicians are encouraged to prescribe naloxone for any patients at risk of opioid overdose from either prescribed opioids or illicit opioids. In a nonrandomized intervention study, clinicians were asked to voluntarily prescribe naloxone to patients on long-term opioid treatment or individuals whom they otherwise judged to be at risk of witnessing or experiencing an overdose. The researchers reported a 63% decline in opioid-related emergency department visits among those who were pre-scribed naloxone compared with those who were not (Coffin et al. 2016). Many insurance plans cover naloxone, and some cover it even for those likely to witness an overdose. The patients' and caregivers' in-structions can be brief, as detailed in Table 12–3.

In most states, pharmacies may dispense naloxone without a patient-specific order, via standing orders, collaborative agreements, and other state-specific models. Through a standing order, individuals can ask for a prescription of naloxone without visiting a clinician who prescribes medication. This allows pharmacists to recommend naloxone to patients who may be at risk, as well as for quick access by people who become aware of a loved one's risk of overdose. However, one perceived barrier to retrieving naloxone from a pharmacy is the copayment expense. In 2017, New York became the first state to implement a naloxone copayment as-sistance program. Through this program, up to $40 of the naloxone co-payment is covered by the New York State Department of Health for anyone with prescription coverage as part of their health insurance.

The increase in fentanyl and fentanyl analogues in the illicit drug market has raised a new set of concerns when responding to opioid overdoses, because fentanyl-related overdoses have been reported to oc-cur much more rapidly (within several minutes) than traditional heroin overdoses (which often occur over the course of an hour or more) (Schumann et al. 2008; Somerville et al. 2017). Evidence from commu-nities with fentanyl-associated overdose outbreaks indicates that nalox-one has been effective in reversing overdoses, although in some cases higher doses may be required (Schumann et al. 2008; Somerville et al. 2017). Because it is nearly impossible, however, to determine whether an overdose is fentanyl related at first point of care or contact, naloxone availability and training for people who use drugs as well as for first re-sponders in the community are critical to ensuring the quickest and most effective response.

Opioid Agonist Treatment With the Harm Reduction Philosophy

Treatments using buprenorphine and methadone, as well as naltrexone, are discussed in detail in Chapter 10, "Medication-Assisted Treatment for Opioid Use Disorder." When naltrexone is included, these treatment modalities are referred to as medication-assisted treatment (MAT), but

TABLE 12–3. Opioid overdose prevention training—essential topics

What effect does naloxone have?

Reverses overdoses from opioids (e.g., heroin, oxycodone, hydrocodone, methadone).

Will not cause harm if it is not an opioid overdose.

How to recognize an overdose

A person will be unconscious, have breathing problems, and turn blue or gray.

What to do

Perform sternal rub to attempt to wake the person.

Call 911.

Naloxone: clinician or trainer to demonstrate assembly (if applicable) and administration.

Give first dose.

If victim is still unresponsive after 2–3 minutes, give second dose.

Put victim in recovery position.

If emergency medical services was not called, assess the victim:

Not walking and talking? Get medical care immediately.

Walking and talking? Stay with the person and monitor for 3 hours.

when only opioid agonists are included, the term is either OAT or opioid replacement therapy. The harm reduction–oriented approach prefers OAT. In this section, the role of opioid agonists with a harm reduction philosophy is discussed. Traditional drug treatment and harm reduction techniques have similar goals: prevention of drug-related deaths and illnesses, reductions in criminal behaviors, and reintegration of people who have been stigmatized and marginalized because of drug use into the community. Traditional drug treatment often considers abstinence from all substances to be crucial to achieving these goals. However, studies have shown that participation in OAT reduces injection frequency, HIV transmission, overdose (Schwartz et al. 2013), and criminal activity (Havnes et al. 2012)—even among those who continue to use and inject opioids and/or other substances (Gjersing and Bretteville-Jensen 2013). The role of opioid agonists has become even more crucial in the face of the current opioid crisis. A recent meta-analysis on the impact of OAT maintenance showed consistent and dramatic decreases in overdose mortality after the first 4 weeks of methadone treatment, in some studies by as much as 80% (Sordo et al. 2017). For these reasons, better access to buprenorphine and methadone is vital to reducing harm from the current opioid emergency in the United States.

Access to methadone or buprenorphine is limited by many factors, but reducing barriers to buprenorphine access is far more feasible in many settings than reducing barriers to methadone access (for reasons discussed in Chapter 10). Kourounis et al. (2016) identified a variety of treatment design factors that serve as barriers to many people intending to access treatment; these factors include but are not limited to required psychosocial interventions, little tolerance for relapse or other drug use while enrolled in programs, and limits on duration of treatment. It is clear from the literature that OAT alone without counseling is highly effective in reducing illicit opioid use and associated harms (Schwartz et al. 2013). The federal regulations regarding buprenorphine require only that a practitioner refer a patient to counseling but not that the practitioner enforce participation. Also, the role of the prescribing clinicians themselves in providing counseling should not be overlooked, particularly for psychiatric practitioners. Harm reduction–oriented agencies often provide or refer participants to counseling, but it should not be a requirement for receiving any service.

Urine drug testing is usually a part of drug treatment; however, the choice of panel to use and the response to the results should be well thought out. OAT is beneficial in preventing overdose deaths and other harms, even in people who use other drugs such as marijuana, stimulants, and benzodiazepines and/or who sometimes continue to use illicit opioids. In some practices, there is little tolerance for any illicit drug use and positive drug screens, which can lead to discontinuation of treatment, increasing the overall likelihood of harm. In 2017, the FDA cautioned against refusing access to or discontinuing use of buprenorphine or methadone even when a patient is using benzodiazepines or other depressants, stating that despite the increased risk involved, the risks of being out of treatment are much greater (U.S. Food and Drug Administration 2017). This approach is also supported by the American Society of Addiction Medicine's (2015) guidelines on the use of medications in the treatment of addiction involving opioids, which recommend that "[t]he use of marijuana, stimulants, or other addictive drugs should not be a reason to suspend opioid use disorder treatment" (p. 5). The risk of using the other drug while on buprenorphine should be weighed against the risk of fatal overdose and other adverse outcomes if treatment is discontinued or not provided. Both of these guidance documents also support the need for long-term treatment with medication for many patients.

Many practitioners are concerned about the diversion of buprenorphine to people other than those for whom it is prescribed. It is important to note that diversion is not unique to buprenorphine; it also occurs with many other controlled psychoactive medications. The barriers preventing unlimited access to buprenorphine are significant predictive factors in diversion; therefore, increasing prescription access might be an effective way to reduce diversion (Lofwall and Havens 2012). Notably, nearly half of all diverted buprenorphine is used to alleviate and self-medicate withdrawal symptoms rather than "to get high" (Lofwall and Havens 2012). In addition, practitioners should be aware that buprenorphine is rarely involved in opioid overdose deaths (Paone et al. 2015). It is not possible to prevent all diversion, even by daily observed dosing. Nevertheless, prescribers should take care to reduce the likelihood of diversion and to ensure that patients are taking at least some of the medication. There are many ways of doing this, including testing urine for buprenorphine metabolites, occasionally observing dosing, and making unscheduled medication counts (Lofwall and Walsh 2014).

Access to Sterile Injecting Equipment

A significant related consequence of the opioid overdose crisis in the United States is the increase in other drug-related harms among people who inject drugs. This includes an emerging epidemic of newly acquired hepatitis C virus (HCV) infections among people who inject drugs, with low levels of awareness among the populations affected (Valdiserri et al. 2014). Adolescents and young adults (under age 30 years) who inject drugs have been particularly impacted, accounting for most newly acquired infections according to surveillance data reports from the Centers for Disease Control and Prevention (2015). Because HCV can be asymptomatic for many years, the majority of people with HCV do not know they have it, and reported data probably significantly underestimate its incidence and prevalence (Centers for Disease Control and Prevention 2015).

The use of sterile injection equipment is essential for the prevention of HCV, HIV, and other blood-borne infections among people who inject drugs (Edlin 2004), and programs that facilitate access to such equipment are called syringe-needle access programs (SNAPs). Countries where access to sterile injecting equipment has been implemented on a large scale have seen reductions in HIV and HCV transmission by reducing the need to share and reuse hypodermic needles (Aspinall et al. 2014). Secondary benefits of SNAPs include increased enrollment in substance use disorder treatment (Hagan et al. 2000; Strathdee et al. 2006), increased retention in HIV treatment, and reduced disease transmission by needle stick injuries among first responders (Groseclose et al. 1995). Facilitating access to sterile injection equipment through harm reduction approaches can be implemented and integrated into several outlets for people who inject drugs, including community-based programs and pharmacies.

The primary purpose of SNAPs is to distribute new, sterile syringe-needles and other injecting equipment, while collecting and disposing of used syringe-needles and equipment. Originally, SNAPs operated as "exchanges" in which the number of syringe-needles that were distributed was limited by the number of syringe-needles that a person brought into the program (Bramson et al. 2015). Although such exchange requirements were intended to maximize syringe-needle collection, they ended up limiting access to new sterile syringe-needles and not decreasing the potential for reuse of syringes (Bramson et al. 2015). Wide distribution of injecting equipment has been associated with safer injection practices and lower incidence rates of infectious diseases compared with more conservative exchange schemes (Bluthenthal et al. 2007). Thus, SNAPs should provide unrestricted and unlimited access to sterile injection equipment for participants. Community-based SNAPs also have the unique opportunity to provide low-threshold access to a variety of health-related and social services, such as HIV, viral hepatitis, and tuberculosis screening; viral hepatitis vaccinations; and on-site referrals, including referrals for substance use disorder treatment and gender-specific services for women. Providing comprehensive case management interventions (including referrals to medical and social services) within SNAPs has been found to increase rates of treatment entry among participants (Strathdee et al. 2006). More recently, many

SNAPs have incorporated overdose prevention training and naloxone kit dispensing as part of the services they offer.

Another feasible option is leveraging pharmacies to provide access to sterile syringes, either over the counter or with an individual prescription. Many states have amended laws to facilitate expanded access to syringes in pharmacies. To find specific state laws on syringe access, visit this page at the Policy Surveillance Program website: http://lawatlas.org/datasets/paraphernalia-laws. Although research on pharmacy-based access to sterile injecting equipment is limited, anticipated barriers may include pharmacy staff attitudes, training needs, and requirements to show identification. Care providers should further explore engagement and collaboration opportunities with pharmacies to reduce perceived barriers.

Syringe-needle prescription is another feasible option. This approach was implemented successfully in Providence, Rhode Island, in 1999, and demonstrated feasibility and acceptability and enhanced communication between people who inject drugs and health care providers (Rich et al. 2004). Prescribers offered syringe-needle prescriptions as part of general medical care, typically prescribing 100 syringes at a time. In addition, individuals received access to a portable disposal container and had discussions on safer injection techniques, recognizing infections, and safe disposal of used equipment. A national survey of a representative sample of U.S. physicians, with a 20% response rate, found that most respondents were unaware of the laws in their state around syringe access. Almost half of the responding prescribers reported that they would consider prescribing syringes to prevent transmission of infections, and 3.4% reported that they had prescribed to individuals who inject drugs for this purpose (Macalino et al. 2009).

Other Innovative Harm Reduction Approaches

Several other harm reduction–oriented interventions, which have been widely used in other countries, are worth highlighting. These include supervised injection facilities (SIFs), syringe-dispensing machines (SDMs), and heroin- or hydromorphone-assisted treatment (HAT). Adopting these emerging innovations in the United States may provide viable options for addressing the opioid overdose crisis.

SIFs, also known as safe consumption spaces, are legally sanctioned facilities where people can go to consume previously obtained drugs under trained supervision in a hygienic environment, with appropriate equipment, and without fear of arrest. The primary goal of SIFs is to improve the health status of the targeted population while also serving as a response to the problem of public injection (e.g., in parks, empty lots, public restrooms) (Potier et al. 2014). The populations primarily targeted for these facilities tend to be the most marginalized and experience high rates of housing insecurity and homelessness.

SIFs were first implemented in Switzerland, Germany, and the Netherlands during the 1980s, and they have since been adopted as an effective approach for reducing deaths from overdoses and other drug-related harms in more than 90 countries (European Harm Reduction Network 2016). SIFs are strongly associated with reductions in overdose fatalities near the facility, with no known overdose deaths reported within a facility as of 2011 (Marshall et al. 2011), and the authors are unaware of any deaths since the 2011 report. One systematic review revealed unambiguous effectiveness of SIFs across studies around the world, including a significant reduction in drug-related health and social harms (i.e., a decrease in syringe sharing, public injection, newly acquired infectious diseases) (Potier et al. 2014). In addition, SIFs were found to increase referrals to drug treatment and access to necessary health services. Moreover, several studies concluded that SIFs have significant positive cost-benefit ratios and are therefore highly cost-effective. There is no evidence that SIFs are associated with an increase in crime, illicit drug trade, or violence in communities where they are located (Potier et al. 2014).

Clean injection equipment can also be distributed via public SDMs. SDMs are designed to be accessible 24 hours a day, 7 days per week, without the fixed overhead and staffing costs of SNAPs, and without requiring that people who inject drugs visit a pharmacy. SDMs have been shown to attract individuals who inject drugs who would not otherwise go to SNAPs or pharmacies, such as younger people, people who more recently started injecting, and people with no contact with addiction service providers. SDMs have been introduced in more than 100 cities in Europe, Australia, and New Zealand (Duplessy and Reynaud 2014), but they remain illegal in the United States.

In Canada, Australia, and many countries throughout Europe, pharmacological heroin, also known as heroin-assisted treatment, has been used successfully for opioid maintenance treatment to reduce the risks of injecting illicit opioids. Several trials have shown effective, positive outcomes using slow-release morphine (Ferri et al. 2013), heroin (Ferri et al. 2011), and hydromorphone (Oviedo-Joekes et al. 2016) in controlled settings for patients who have not done well with methadone. As with other harm reduction approaches, positive outcomes for pharmacological heroin include reductions in illicit drug use, crime, disease, and overdose, as well as improvements in health, well-being, social reintegration, and treatment retention (Ferri et al. 2011, 2013; Oviedo-Joekes et al. 2016).

Gender-responsive or women-specific services in harm reduction approaches and traditional drug treatment are often overlooked and underemphasized. Although the prevalence of injecting drugs is lower in women than in men, women who inject drugs often have higher rates of HIV and HCV infection (Iversen et al. 2015). In addition, gender-based violence in combination with past traumatic life experiences disproportionately affects women who inject drugs (Gilbert et al. 2015). For women of reproductive age, consistent opioid use may delay or stop the menstrual cycle, and then women may be unaware if they become pregnant (Pinkham and Malinowska-Sempruch 2008). Redesigning harm reduction approaches to make them more gender responsive can be accomplished through adapting programs in a variety of ways, such as facilitating women-only hours, providing free contraceptives, offering pregnancy testing, providing child care, and helping women to navigate referrals for services such as domestic violence shelters or reproductive health providers.

Future Directions for Harm Reduction in the United States

The harm reduction movement is based on a commitment to ensure the health and human rights for people who use drugs. Therefore, harm reduction techniques should be incorporated into all aspects of care and treatment for individuals who use drugs. The normalization of harm reduction practices and an understanding of the philosophy of harm reduction are a necessary response to the current opioid overdose crisis. The strategies and evidence outlined in this chapter provide numerous ways in which common risks for overdose can be reduced and lives can be saved. Without rapid uptake of various harm reduction interventions, the opioid overdose crisis will continue to result in a substantial and increasing number of preventable deaths. Clinicians and advocates should continue to consider ways in which harm reduction can be implemented through effective, innovative health approaches to drug use, drug treatment, and drug policy that are based on science and research.

Key Chapter Points

▶ Harm reduction is a set of public health strategies and ideas aimed at reducing negative consequences associated with drug use. Harm reduction is also a movement for social justice built on a belief in, and respect for, the rights of people who use drugs.

▶ Health care providers can integrate harm reduction approaches into the continuum of care and treatment for patients who use drugs. Clinicians should ensure that their language and practice with individuals who use drugs is nonjudgmental and person centered. Known or suspected active drug use should never be a justification for withholding or discontinuing care.

▶ Clinicians should locate within their communities any harm reduction–oriented resources, such as syringe-needle access programs and opioid overdose prevention programs. Alternatively, clinicians can furnish or prescribe syringes and/or discuss safe injecting practices. The authors have found it helpful to say, "I hope you never inject again, but if you or your friends do, I want you to know how to do it as safely as possible."

▶ Provision of naloxone to patients at risk of overdose is a feasible and evidence-based intervention. All states allow prescribing of naloxone to people at risk of overdose; many explicitly allow it for people at risk of witnessing an overdose. Patients prescribed or misusing opioids should be counseled on recognition and response to an opioid overdose and be offered take-home naloxone.

▶ Opioid agonist treatment can prevent morbidity and mortality, even in patients who are not able or willing to pursue abstinence from drug use or participate in counseling. All eligible clinicians should obtain a waiver to prescribe buprenorphine, which is associated with dramatic decreases in opioid overdose deaths. Even if a practitioner is not prepared to treat OUD, the waiver can be useful in urgent situations, such as initiating or continuing a patient in need of buprenorphine until he or she is transitioned to another practice or program.

▶ Provision of sterile syringes is effective in preventing infections, including HIV and hepatitis C virus infection. Community-based syringe-needle access programs are low-threshold services for people who inject drugs to help them access sterile injecting equipment and properly dispose of used equipment. Additional benefits may include increased enrollment in medical care or retention in treatment (e.g., HIV treatment, substance use disorder treatment).

▶ Other evidence-based, emerging harm reduction approaches discussed among advocates in the United States include supervised injection facilities, public syringe-dispensing machines, heroin-assisted treatment, and gender-responsive harm reduction approaches.

References

American Society of Addiction Medicine: National Practice Guideline for the Use of Medications in the Treatment of Addiction Involving Opioid Use. 2015. Available at: https://www.asam.org/docs/default-source/practice-support/guidelines-and-consensus-docs/asam-national-practice-guideline-supplement.pdf. Accessed April 4, 2018.

Aspinall EJ, Nambiar D, Goldberg DJ, et al: Are needle and syringe programmes associated with a reduction in HIV transmission among people who inject drugs: a systematic review and meta-analysis. Int J Epidemiol 43(1):235–248, 2014 24374889

Bertram E, Blachman M, Sharpe K, et al: Drug War Politics: The Price of Denial. Berkeley, University of California Press, 1996

Bluthenthal RN, Ridgeway G, Schell T, et al: Examination of the association between syringe exchange program (SEP) dispensation policy and SEP client-level syringe coverage among injection drug users. Addiction 102(4):638–646, 2007 17286637

Bramson H, Des Jarlais DC, Arasteh K, et al: State laws, syringe exchange, and HIV among persons who inject drugs in the United States: history and effectiveness. J Public Health Policy 36(2):212–230, 2015 25590514

Burris S, Norland J, Edlin BR: Legal aspects of providing naloxone to heroin users in the United States. Int J Drug Policy 12(3):237–248, 2001

Centers for Disease Control and Prevention: Viral hepatitis surveillance—United States, 2015. 2015. Available at: https://www.cdc.gov/hepatitis/statistics/2015surveillance/pdfs/2015HepSurveillanceRpt.pdf. Accessed April 4, 2018.

Clark AK, Wilder CM, Winstanley EL: A systematic review of community opioid overdose prevention and naloxone distribution programs. J Addict Med 8(3):153–163, 2014 24874759

Coffin PO, Behar E, Rowe C, et al: Nonrandomized intervention study of naloxone coprescription for primary care patients on long term opioid therapy for pain. Ann Intern Med 165(4):245–252, 2016 27366987

Duplessy C, Reynaud EG: Long-term survey of a syringe-dispensing machine needle exchange program: answering public concerns. Harm Reduct J 11:16, 2014 24885902

Edlin BR: Hepatitis C prevention and treatment for substance users in the United States: acknowledging the elephant in the living room. Int J Drug Policy 15(2):81–91, 2004

Enteen L, Bauer J, McLean R, et al: Overdose prevention and naloxone prescription for opioid users in San Francisco. J Urban Health 87(6):931–941, 2010 20967505

European Harm Reduction Network: Drug consumption rooms: an overview of provision and evidence. 2016. Available at: http://www.emcdda.europa.eu/topics/pods/drug-consumption-rooms. Accessed April 4, 2018.

Fairbairn N, Coffin PO, Walley AY: Naloxone for heroin, prescription opioid, and illicitly made fentanyl overdoses: challenges and innovations responding to a dynamic epidemic. Int J Drug Policy 46:172–179, 2017 28687187

Ferri M, Davoli M, Perucci CA: Heroin maintenance for chronic heroin-dependent individuals. Cochrane Database Syst Rev 7(12):CD003410, 2011 22161378

Ferri M, Minozzi S, Bo A, Amato L: Slow-release oral morphine as maintenance therapy for opioid dependence. Cochrane Database Syst Rev 5(6):CD009879, 2013 23740540

Friedman SR, De Jong W, Wodak A: Community development as a response to HIV among drug injectors. AIDS 7 (suppl 1):S263–S269, 1992 8363797

Gammon DL, Su S, Jordan S, et al: Alteration in prehospital drug concentration after thermal exposure. Am J Emerg Med 26(5):566–573, 2008 18534286

Gilbert L, Raj A, Hien D, et al: Targeting the SAVA (substance abuse, violence and AIDS) syndemic among women and girl. J Acquir Immune Defic Syndr 69 (suppl 2):5118–5127, 2015 25978478

Gjersing L, Bretteville-Jensen AL: Is opioid substitution treatment beneficial if injecting behaviour continues? Drug Alcohol Depend 133(1):121–126, 2013 23773951

Groseclose SL, Weinstein B, Jones TS, et al: Impact of increased legal access to needles and syringes on practices of injecting-drug users and police officers—Connecticut, 1992–1993. J Acquir Immune Defic Syndr Hum Retrovirol 10(1):82–89, 1995 7648290

Hagan H, McGough JP, Thiede H, et al: Reduced injection frequency and increased entry and retention in drug treatment associated with needle-exchange participation in Seattle drug injectors. J Subst Abuse Treat 19(3):247–252, 2000 11027894

Havnes I, Bukten A, Gossop M, et al: Reductions in convictions for violent crime during opioid maintenance treatment: a longitudinal national cohort study. Drug Alcohol Depend 124(3):307–310, 2012 22382045

Hawk M, Coulter RWS, Egan JE, et al: Harm reduction principles for healthcare settings. Harm Reduct J 14(1):70, 2017 29065896

Iversen J, Page K, Madden A, et al: HIV, HCV, and health-related harms among women who inject drugs: implications for prevention and treatment. J Acquir Immune Defic Syndr 69 (suppl 2):S176–S181, 2015 25978485

Kelly JF, Saitz RD, Wakeman S: Language, substance use disorders, and policy: the need to reach consensus on an "addiction-ary." Alcohol Treat Q 34(1):116–123, 2016

Kourounis G, Richards BD, Kyprianou E, et al: Opioid substitution therapy: lowering the treatment thresholds. Drug Alcohol Depend 161:1–8, 2016 26832931

Lim JK, Bratberg JP, Davis CS, et al: Prescribe to prevent: overdose prevention and naloxone rescue kits for prescribers and pharmacists. J Addict Med 10(5):300–308, 2016 27261669

Lofwall MR, Havens JR: Inability to access buprenorphine treatment as a risk factor for using diverted buprenorphine. Drug Alcohol Depend 126(3):379–383, 2012 22704124

Lofwall MR, Walsh SL: A review of buprenorphine diversion and misuse: the current evidence base and experiences from around the world. J Addict Med 8(5):315–326, 2014 25221984

Macalino GE, Sachdev DD, Rich JD, et al: A national physician survey on prescribing syringes as an HIV prevention measure. Subst Abuse Treat Prev Policy 4(1):13, 2009 19505336

Marshall BD, Milloy MJ, Wood E, et al: Reduction in overdose mortality after the opening of North America's first medically supervised safer injecting facility: a retrospective population-based study. Lancet 377(9775):1429–1437, 2011 21497898

Maxwell S, Bigg D, Stanczykiewicz K, et al: Prescribing naloxone to actively injecting heroin users: a program to reduce heroin overdose deaths. J Addict Dis 25(3):89–96, 2006 16956873

McDonald R, Strang J: Are take-home naloxone programmes effective? Systematic review utilizing application of the Bradford Hill criteria. Addiction 111(7):1177–1187, 2016 27028542

Oviedo-Joekes E, Guh D, Brissette S, et al: Hydromorphone compared with diacetylmorphine for long-term opioid dependence: a randomized clinical trial. JAMA Psychiatry 73(5):447–455, 2016 27049826

Paone D, Tuazon E, Stajic M, et al: Buprenorphine infrequently found in fatal overdose in New York City. Drug Alcohol Depend 155:298–301, 2015 26305073

Pinkham S, Malinowska-Sempruch K: Women, harm reduction and HIV. Reprod Health Matters 16(31):168–181, 2008 18513618

Potier C, Laprévote V, Dubois-Arber F, et al: Supervised injection services: what has been demonstrated? A systematic literature review. Drug Alcohol Depend 145:48–68, 2014 25456324

Rich JD, McKenzie M, Macalino GE, et al: A syringe prescription program to prevent infectious disease and improve health of injection drug users. J Urban Health 81(1):122–134, 2004 15047791

Schumann H, Erickson T, Thompson TM, et al: Fentanyl epidemic in Chicago, Illinois and surrounding Cook County. Clin Toxicol (Phila) 46(6):501–506, 2008 18584361

Schwartz RP, Gryczynski J, O'Grady KE, et al: Opioid agonist treatments and heroin overdose deaths in Baltimore, Maryland, 1995–2009. Am J Public Health 103(5):917–922, 2013 23488511

Somerville NJ, O'Donnell J, Gladden RM, et al: Characteristics of fentanyl overdose—Massachusetts, 2014–2016. MMWR Morb Mortal Wkly Rep 66(14):382–386, 2017 28406883

Sordo L, Barrio G, Bravo MJ, et al: Mortality risk during and after opioid substitution treatment: systematic review and meta-analysis of cohort studies. BMJ 357:j1550, 2017 28446428

Sporer KA: Acute heroin overdose. Ann Intern Med 130(7):584–590, 1999 10189329

Sporer KA: Strategies for preventing heroin overdose. BMJ 326(7386):442–444, 2003 12595388

Stancliff S, Phillips BW, Maghsoudi N, et al: Harm reduction: front line public health. J Addict Dis 34(2–3):206–219, 2015 26080038

Strachdee SA, Ricketts EP, Huettner S, et al: Facilitating entry into drug treatment among injection drug users referred from a needle exchange program: results from a community-based behavioral intervention trial. Drug Alcohol Depend 83(3):225–232, 2006 16364566

U.S. Food and Drug Administration: FDA Drug Safety Communication: FDA urges caution about withholding opioid addiction medications from patients taking benzodiazepines or CNS depressants: careful medication management can reduce risks. September 26, 2017. Available at: https://www.fda.gov/Drugs/DrugSafety/ucm575307.htm. Accessed April 4, 2018.

Valdiserri R, Khalsa J, Dan C, et al: Confronting the emerging epidemic of HCV infection among young injection drug users. Am J Public Health 104(5):816–821, 2014 24625174

van Boekel LC, Brouwers EP, van Weeghel J, et al: Stigma among health professionals towards patients with substance use disorders and its consequences for healthcare delivery: systematic review. Drug Alcohol Depend 131(1–2):23–35, 2013 23490450

Walley AY, Xuan Z, Hackman HH, et al: Opioid overdose rates and implementation of overdose education and nasal naloxone distribution in Massachusetts: interrupted time series analysis. BMJ 346:f174, 2013 23372174

Wheeler E, Jones TS, Gilbert MK, et al; Centers for Disease Control and Prevention: Opioid overdose prevention programs providing naloxone to laypersons—United States, 2014. MMWR Morb Mortal Wkly Rep 64(23):631–635, 2015 26086633

White WL: Medication-assisted recovery from opioid addiction: historical and contemporary perspectives. J Addict Dis 31(3):199–206, 2012 22873182

13

Prevention of Opioid Misuse and Addiction Through Policy Approaches

Tauheed Zaman, M.D.
Leo Beletsky, J.D., M.P.H.
Keith A. Hermanstyne, M.D., M.P.H., M.S.H.P.M.

Clinical Vignette: Opioids and a New Patient Evaluation for James

Dr. Hirschfield is an outpatient psychiatrist working in an urban academic center. She has a new patient evaluation scheduled, and she begins reviewing the referral notes from the intake office. James is a 54-year-old man with a history of chronic back pain who has been reporting problems with his mood, appetite, and energy over the past 3 months. When he arrives for his initial appointment, he reports his reluctance to engage in psychiatric care, stating that he had a negative encounter with a previous psychiatrist at another clinic.

He endorses a 6-month history of depressed mood, decreased appetite, low motivation, and occasional suicidal thoughts. When reviewing his medical history, James mentions that he has suffered from chronic

361

back pain ever since he sustained a workplace injury (he is a construction worker) 1 year ago. He is reluctant to discuss whether he has a current primary care doctor, saying that it has no relationship to his depressive symptoms while also stating that he has had some problems with his primary care physician. When pressed about what is causing this rift, he says that his primary care physician refuses to refill his OxyContin (extended-release oxycodone) prescription from last year despite his chronic pain. He denies any heroin use but states that he sometimes buys Vicodin (hydrocodone-acetaminophen) and Percocet (oxycodone-acetaminophen) from friends. When he runs out of opioids, he starts to feel sweaty, anxious, and nauseated. Near the end of the visit, Dr. Hirschfield conveys that the client may have a diagnosis of major depressive disorder and highlights her concerns that James may also have opioid use disorder (OUD). The client denies that he has any problems with opioids and angrily walks out of the office, stating that he may never return. He later calls and apologizes for ending his appointment early and agrees to return next week for a follow-up visit.

Once James leaves, Dr. Hirschfield starts considering her next steps and the policies that might inform her management should he return to her care. She could log into her state's prescription drug monitoring database to see her patient's opioid prescription history. However, she has questions: Are prescription drug monitoring programs effective? How could she use these data to better care for James? She recalls that the patient was obtaining opioids prescribed to others. What are local, state, and federal policies that affect opioid drug supply? She is also aware that although James denied heroin use, patients with OUD may transition from prescription opioids to injected heroin use. What are the statutes that govern programs that reduce the negative sequelae of opioid injection drug use? Are there educational requirements for treatment providers around pain management and opioid use? If James is willing, she plans to further explore his history of opioid use, complete a full OUD evaluation, and offer treatment as appropriate. What are the regulations that affect availability of medication-assisted treatment (MAT) such as buprenorphine?

As the vignette demonstrates, policy related to the opioid crisis can target reducing opioid supply, decreasing opioid demand, and instituting harm reduction strategies to mitigate the harmful consequences of opioid misuse. Following a brief review of the different federal organizations that have implemented recent policies in response to the opioid crisis, this chapter provides an in-depth exploration of initiatives that have targeted provider education, prescription drug monitoring programs (PDMPs), availability of medications used to treat or prevent opioid misuse, and access to harm reduction programs including syringe-needle access programs and safe injection facilities.

Federal Efforts Directed Toward the Current Opioid Crisis

Several federal organizations have implemented policy changes in a direct response to the current opioid crisis. The Drug Enforcement Administration (DEA) has initiated recent changes in an effort to limit the national opioid supply. In 2014, the DEA reclassified all hydrocodone-containing pain medications from Schedule III (drugs considered to have low to moderate potential for physical and psychological dependence) to Schedule II (drugs with currently accepted medical use that are deemed to have high potential for abuse); this reclassification led to a mandatory 30-day supply limit on this class of medications. In a recent analysis examining how this policy change impacted a sample of privately insured adults ages 18–64, Raji and colleagues (2017) found that between 2013 and 2015, prescriptions for hydrocodone-containing pain medications decreased by approximately 26% and prescriptions for any opioid decreased by 11%, although there was a small concurrent increase in non-hydrocodone-based products, primarily medications involving codeine. The study's authors hypothesized that variations in PDMPs and state laws that target opioid regulation could have contributed to differences observed across states.

The U.S. Food and Drug Administration (FDA) has also taken on a key role in attempts to reduce opioid misuse. In recent years, the FDA has implemented revised medication label warnings highlighting the risk of opioid addiction and the danger of combining opioids with benzodiazepines and has clarified the risks associated with opioids in medication guides included with a medication. The FDA has developed a risk evaluation and mitigation strategy (REMS) for extended-release opioids and has supported pharmaceutical efforts to create new abuse-deterrent opioid formulations (Aschenbrenner 2018). However, research on the real-world efficacy of abuse-deterrent opioids has been mixed. For example, postmarketing analysis of modified extended-release oxycodone (OxyContin) has shown decreases in diversion, overdose deaths, and prescription shopping, whereas other studies have found that decreases in prescription opioid access due to abuse-deterrent formulations may coincide with an increase in heroin and other opioid use (Pergolizzi et al. 2018). Further changes in FDA policy occurred in 2017, including increased external advisory input in regard to opioid medication approval, new requirements for data collection related to long-term use of extended-release opioids, and modification to REMS to enhance continuing medical education (CME) training (e.g., targeting providers who prescribe immediate-release opioids, providing content on safe prescribing methods, promoting use of nonopioid medications, broadening the audience for education efforts to include pharmacists and nurses) (Aschenbrenner 2018). There will also be increased efforts to create generic versions of opioids with abuse-deterrent technology given that only brand name versions currently exist (Aschenbrenner 2018). Most recently, the FDA has announced intentions to invest in expanded access to opioid agonist treatment (OAT).

Although these DEA and FDA policy changes may reduce opioid supply, they may also contribute to negative consequences in regard to the illicit opioid market. A recent article examined the effects of opioid prescription reduction and suggested that this decrease in supply could contribute to a lack of pain management and people using unregulated black market products such as heroin, which could then lead to increased injection drug use (Beletsky and Davis 2017). This transition to black market opioids can increase overdose death risk, and emphasizing policies that focus on supply reduction and increasing law enforcement can limit resources dedicated to addressing the structural determinants that lead to opioid misuse, including economic challenges, trauma, and reduced social capital (Dasgupta et al. 2018).

Although specific federal organizations and their respective policies have important implications for targeting opioid misuse, the current presidential administration has also recently initiated efforts focused on the opioid crisis. The Trump administration appointed an opioid commission in March 2017 that subsequently recommended that the president declare a national emergency (Davis 2017). President Trump later declared the opioid crisis a "health emergency" under the Public Health Service Act (section 319), which is an important distinction: a national emergency declared under the Robert T. Stafford Disaster Relief and Emergency Assistance Act (P.L. 100-707), commonly called the Stafford Act, would have allowed for fund allocation via the Federal Emergency Management Agency (FEMA), which the current designation does not. However, the president's declaration and the formal designation by acting Health Secretary Eric D. Hargan of a public health crisis allowed for limited opioid-specific grant funding, including support for increased use of telemedicine in rural regions.

Whereas these changes in federal policy may have long-term impacts on the current opioid crisis, local and state jurisdictions can also make changes that directly affect education on pain management and safe opioid prescribing for medical providers, providers' ability to monitor their patients' use of prescribed opioids, the availability of MAT and naloxone, and harm reduction programs that target persons who inject opioids. The following sections examine how policy can affect these key components of addressing the crisis.

Policies to Improve Provider Education on Opioid Use

As the opioid crisis has become increasingly visible in American media, there have been concurrent efforts to improve provider education around opioid usage aimed at medical students, resident trainees, and attending physicians. Although there are no current guidelines for medical school curricula regarding opioids, more attention has been paid to improved training of medical students regarding pain management and safe opioid prescribing. Since the 2016 publication of guidelines on pain management from the Centers for Disease Control and Prevention (CDC; www.cdc.gov/mmwr/volumes/65/rr/rr6501e1.htm) centered on safe opioid use, many medical schools have pledged to integrate these guidelines into their curricula (Brinkley 2016). This CDC publication reviewed best practices on when to use opioids for chronic pain, provided information on how to select between different opioid medications, and guided primary care clinicians on the potential dangers of opioid use (Dowell et al. 2016). The guidelines emphasized not using opioid medications as a first-line treatment for chronic pain while also encouraging providers to monitor for addiction risk.

For psychiatry residents, the Accreditation Council for Graduate Medical Education has general requirements that include teaching about addiction psychiatry, and residents must receive training in evaluating and treating substance use disorders (SUDs) (Accreditation Council for Graduate Medical Education 2017). This training includes managing overdoses and the use of pharmacotherapy in SUD treatment. At this time, there are no specific training requirements that focus on opioid use. However, following residency, providers may have CME requirements related to pain management and opioid prescribing in order to receive state medical board licensure. Recently, the Georgia state medical board required that beginning in 2018, all physicians must attend a 3-hour training program on opioid prescribing prior to renewing their medical license (Yu 2017). Similarly, Pennsylvania now has a requirement for a 2-hour CME course in pain management, identifying SUDs, and safe prescribing of opioid medication as a prerequisite for medical license renewal (Harvan 2018). Several other states have similar requirements, and future efforts may lead to additional states requiring that active physicians demonstrate that they have acquired CME or similarly updated training around opioid prescribing prior to medical board licensing renewal.

Prescription Drug Monitoring Programs

PDMPs are electronic databases that track controlled substance prescriptions, including opioid medications, at the state level (Figure 13–1; Centers for Disease Control and Prevention 2017). These programs aim to improve the safety of opioid prescribing by giving clinicians information on patients' prescription history, including a list of prescribed controlled substances, dates, dosages, and prescribers. All U.S. states, the District of Columbia, and the U.S. territory of Guam have operational PDMPs (Brandeis University Prescription Drug Monitoring Program Training and Technical Assistance Center 2018). Agencies administering PDMPs vary by state and include boards of pharmacy, state departments of health, professional licensing organizations, law enforcement, substance abuse authorities, and consumer protection agencies (National Alliance for Model State Drug Laws 2016). There is currently no integrated database that contains controlled substance prescription data from all states; however, the majority of states share their data with other individual PDMPs (e.g., neighboring states) or with authorized users in other states.

As with any tool, PDMPs can affect outcomes only if opioid prescribers use the databases in the course of clinical care. However, only a minority of providers who prescribe controlled substances are registered to

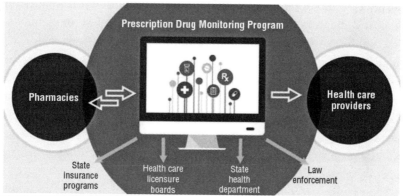

FIGURE 13–1.   Diagram of a prescription drug monitoring program (PDMP).

Source.   Reprinted from Centers for Disease Control and Prevention: "What States Need to Know About PDMPs." October 3, 2017. Available at: https://www.cdc.gov/drugoverdose/pdmp/states.html. Accessed April 5, 2018.

access their state's PDMP, with only 35% registered as of December 2013 (Brenwald 2013). Some states have responded by mandating prescribers to check the database prior to writing controlled substance prescriptions. Thirty states and the territory of Guam mandate that practitioners check the database under certain circumstances, although the class of providers, practice setting, and circumstances vary by state. These laws have faced some opposition due to potential drawbacks including the burdens of gaining and maintaining access to the databases, ambiguous guidance on how data should affect prescribing, and provider concerns regarding penalties related to the mandates (Haffajee et al. 2015). Early data gathered after Kentucky, Tennessee, New York, and Ohio passed PDMP mandates indicate that these laws are associated with increased utilization of the databases, as well as declines in opioid prescribing (Brandeis University Prescription Drug Monitoring Program Center of Excellence 2016). Notably, in several states, laws around PDMP monitoring have been tailored to address the concerns of prescriber organizations, indicating the importance of such collaboration before institution of regulations affecting prescriber practices.

State PDMPs have been studied in terms of their effects on opioid prescribing, diversion and supply, misuse, and opioid-related morbidity and mortality with mixed results thus far (Finley et al. 2017). Much of the data remain observational and state-specific, with trends suggesting modest decreases in opioid prescribing following PDMP implementation and high-risk prescribers and patients being disproportionately responsive (Chang et al. 2016; Rutkow et al. 2015). Variability in the provisions of PDMP laws by state makes it particularly challenging to draw conclusions from data on a national scale. Early evidence points to U.S. states with more robust programs having fewer prescription opioid overdose deaths than those with weaker programs (Pardo 2017). However, data on overall overdose morbidity and mortality outcomes are mixed (Beletsky 2018; Fink et al. 2018).

Overall, limited data thus far support the utility of PDMPs as tools for reducing supplies of prescribed opioids. It remains crucial to ensure a standard set of expectations around PDMP monitoring, ease and reliability of access to the database, and clear guidelines on how to interpret and use the information provided. Such consistency may allow providers to prescribe more safely and may reduce risks associated with vulnerable pain patients inappropriately losing access to needed prescriptions. Further study is required to determine whether PDMPs contribute to several important outcomes, such as decreased rates of OUD, reduced morbidity and mortality related to opioid misuse, and lower rates of heroin use.

Policy Effects on Buprenorphine and Naloxone Access

Access to Buprenorphine

MAT is the first-line approach for treating OUD, and buprenorphine is one of the main pharmacotherapies used, in addition to methadone and long-acting extended-release naltrexone (XR-naltrexone). As Chapters 10 ("Medication-Assisted Treatment for Opioid Use Disorder") and 12 ("Harm Reduction: Caring for People Who Misuse Opioids") describe in depth, OAT (i.e., methadone or buprenorphine) has a larger and stronger supporting evidence base than XR-naltrexone, and because buprenorphine can be prescribed in office-based settings, its use potentially is more flexible and has fewer barriers when compared with methadone delivery in opioid treatment programs. Therefore, increasing buprenorphine access may be particularly strategic for MAT-related policies. Buprenorphine first became an available treatment when it received FDA approval in

2002, and following the Drug Addiction Treatment Act in 2000 (DATA 2000; Title XXXV, Section 3502 of the Children's Health Act of 2000 [P.L. 106-310]), which allowed trained physicians to apply for a waiver to treat OUD with Schedule III–V controlled substances without requiring separate DEA registration under a narcotic treatment program certification (Drug Enforcement Administration 2018). Once physicians received this level of certification, they could treat an initial total of 30 patients and subsequently apply for further authorization to treat a greater number of patients after 1 year. Although DATA 2000 provided an important tool to treat OUD, access to prescribing buprenorphine was limited to physicians, and the patient quotas limited how many patients could receive this office-based treatment.

Since the approval of DATA 2000, there have been several attempts to increase access to buprenorphine. Initially, physicians who received buprenorphine certification could apply to increase the census from 30 to 100 patients; however, in 2016, the U.S. Department of Health and Human Services authorized an increase in this maximum patient panel to 275 (Gutkind 2016). In addition, the 2016 Comprehensive Addiction and Recovery Act allowed nurse practitioners and physician assistants to prescribe buprenorphine after completing a 24-hour training course (American Society of Addiction Medicine 2016b).

Although these recent changes will potentially have a significant impact on the number of patients who can receive buprenorphine in the United States, there are several persistent challenges that can affect access. There are not enough buprenorphine prescribers, with one study stating that if every currently buprenorphine-waivered physician were prescribing at capacity, there would still be a gap of almost 1 million people who were not receiving treatment in the United States (Jones et al. 2015). Despite the training required to receive a buprenorphine waiver, providers have cited difficulties feeling comfortable prescribing buprenorphine. Cost can also be a barrier, because clients who have low income or are uninsured may not be able to afford out-of-pocket costs for the medication (Abraham et al. 2017). Funding can also affect buprenorphine access in a more global way, as almost 66% of specialty treatment programs rely on Substance Abuse and Mental Health Services Administration (SAMHSA) funding administered via a single-state agency within each state (Abraham et al. 2017). Through contract specifications, single-state agencies can influence the adoption of specific medication strategies by each state's treatment programs, and a recent study of state-specific funding showed how state policies influence how often treatment programs provide buprenorphine to clients. Using data from the National Drug Abuse Treatment System Survey collected in 2013–2014, Abraham and colleagues (2017) found that treatment programs had a significantly higher likelihood of adopting buprenorphine if states provided block grant funding and technical assistance. However, overall uptake of buprenorphine was relatively low, with less than 30% of treatment programs offering this medication. These findings suggest that specific state funding and technical assistance are crucial. The study's authors suggested that increased funding from the 21st Century Cures Act of 2016 dedicated to the opioid crisis and additional SAMHSA-driven initiatives may help to steer more programs to improve medication access. In addition, further state subsidies can supplement Medicaid and SAMHSA block grant funding, which can facilitate greater buprenorphine access, especially because fewer than half of the states with the highest rates of opioid-related overdose deaths currently have additional state funding in place.

Medicaid is also a significant driver in terms of buprenorphine access, with a study finding that whether a state's Medicaid program covered buprenorphine impacted whether the medication was used in SUD treatment programs (Sharma et al. 2017). State variability with regard to buprenorphine's availability on a Medicaid formulary could have drastic effects on whether or not people with limited or low income can obtain this medication (Sharma et al. 2017). In addition, even when Medicaid allows clients to receive buprenorphine, differences in Medicaid managed care programs can limit whether patients can afford the medication. Some plans may require preauthorization before approving insurance payment for buprenorphine or necessitate nonphysician counseling in conjunction with the medication prescription. High co-payment costs may make acquiring buprenorphine functionally impossible for some Medicaid recipients.

In contrast, there is evidence that Medicaid expansion via the Patient Protection and Affordable Care Act of 2010 (ACA; P.L. 111-148) can increase Medicaid coverage for buprenorphine. A study of Medicaid drug utilization files between 2011 and 2014 looked at expansion (both immediate and late expansion) and nonexpansion states, demonstrating a significant increase in both Medicaid-covered buprenorphine prescriptions and Medicaid-related buprenorphine spending (Wen et al. 2017) in expansion states. States that had expanded Medicaid in 2014 had an almost 70% increase in prescriptions along with 50% higher buprenorphine spending, whereas states that did not expand Medicaid or expanded Medicaid later than 2014 did not show similar trends. These findings suggest the importance of Medicaid in ensuring that more patients have access to buprenorphine-assisted treatment for OUD.

Access to Naloxone

Naloxone, a μ opioid receptor antagonist, is well established as a safe and effective means of reversing opioid overdoses. As Chapter 12 details, the medication has been identified as an important harm reduction tool in the context of the opioid crisis. SAMHSA has encouraged the use of naloxone as a part of its Opioid Overdose Prevention Toolkit (Substance Abuse and Mental Health Services Administration 2016), and the American Society of Addiction Medicine has advocated for expanding access to the medication and reducing legislative barriers to its prescription (American Society of Addiction Medicine 2016a). Even as medical providers have moved toward prescribing naloxone for at-risk opioid-using patients, law enforcement agencies are increasingly encouraging naloxone training for officers. The U.S. Bureau of Justice Assistance recently developed the Law Enforcement Naloxone Toolkit, aimed at educating first responders about the use of naloxone and appropriate treatment of overdose (Bureau of Justice Assistance National Training and Technical Assistance Center 2018). In addition, many states have Good Samaritan laws that protect those administering naloxone or bystanders who summon emergency responders from arrest or other legal consequences (Network for Public Health Law 2017). The combined efforts of medical professionals and law enforcement agencies aim to increase access to naloxone. Additionally, community-based harm reduction coalitions across the country are attempting to expand laypersons' access to naloxone in a variety of nonmedical settings. Results from a survey conducted by the Harm Reduction Coalition of 136 community-based organizations reporting about 644 sites across the United States showed an exponential increase in the provision and/or prescribing of naloxone to laypersons between 1996 and 2014 (Figure 13–2; Wheeler et al. 2015). Further study is required to determine the efficacy and cost-effectiveness of expanding naloxone prescribing via medical pro-

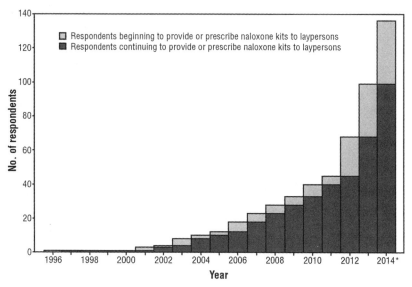

FIGURE 13–2. Naloxone access for laypersons between 1996 and 2014.

*As of June 2014.

Source.   Reprinted from Wheeler E, Jones TS, Gilbert MK, et al; Centers for Disease Control and Prevention: "Opioid Overdose Prevention Programs Providing Naloxone to Laypersons—United States, 2014." *Morbidity and Mortality Weekly Report* 64(23):631–635, 2015 26086633.

fessionals and law enforcement use versus such community-based efforts (Townsend et al. 2017).

Policy and Harm Reduction Programs: Supervised Injection Facilities and Needle Exchange Programs

Supervised Injection Facilities

As described in Chapter 12, supervised injection facilities (SIFs), or safe consumption spaces, are legally sanctioned facilities where people can inject drugs, including heroin or other opioids, under the supervision of medical professionals. There are approximately 100 SIFs operating in 66 cities around the world, but no such facilities are authorized in the United States (Drug Policy Alliance 2018). The movement for SIFs in the United States has gained momentum in the wake of the opioid epidemic. At the time of this writing, San Francisco was poised to become the first U.S. city to create SIFs, after a task force of the San Francisco Department of Public Health voted unanimously in favor of it upon completing a thorough review of safety, efficacy, and cost-effectiveness (Lieber 2018; San Francisco Department of Public Health 2017). Other cities, including Seattle, Baltimore, and Philadelphia, have also taken steps toward providing SIFs through a mixture of public and private funding, although cities must contend with state and federal laws that may be at odds with the creation of such facilities.

SIFs aim to connect with hard-to-reach and marginalized populations; reduce morbidity and mortality related to overdose; reduce infections, including human immunodeficiency virus (HIV) and hepatitis C virus (HCV) infection; and reduce use of injected drugs in public areas such as shooting galleries (places that are frequently used as an injection site by injection drug users) (Beletsky et al. 2008). At the same time, such facilities aim to provide access to clean syringes and paraphernalia ("works"), health education, and referrals (to addiction treatment, medical care, social support, and work/reintegration projects), alongside other services (Woods 2014). Early studies of SIFs have demonstrated their success in reaching marginalized populations, improving rates of safe and hygienic use, reducing drug-related deaths and emergency department visits, and increasing referrals to detoxification and SUD treatment services (European Monitoring Centre for Drugs and Drug Addiction 2017). Population-level effects of SIFs on rates of HIV, HCV, and other infectious disease transmission remain unclear. Despite the controversy and legal hurdles to creating such facilities, no studies have demonstrated that SIFs encourage substance use or adversely affect communities and public health outcomes.

Syringe Service Programs

Some of the challenges faced by SIFs mirror those of needle-syringe exchange programs, which are known by several other names, including needle exchange programs, syringe exchange programs, and syringe-needle access programs (SNAPs) (Centers for Disease Control and Prevention 2018). First established in the 1980s in response to the HIV epidemic, these community-based programs provide access to sterile needles, syringes, alcohol swabs, clean water, and other HIV and HCV prevention methods, including condoms. Many also provide education and connection to ongoing medical or substance-related treatment and social services. Despite initially being developed in the context of HIV prevention and treatment, many current SNAPs provide services specific to opioid use, including primary prevention of overdoses, provision of naloxone for overdose reversals, and connection to substance abuse treatment (U.S. Department of Health and Human Services 2016). Studies have demonstrated that SNAPs can effectively connect patients to and help retain them in comprehensive SUD treatment (Brooner et al. 1998; Gjersing and Bretteville-Jensen 2013).

Despite the proven benefits of SNAPs, they are not universally accessible in the United States, although the opioid epidemic has prompted more states and jurisdictions to approve such programs (Nadelmann and LaSalle 2017). As of 2017, there were 196 cities in the United States, primarily on the east and west coasts, that offered such programs. In response to the opioid epidemic, Congress lifted the ban on federal funding for SNAPs in 2015. This has raised the possibility that more such programs may become accessible as part of a broader public health effort to curb the morbidity and mortality related to the opioid epidemic. However, state-level barriers remain, including laws that limit funding and access based on the misperception that SNAPs may encourage opioid misuse.

Key Chapter Points

▶ Several federal agencies, including the Drug Enforcement Administration and U.S. Food and Drug Administration, have implemented new policies in response to the opioid crisis, including attempts to reduce opioid prescription supplies, improve prescription labeling, and support a greater number of abuse-deterrent opioid formulations.

▶ Policy efforts that target opioid supply reduction without adequate attention to demand and harm reduction may have negative consequences, such as increased use of heroin and overdose death risk, and may de-emphasize tackling structural causes of opioid use.

▶ Some states have implemented continuing medical education requirements on pain management and safe opioid prescribing prior to state medical licensing renewal. Medical schools have dedicated increased attention to these topics as well.

▶ Prescription drug monitoring programs (PDMPs) can track a patient's opioid prescriptions, although state requirements around their use vary. Current evidence suggests that PDMPs can help reduce opioid supply and may correlate with reduced overdose mortality, but data are mixed.

▶ Expanding access to buprenorphine represents a key medication-assisted treatment–related strategy in mitigating the opioid epidemic. Changes to the DATA 2000 legislation have attempted to increase the number of buprenorphine providers available and expand the maximum patient census allowed per waivered clinician. However, variability in state funding and insurance barriers can limit patients' access to buprenorphine.

▶ There have been efforts to increase access to naloxone via Good Samaritan laws, medical provider prescribing, law enforcement training, and community-based programs.

▶ The potential benefits of proven harm reduction strategies, including supervised injection facilities and syringe-needle access programs, are limited by local, state, and federal laws.

References

Abraham AJ, Andrews CM, Grogan CM, et al: State-targeted funding and technical assistance to increase access to medication treatment for opioid use disorder. Psychiatr Serv 69(4):448–455, 2017 29241428

Accreditation Council for Graduate Medical Education: ACGME program requirements for graduate medical education in psychiatry. July 1, 2017. Available at: https://www.acgme.org/Portals/0/PFAssets/ProgramRequirements/400_psychiatry_2017-07-01.pdf. Accessed February 13, 2018.

American Society of Addiction Medicine: Public policy statement on the use of naloxone for the prevention of opioid overdose deaths. 2016a. Available at: https://www.asam.org/docs/default-source/public-policy-statements/use-of-naloxone-for-the-prevention-of-opioid-overdose-deaths-final.pdf. Accessed February 11, 2018.

American Society of Addiction Medicine: Summary of the Comprehensive Addiction and Recovery Act. 2016b. Available at: https://www.asam.org/advocacy/issues/opioids/summary-of-the-comprehensive-addiction-and-recovery-act. Accessed February 13, 2018.

Aschenbrenner DS: The FDA's latest response to opioid abuse and overdose. Am J Nurs 118(1):22–23, 2018 29280800

Beletsky L: Deploying prescription drug monitoring to address the overdose crisis: Ideology meets reality. Indiana Health Law Rev 15(2):139–187, 2018

Beletsky L, Davis CS: Today's fentanyl crisis: Prohibition's Iron Law, revisited. Int J Drug Policy 46:156–159, 2017 28735773

Beletsky L, Davis CS, Anderson E, et al: The law (and politics) of safe injection facilities in the United States. Am J Public Health 98(2):231–237, 2008 18172151

Brandeis University Prescription Drug Monitoring Program Center of Excellence: PDMP prescriber use mandates: characteristics, current status, and outcomes in selected states. May 2016. Available at: http://www.pdmpassist.org/pdf/Resources/Briefing_on_mandates_3rd_revision_A.pdf. Accessed February 11, 2018.

Brandeis University Prescription Drug Monitoring Program Training and Technical Assistance Center: Prescription drug monitoring frequently asked questions (FAQ). 2018. Available at: http://www.pdmpassist.org/content/prescription-drug-monitoring-frequently-asked-questions-faq. Accessed February 11, 2018.

Brenwald S: U.S. Department of Justice Bureau of Justice Assistance: Prescription drug monitoring program performance report. January–December 2013. Available at: https://www.bja.gov/Publications/PDMP_PPR_Jan-Dec13.pdf. Accessed February 11, 2018.

Brinkley C: U.S. medical schools expand training to curb painkiller abuse. June 28, 2016. Available at: https://apnews.com/a0a7596187b7437dbd2aaf21cf4b4b17/us-medical-schools-expand-training-curb-painkiller-abuse. Accessed February 13, 2018.

Brooner R, Kidorf M, King V, et al: Drug abuse treatment success among needle exchange participants. Public Health Rep 113 (suppl 1):129–139, 1998 9722818

Bureau of Justice Assistance National Training and Technical Assistance Center: Law Enforcement Naloxone Toolkit. 2018. Available at: https://www.bjatraining.org/tools/naloxone/Naloxone-Background. Accessed February 11, 2018.

Centers for Disease Control and Prevention: What states need to know about PDMPs. October 3, 2017. Available at: https://www.cdc.gov/drugoverdose/pdmp/states.html. Accessed February 11, 2018.

Centers for Disease Control and Prevention: Syringe services programs. February 27, 2018. Available at: https://www.cdc.gov/hiv/risk/ssps.html. Accessed February 12, 2018.

Chang HY, Lyapustina T, Rutkow L, et al: Impact of prescription drug monitoring programs and pill mill laws on high-risk opioid prescribers: a comparative interrupted time series analysis. Drug Alcohol Depend 165:1–8, 2016 27264166

Dasgupta N, Beletsky L, Ciccarone D: Opioid crisis: no easy fix to its social and economic determinants. Am J Public Health 108(2):182–186, 2018 29267060

Davis JH: Trump declares opioid crisis a "health emergency" but requests no funds. The New York Times, October 26, 2017. Available at: https://www.nytimes.com/2017/10/26/us/politics/trump-opioid-crisis.html. Accessed February 13, 2018.

Dowell D, Haegerich TM, Chou R: CDC guideline for prescribing opioids for chronic pain—United States, 2016. MMWR Recomm Rep 65(1):1–49, 2016 26987082

Drug Enforcement Administration: DEA requirements for DATA waived physicians (DWPs). 2018. Available at: https://www.deadiversion.usdoj.gov/pubs/docs/dwp_buprenorphine.htm. Accessed February 13, 2018.

Drug Policy Alliance: Supervised consumption facilities. 2018. Available at: http://www.drugpolicy.org/issues/supervised-injection-facilities. Accessed February 11, 2018.

European Monitoring Centre for Drugs and Drug Addiction: Drug consumption rooms: an overview of provision and evidence. June 2017. Available at: http://www.emcdda.europa.eu/topics/pods/drug-consumption-rooms. Accessed February 11, 2018.

Fink DS, Schleimer JP, Sarvet A, et al: Association between prescription drug monitoring programs and nonfatal and fatal drug overdoses: a systematic review. Ann Intern Med 168(11):783–790, 2018 29801093

Finley EP, Garcia A, Rosen K, et al: Evaluating the impact of prescription drug monitoring program implementation: a scoping review. BMC Health Serv Res 17(1):420, 2017 28633638

Gjersing L, Bretteville-Jensen AL: Is opioid substitution treatment beneficial if injecting behaviour continues? Drug Alcohol Depend 133(1):121–126, 2013 23773951

Gutkind S: Changes to buprenorphine prescriber limits. July 21, 2016. Available at: https://cherishresearch.org/2016/07/changes-buprenorphine-prescriber-limits. Accessed February 13, 2018.

Haffajee RL, Jena AB, Weiner SG: Mandatory use of prescription drug monitoring programs. JAMA 313(9):891–892, 2015 25622279

Harvan A: Physician license renewal in Pennsylvania: what you need to know. 2018. Available at: https://www.pamedsoc.org/detail/article/medical-license-renewal-pennsylvania. Accessed February 13, 2018.

Jones CM, Campopiano M, Baldwin G, et al: National and state treatment need and capacity for opioid agonist medication-assisted treatment. Am J Public Health 105(8):e55–e63, 2015 26066931

Lieber M: Safe injection sites in San Francisco could be the first in the U.S. February 7, 2018. Available at: https://www.cnn.com/2018/02/07/health/safe-injection-sites-san-francisco-opioid-epidemic-bn/index.html. Accessed February 11, 2018.

Nadelmann E, LaSalle L: Two steps forward, one step back: current harm reduction policy and politics in the United States. Harm Reduct J 14(1):37, 2017 28606093

National Alliance for Model State Drug Laws: Compilation of prescription monitoring program maps. May 2016. Available at: http://www.namsdl.org/library/CAE654BF-BBEA-211E-694C755E16C2DD21/. Accessed February 11, 2018.

Network for Public Health Law: Legal interventions to reduce overdose mortality: naloxone access and overdose Good Samaritan laws. July 2017. Available at: https://www.networkforphl.org/_asset/qz5pvn/legal-interventions-to-reduce-overdose.pdf. Accessed February 11, 2018.

Pardo B: Do more robust prescription drug monitoring programs reduce prescription opioid overdose? Addiction 112(10):1773–1783, 2017 28009931

Pergolizzi JV Jr, Raffa RB, Taylor R Jr, Vacalis S: Abuse-deterrent opioids: an update on current approaches and considerations. Curr Med Res Opin 34(4):711–723, 2018 29262730

Raji MA, Kuo Y-F, Adhikari D, et al: Decline in opioid prescribing after federal rescheduling of hydrocodone products. Pharmacoepidemiol Drug Saf Dec 21, 2017 [Epub ahead of print] 29271049

Rutkow L, Chang HY, Daubresse M, et al: Effect of Florida's drug monitoring program and pill mill laws on opioid prescribing and use. JAMA Intern Med 175(10):1642–1649, 2015 26280092

San Francisco Department of Public Health: Safe Injection Services Task force—final report. September 2017. Available at: https://www.sfdph.org/dph/files/SIStaskforce/SIS-Task-Force-Final-Report-2017.pdf. Accessed February 11, 2018.

Sharma A, Kelly SM, Mitchell SG, et al: Update on barriers to pharmacotherapy for opioid use disorders. Curr Psychiatry Rep 19(6):35, 2017 28526967

Substance Abuse and Mental Health Services Administration: Opioid Overdose Prevention Toolkit. March 3, 2016 (revised). Available at: https://store.samhsa.gov/product/Opioid-Overdose-Prevention-Toolkit/SMA18-4742. Accessed August 2018.

Townsend T, Doan T, Blostein F, et al: Cost-effectiveness of alternative naloxone distribution strategies: first responder and layperson distribution. Paper presented at AcademyHealth Annual Research Meeting, New Orleans, LA, 2017. Available at https://academyhealth.confex.com/academyhealth/2017arm/meetingapp.cgi/Paper/19853. Accessed August 2018

U.S. Department of Health and Human Services: Department of Health and Human Services implementation guidance to support certain components of syringe services programs. 2016. Available at: https://www.hiv.gov/sites/default/files/hhs-ssp-guidance.pdf. Accessed February 11, 2018.

Wen H, Hockenberry JM, Borders TF, et al: Impact of Medicaid expansion on Medicaid-covered utilization of buprenorphine for opioid use disorder treatment. Med Care 55(4):336–341, 2017 28296674

Wheeler E, Jones TS, Gilbert MK, et al; Centers for Disease Control and Prevention: Opioid overdose prevention programs providing naloxone to laypersons—United States, 2014. MMWR Morb Mortal Wkly Rep 64(23):631–635, 2015 26086633

Woods S: Drug consumption rooms in Europe: organisational overview. 2014. Available at: http://www.drugconsumptionroom-international.org/images/pdf/dcr_in_europe.pdf. Accessed February 11, 2018.

Yu E: Ga. doctors required to get opioid prescription training. August 14, 2017. Available at: https://www.wabe.org/ga-doctors-required-get-opioid-prescription-training/. Accessed February 13, 2018.

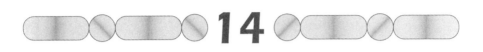

14

Performance Measures and Quality Improvement for the Opioid Epidemic

Arthur Robin Williams, M.D., M.B.E.

Case Vignette: Clara Takes on the Opioid Epidemic

Clara is the director of her state's addiction services office in the Department of Mental Health and has been charged with tackling the opioid crisis. She works in a large midwestern state that has observed a 250% increase in the annual opioid-related overdose death rate in the past decade. Owing to increasing political pressure, the governor's office has been requesting information on what can be done to lower overdose mortality. Political pressure has mounted in part because of recent news articles in local and national media characterizing suspicious practices among some treatment providers and sober living facilities, as well as growing public awareness of high rates of overdose following treatment at detoxification facilities in the state. The governor's chief of staff is proposing a "score card system" to evaluate treatment programs in order to inform consumer choice and redirect public funding in the state to opioid use disorder (OUD) treatment programs that are "evidence-based" and that have the best outcomes.

> To begin to tackle this problem, Clara has instructed her staff to look into quality measure development for the treatment of OUD to determine if existing measures are sufficient for her state's use or if she will need to create measures tailored to the state's population.

This chapter provides a brief overview of quality measure development, key measure characteristics and implications for measure use, and data collection and reporting necessary for analysis. Specifically, it will address several key questions: How are quality measures generally developed? What are key components of measures and how do they affect quality measure use? What is needed to evaluate quality of care across different kinds of programs that may treat varying populations of patients with OUD?

Approaches to Framing the Opioid Epidemic

Scale of Opioid Use Disorder and Overdose Rates

The United States is facing the largest epidemic of opioid overdose deaths in its history, and mortality rates continue to climb at an accelerating pace. In 2016, annual unintentional overdose fatalities from opioids amounted to 42,249 deaths (over 115 per day), which may be an underestimate (Han et al. 2015; National Center for Health Statistics 2017; Ruhm 2017). This staggering number of overdose deaths is often a downstream consequence of the burden of untreated and undertreated OUD, reflecting a long-standing addiction treatment gap in the United States (Garnick et al. 2009; Ghitza and Tai 2014). In fact, overdoses frequently occur among persons who have recently been discharged from detoxification programs or treatment (Sordo et al. 2017; Strang et al. 2003).

Despite U.S. Food and Drug Administration (FDA) approval of three medications (methadone, buprenorphine, and extended-release naltrexone [XR-naltrexone]), all of which have been shown to reduce overdose among patients with OUD (Degenhardt et al. 2011; Lee et al. 2016, 2018), there remain low rates of medication initiation and retention (i.e., beyond 6 months) with these medication-assisted treatment (MAT) pharmacotherapies (Williams and Bisaga 2016). As a result, among approximately 2.5 million individuals addicted (1.9 million to prescription opioids and 0.6 million to heroin) (Rudd et al. 2016), only one-fifth receive treatment in a given year (Saloner and Karthikeyan

2015; Substance Abuse and Mental Health Services Administration 2012; Wu et al. 2016), with roughly one-third of those receiving evidence-based care with FDA-approved medication in a given treatment episode (Substance Abuse and Mental Health Services Administration 2017a; Volkow et al. 2014).

Effective treatment of OUD presents a series of clinical challenges; development of quality measures should systematically target several points of intervention and should be informed by goal setting and tracking of progress at each stage with feasible, reliable, and valid measures under a unified framework. However, measures can only perform as well as the longitudinal data collection and reporting systems that contribute to their use. Public health and health care systems must characterize available data sources, summarize current estimates, and create recommendations for data needed to operationalize quality measures to improve outcomes for individuals with OUD.

Prevalence Estimates and Identification of Opioid Use Disorder

For several years, the estimated prevalence of OUD in the United States has been reported as approximately 2.4–2.5 million individuals (Rudd et al. 2016). This number is derived from the National Survey on Drug Use and Health (NSDUH) and is increasingly recognized as likely underestimating the true burden of OUD (Compton et al. 2010; Ruhm 2017). For instance, the NSDUH, administered by the Substance Abuse and Mental Health Services Administration (SAMHSA), surveys approximately 67,500 noninstitutionalized residents each year, with a response rate of approximately 70% (Hunter et al. 2005; Substance Abuse and Mental Health Services Administration 2012); as a result, many individuals at highest risk of OUD (incarcerated and institutionalized individuals, the chronically homeless, and nonrespondents) are not included in the count (Compton et al. 2010). Recent fieldwork has shown that rates of heroin use have been increasing more rapidly than may be reflected in national surveys (Cicero et al. 2017). Such national surveys (listed in Table 14–1 with descriptions, strengths, and limitations) often include large sample sizes and can track trends over time nationally and (for some covariates and outcomes) at the state level. However, they are subject to limitations, as listed in Table 14–1, which warrant caution regarding interpretation of their findings.

TABLE 14–1.   National surveys for monitoring the prevalence of opioid use disorder

Survey	Description	Strengths	Limitations
Monitoring the Future (MTF)	Survey administered directly to students in grades 8, 10, and 12	Administered annually; can detect changing trends among adolescent drug-taking behaviors and perceptions of risk	Misses students who have dropped out of school or are institutionalized
National Comorbidity Survey (NCS)	Emphasizes mental health and comorbidity; found that 1.4% of adults have a drug use disorder other than alcohol (Compton et al. 2007)	Captures substance use disorder status generally in relation to comorbid mental illness	Not specific to classes of drugs (i.e., opioids)
National Epidemiologic Survey on Alcohol and Related Conditions (NESARC)	Three large national surveys: the first two occurred among the same sample of respondents (years 2002 and 2013) and the third among a new group	Panel data (samples same individuals across multiple time points) between the first two waves	Not administered annually
National Health and Nutrition Examination Survey (NHANES)	Assesses health and nutritional status of all age groups	Unique in that it combines surveys with physical exams; reflects self-reported drug use and frequency of use among participants ages 12–59 years	Does not assess for diagnostic criteria or history of disorder or treatment

TABLE 14–1. National surveys for monitoring the prevalence of opioid use disorder *(continued)*

Survey	Description	Strengths	Limitations
National Survey on Drug Use and Health (NSDUH)	Nationwide and state-representative household survey conducted annually (*N*=67,500), 2016 results estimation of 2.1 million individuals with past-year OUD (Substance Abuse and Mental Health Services Administration 2017b)	Highly powered; oversamples youth and young adults ages 12–25 years	Does not reach institutionalized (e.g., incarcerated) individuals
Youth Risk Behavior Survey (YRBS)	Began in the early 1990s by CDC as a biennial survey to assess for risk factors for HIV infection, including drug use by youth	Biennial data dating to 1990s capturing high-risk drug and sexual behaviors among youth	Misses high-risk (e.g., incarcerated) youth

Note. CDC=Centers for Disease Control and Prevention; HIV=human immunodeficiency virus; OUD=opioid use disorder.

In addition to national surveys, which are used to estimate the prevalence of opioid use and OUD, other data sources can give clues as to whether a diagnosis such as OUD is likely increasing or decreasing in prevalence from year to year. Mortality statistics and drug overdose rates can be used to estimate changes in the prevalence of OUD over time; for example, if there is upward of a 1%–2% annual mortality rate for persons with OUD (Degenhardt et al. 2011) and half of deaths are overdose related (Hser et al. 2015), then 33,000 opioid overdose deaths would correspond to approximately 4.4 million individuals with OUD. Like national survey data, estimates of overdose rates must be interpreted with caution. For instance, the Centers for Disease Control and Prevention, SAMHSA, the Office of National Drug Control Policy, and the Department of Justice all have different methodologies for categorizing deaths and characterizing mortality trends. There is widespread variation across states and municipalities in postmortem toxicology practices (e.g., how frequently toxicology is performed, which classes of substances [e.g., fentanyl] are assayed) and reporting, leading to missing and incomplete data.

Other less direct data sources can also help track trends in opioid use over time. For instance, the Department of Justice and law enforcement offices often monitor seizures of illicit substances; drug involvement among arrestees, prisoners, and parolees; and pharmaceutical prescribing activity. Pharmacy, pharmaceutical, physician, and health research associations also track prescription opioid use, including prescription opioids and treatment with Drug Enforcement Administration (DEA)–scheduled medications such as buprenorphine (Cicero et al. 2007; Researched Abuse, Diversion and Addiction-Related Surveillance System website, www.radars.org). Prescription drug monitoring programs (PDMPs) also offer opportunities for surveying trends in controlled substance use (Haffajee et al. 2015; Rutkow et al. 2015).

Treatment data (e.g., change in demand for treatment for OUD, variation in reported drug/s of choice at intake) based on intakes for substance abuse treatment and substance-related hospitalizations suggest changes in problems from drug activity but are inconsistently reported across treatment systems and states (see more information on Treatment Episode Data Sets in the next subsection). More novel surveillance methodologies include analyses of Google search terms and social media (e.g., Facebook, Twitter) activity, which can be analyzed through natural language processing and key word search methodologies to track patterns over time (Curtis et al. 2018; Hanson et al. 2013; Kazemi et al. 2017).

On the basis of available data sources, estimates of the national prevalence of OUD vary widely but seem to cluster around 2.4–2.5 million, with some analyses suggesting up to 4.4 million (Kolodny et al. 2015; Williams 2017). State-level estimates are even more difficult to derive, although it is clear that a handful of states (e.g., Ohio, Kentucky, West Virginia, New Hampshire) have been hit especially hard.

Treatment Initiation and Retention

Major deficits exist in the ability to track the numbers of patients entering care for OUD. The largest source of data on treatment services in the United States, SAMHSA's annual National Survey of Substance Abuse Treatment Services (N-SSATS; Substance Abuse and Mental Health Services Administration 2017a), evaluates only programs that are accredited (via third parties approved by SAMHSA) and funded by SAMHSA on a single day in a given year. As a result, N-SSATS is not designed to monitor treatment provided privately, such as office-based MAT with buprenorphine or XR-naltrexone outside opioid treatment programs (OTPs; formerly known as methadone maintenance programs), such as in federally qualified health centers and other primary care settings. N-SSATS also cannot follow longitudinal outcomes (e.g., how many patients are retained in care) or patients lost to follow-up (e.g., dropouts who have presumably returned to active opioid use).

All publicly funded treatment programs are required to submit data characterizing patients at intake (e.g., first, second, and third drugs of choice; addiction treatment history; demographics) to Treatment Episode Data Sets (TEDS), and a self-selected subset of programs also submits treatment completion reports to TEDS, although this varies across states. TEDS thus captures data differently than N-SSATS but faces similar limitations in that most private providers (especially individual clinicians) do not track or report TEDS data, there is often no follow-up data for individual patient trajectories, and no information is available for patients who leave treatment.

It is estimated that many more patients with OUD receive buprenorphine through private offices (some estimates indicate upward of 800,000 unique individuals receive at least one prescription in a given year, however, some of these may be only for detoxification purposes rather than treatment of OUD) than receive treatment in SAMHSA-accredited programs (i.e., methadone or buprenorphine at an OTP). However, no office within the U.S. Department of Health and Human Services has historically tracked how many patients receive buprenorphine (i.e., initiate treatment) or characterized those who do (e.g., retention rates at 6 months, 1 year, and 2 years) nationally across all treatment settings. A small handful of studies (e.g., those examining insurance claims data for prescription fills) have suggested that the average patient who receives buprenorphine only does so for 30–60 days (Gordon et al. 2015; Stein et al. 2016), falling far short of a minimum threshold of 6–12 months thought to be necessary to confer long-term benefit (Kampman and Jarvis 2015; National Quality Forum 2017). For instance, the Surgeon General's 2016 report on substance use disorders (SUDs) pointed out that patients who receive fewer than 90 days of MAT generally show no long-term benefit (U.S. Department of Health and Human Services 2016).

Even greater challenges limit knowledge of the number of individuals receiving XR-naltrexone, because it is not a controlled substance and therefore fewer monitoring efforts characterize prescription activity. Most published studies of XR-naltrexone characterize outcomes from clinical trials and other settings whereby medications are provided as part of study participation or are court mandated or part of alternative sentencing programs, which do not reflect population-level use (in terms of initiation and retention) in community-based settings (Jarvis et al. 2018).

Although patients receiving methadone must do so through SAMHSA-accredited OTPs and thus are tracked annually (e.g., on March 31, 2015, there were roughly 356,000 patients receiving methadone in an OTP according to N-SSATS), within each state, limited information is available to systematically track the numbers of patients initiating buprenorphine or XR-naltrexone, and even less information is available on the percentage who manage to adhere beyond 6 months, irrespective of MAT modality.

By extension, there are limited data estimating the number of patients with OUD who achieve long-term recovery with or without specialized treatment services (including the use of MAT), because few longitudinal studies exist that follow patients more than 6–12 months. Two large studies are exceptions: the Starting Treatment with Agonist

Replacement Therapies (START) study and the Prescription Opioid Addiction Treatment Study (POATS) by the National Institute on Drug Abuse Clinical Trials Network (Hser et al. 2015; Weiss et al. 2015). Other longitudinal studies from overseas offer additional data to contextualize the findings from START and POATS, which generally found that the majority of patients who remain continuously free of opioid use do so while adherent to a MAT pharmacotherapy such as methadone or buprenorphine. Relapses and overdoses are much more common when patients stop a MAT pharmacotherapy (Hser et al. 2015; Sordo et al. 2017; Strang et al. 2003). To date, no published studies have shown benefit for cessation of MAT. However, data are lacking as to critical inflection points beyond an emphasis on a minimum of 6–12 months of MAT maintenance to achieve long-term benefits (McLellan et al. 2000; National Quality Forum 2017). Expert consensus is that a minimum of 1–2 years of adherence is often necessary before cautiously attempting a taper if one is requested by patients and not clinically contraindicated (National Consensus Development Panel on Effective Medical Treatment of Opiate Addiction 1998).

Data are also lacking regarding which patients do best on which MAT pharmacotherapies, in addition to which patients require longer (e.g., more than 2 years) rather than relatively shorter durations of treatment with MAT. In general, published studies suggest that demographics (e.g., age, race, sex) are less important than addiction severity (e.g., progression to heroin use, injection, overdose history, comorbid cocaine use) and treatment history (e.g., multiple failed attempts at tapers in the past) when predicting long-term retention and outcomes. The OUD Treatment Cascade framework, described later in this chapter, coupled with standardized reporting of quality measures, could help identify which patients struggle at which stages of the cascade to allow for the development of high-impact interventions for specific subpopulations and settings.

Barriers to Care and Risk Factors for Overdose

Despite a strong evidence base for effective treatment with MAT, there remain low rates of initiation and retention because of many barriers impeding access to these medications (American Society of Addiction Medicine 2013; Timko et al. 2016). Current estimates are that only about 20% of the roughly 2.4 million individuals with OUD are engaged in care each year (Saloner and Karthikeyan 2015; Wu et al. 2016). With only 35% of those in care estimated to receive evidence-based treatment (i.e., initiation of one of the three MAT medications) during a given care episode, and considering that the 6-month retention rate is under 30%–50% in most settings, only a fraction of individuals with OUD achieve long-term remission in the United States following a single episode of care, contributing to the escalating overdose mortality rate (Williams et al. 2017).

At present, barriers to receiving evidence-based care with MAT span many aspects of the drug treatment system (Table 14–2). Seventeen states have Medicaid programs that do not cover methadone maintenance, and publicly funded programs often arbitrarily limit treatment duration (American Society of Addiction Medicine 2013). Although addiction treatment has been deemed one of 10 "essential health benefits" under the Patient Protection and Affordable Care Act of 2010 (P.L. 111-148), methadone or buprenorphine maintenance has not yet been included in the mandate. Recently, professional and consumer advocacy groups have been petitioning the Centers for Medicare and Medicaid Services to explicitly mandate MAT coverage under essential health benefits for substance abuse treatment.

Even with private or public insurance coverage, patients with OUD are often difficult to engage in treatment. Many patients in need of substance abuse treatment lack insight into the severity of their condition and do not willingly seek treatment (Substance Abuse and Mental Health Services Administration 2017a; Williams et al. 2015). Many primary care settings are ill equipped to treat psychiatric comorbidity among patients with OUD or lack the resources for comprehensive services to engage patients in care. Given these challenges, for the foreseeable future, specialized addiction services provided through publicly funded substance abuse treatment programs (both outpatient and residential) are likely to remain vital to the care of patients who are addicted to opioids. Yet, institutionalized ideology favoring medication-free ("abstinence only") approaches modeled on treating alcoholism in the mid-twentieth century persists throughout these programs, and some patients feel stigmatized for using MAT.

There is a critical opportunity to develop quality measures for effectively engaging patients with OUD in specialty care under a unified framework. Effective treatment of OUD presents a series of clinical

TABLE 14–2. Barriers to accessing evidence-based care with medication-assisted treatment

Barriers	Methadone	Buprenorphine	Extended-release naltrexone
Medicaid coverage limitations	17 states do not cover methadone maintenance. Methadone maintenance is not included under the "essential health benefit" designation by the Centers for Medicare and Medicaid Services.	Some states limit lifetime use (e.g., capped at 1–3 years).	10+ states cover as a medical benefit (rather than pharmacy benefit). Physicians are required to purchase the medication up front and bill ("buy and bill") after it is administered.
Medicaid prior authorization restrictions	Some states have treatment duration limits or require copayments for treatment beyond 3–6 months.	48 states require prior authorizations, restricting access (e.g., through burdens on providers, requiring documentation of counseling for approval).	"Step therapy" requires patients to have failed other treatments prior to approval.

TABLE 14–2. Barriers to accessing evidence-based care with medication-assisted treatment *(continued)*

Barriers	Methadone	Buprenorphine	Extended-release naltrexone
Commercial insurance coverage barriers	Coverage of methadone maintenance under "essential health benefit" designation is extremely rare.	Many plans require "step therapy," prior authorizations, and documentation of counseling. Some plans limit use to temporary detoxification only. Some plans require laboratory documentation of opioid use (i.e., urine toxicology).	Plans may no longer pay for "medically necessary" treatment once the patient is stable. Providers are required to "buy and bill" and administer as a medical benefit.
Provider capacity	Physicians cannot prescribe in office-based settings or dispense via local pharmacies because of federal regulations.	More than 40% of U.S. counties do not have a single buprenorphine-waivered physician, and around half of waivered physicians do not prescribe.	Virtually no physicians administer it as part of standard residency/training programs.
Accessibility and finding a provider	Patients in rural areas spend upward of $50/week just on travel costs to attend daily; patients often face long waiting lists of several months.	One-third of states have fewer than half of waivered physicians listed on the national buprenorphine treatment locator; in rural areas, waivered physicians often have full practices and cannot legally accept new patients.	Providers are exceptionally hard to find.

TABLE 14–2. Barriers to accessing evidence-based care with medication-assisted treatment *(continued)*

Barriers	Methadone	Buprenorphine	Extended-release naltrexone
Addiction treatment programs	Most substance abuse treatment programs are not affiliated with methadone programs; many residential treatment programs refuse patients taking methadone.	Some treatment programs pressure patients to discontinue buprenorphine under a medication-free, abstinence-only model.	Many programs lack medical professionals to prescribe and administer.

Source. Data from American Society of Addiction Medicine 2013; Substance Abuse and Mental Health Services Administration 2017a.

challenges; development of quality measures provides opportunities to systematically target several points of intervention and could be informed by goal setting and tracking of progress at each stage with feasible, reliable, and valid measures.

Existing Quality Measure Frameworks

Quality measures for effectively engaging patients affected by OUD in specialty care are needed at the structural, process, and outcome levels (Donabedian 1988). *Structural measures* refer to quality measures at the system and provider level, such as the percentage of emergency departments with an addiction specialist available during all hours of operation or the percentage of OUD specialty treatment programs with at least one physician qualified to prescribe buprenorphine (i.e., under a DEA waiver per the Drug Addiction Treatment Act of 2000 [DATA 2000; PL 106-310]). Structural measures can be incorporated into accreditation standards and funding algorithms for value-based care reimbursement models such as the Merit-based Incentive Payment System. *Process measures* refer to metrics pertaining to service delivery, such as the percentage of patients who receive a urine drug screen on presentation to an emergency department or the percentage of patients offered MAT upon intake to specialty treatment. Process measures are relatively easy to track in real time (i.e., through an electronic health record) and can serve as a proxy for quality of care (Garnick et al. 2006). *Outcome measures* typically refer to patients' clinical outcomes, such as results from urine toxicology or the percentage of patients retained on MAT with clinically meaningful improvements in health and quality of life (e.g., measured with short questionnaires or other standardized assessment tools [Bray et al. 2017]) in addition to patterns of drug use. However, outcome measures require risk adjustment based on patient characteristics that often impact outcomes (Harris et al. 2007) and can be more difficult to track through electronic health records.

Despite a burgeoning movement for quality measures across the health care landscape, measures specific for SUDs, much less OUD, are scarce (Williams et al. 2018). The National Committee for Quality Assurance (NCQA) has adopted two measures as Healthcare Effectiveness Data Information Set (HEDIS) measures related to SUDs generally: an Initiation measure assessing the percentage of patients who have a treatment intake within 14 days of a new SUD diagnosis and an Engagement measure that assesses the percentage of patients who initiate treatment who have a minimum of two additional visits in the subsequent 30 days (National Committee for Quality Assurance 2017). Both are process measures. The NCQA has recently decided to include receipt of MAT as a qualifying service for satisfying these two measures' requirements. Although such HEDIS measures are used by the great majority of managed care insurance plans to evaluate quality, they do not offer the level of granular detail needed to track patient progression through OUD Treatment Cascade stages (Williams et al. 2018), which are described in the following section. A new National Quality Forum (NQF)–endorsed outcome measure developed by the RAND Corporation in 2017 assesses the percentage of MAT patients who adhere for at least 180 days and is a rare example of a quality measure that is built upon the evidence base for treatment specific to OUD (National Quality Forum 2017).

The Agency for Healthcare Research and Quality (AHRQ) is a federal agency with a mission to produce evidence to make health care safer, higher quality, and more accessible, equitable, and affordable. AHRQ maintains a National Quality Measure Clearinghouse. The NQF is a "not-for-profit, nonpartisan, membership-based organization that works to catalyze improvements in healthcare" (www.qualityforum.org/About_NQF/) and endorses measures developed by other parties such as the NCQA, the Joint Commission, and professional guilds such as the American Psychiatric Association, as well as health care policy nonprofit research groups such as the RAND Corporation. Both the NQF and AHRQ maintain comprehensive databases cataloging over 3,000 quality measures, including their original developers, specifications, and endorsement statuses spanning all fields of medicine (however, under the Trump administration, funding for the AHRQ website has been eliminated and the website has been shut down).

Across the two clearinghouses, there are seven unique quality measures (Table 14–3) that address the treatment of OUD directly (Williams et al. 2018); each is a process measure reflecting patterns of service delivery (i.e., percentage of patients with OUD engaged in care). Two are specific to the treatment of OUD (rather than SUDs generally). One is the 2017 measure developed by RAND (#3715 Continuity of MAT for OUD) for tracking the percentage of patients who initiate MAT who continue to take the medication for a minimum of 180 days (National Quality Forum 2017). It is the only identified measure that could serve as an outcome

TABLE 14–3. Existing quality measures related to the treatment of opioid use disorder

Clearinghouse	Endorsement year by NQF	Quality measure	Measure developer	Category
NQF Clearinghouse	2017	#3715 Continuity of pharmacy for OUD (percentage with 180+ days taking MAT among those who initiate MAT)	RAND	Outcome
NQF Clearinghouse	2015	#2605 Follow-up AOD service after emergency department visit for AOD (percentage within 7 days and percentage within 30 days)	NCQA	Process
AHRQ NQMC and NQF Clearinghouse	2014	#010148 Percentage with AOD diagnosis that receives *or refuses* a MAT or referral at hospital discharge (AOD treatment provided or offered at discharge from inpatient hospitalization)	TJC	Process
AHRQ NQMC and NQF Clearinghouse	2014	#010149 Percentage with AOD diagnosis that receives a MAT or referral at hospital discharge (AOD treatment provided or offered at discharge from inpatient hospitalization)	TJC	Process

TABLE 14–3. Existing quality measures related to the treatment of opioid use disorder *(continued)*

Clearinghouse	Endorsement year by NQF	Quality measure	Measure developer	Category
AHRQ_NQMC and NQF Clearinghouse	2009	#009966 (#010574) Percentage with initiation of AOD treatment within 14 days of new SUD diagnosis (comparable to NQF #0004 Initiation and engagement of AOD treatment)	NCQA	Process
AHRQ_NQMC and NQF Clearinghouse	2009	#009967 (#010575) Percentage with engagement in AOD treatment (2 + visits) within 30 days of initiation (comparable to NQF #0004 Initiation and engagement of AOD treatment)	NCQA	Process
AHRQ_NQMC	N/A	#004208 Percentage >18 years with current opioid addiction counseled on psychosocial and pharmacological treatments	APA, NCQA, PCPI	Process

Note. AHRQ_NQMC=Agency for Healthcare Research and Quality's National Quality Measure Clearinghouse; AOD=alcohol or other drug; APA=American Psychiatric Association; NCQA=National Committee for Quality Assurance; NQF=National Quality Forum; OUD=opioid use disorder; PCPI=Physician Consortium for Performance Improvement (American Society of Addiction Medicine 2014); SUD=substance use disorder; TJC=The Joint Commission.
Source. Adapted from Williams et al. 2018.

measure rather than a process measure, although it was not originally developed as an outcome measure. A second measure, #004208, reflects the percentage of patients with OUD counseled on the existence of available treatments but does not actually track receipt of evidence-based treatments. It is a measure that has not been endorsed by the NQF, likely in part because of its limited clinical meaningfulness because of its difficult use in clinical settings.

Organizing efforts to respond to the opioid overdose epidemic around a framework of quality measures, akin to the human immunodeficiency virus (HIV) cascade of care, could significantly improve outcomes and reduce mortality (Gardner et al. 2011; Socías et al. 2016; Williams et al. 2017). The HIV cascade of care was initially organized around a primary outcome of viral suppression, in part to minimize risk of further transmission of HIV to others in addition to maximizing patient health. The HIV cascade framework establishes key stages (diagnosis, engagement in care, initiation of antiretrovirals, viral suppression, and retention in care) through which HIV-infected persons can progress to successfully achieve viral suppression, thereby improving individual health and eliminating transmission risk to others (Gardner et al. 2011). For instance, the United Nations has established a 90-90-90 goal aiming to successfully diagnose 90% of all HIV-infected persons worldwide, successfully engage 90% of those diagnosed in treatment, and virally suppress at least 90% of those in treatment by the year 2020.

Translating the 90-90-90 goal to the opioid overdose epidemic would require identifying 2.25 million individuals with OUD (of the approximately 2.5 million affected), engaging more than 2.025 million of those in evidence-based treatment, and assisting 1.82 million into long-term recovery. Identifying such an ambitious goal can inform the development of quality measures and direct resources to best satisfy them. Given differences between the nature of detecting HIV and OUD (i.e., many individuals infected with HIV can go for many years before becoming symptomatic and must be diagnosed with a laboratory test) and treating patients (HIV viral suppression requires daily medication adherence, whereas some patients with OUD can intermittently cease opioid use without MAT), the OUD Treatment Cascade model does not seamlessly translate. However, it models the opportunities that a unified framework can provide to clinicians, researchers, and policy makers.

The HIV cascade of care has demonstrated benefits across settings and populations. Given that the cascade offers a common model, it allows for comparisons both over time and in various settings to trend outcomes, identify critical gaps in care and resulting disparities, and develop interventions at the population level (Horberg et al. 2015; Mugavero et al. 2013; Zanoni and Mayer 2014). Because of its simple and standardized structure, it more easily allows for comparisons across locations and time. The model has also been successfully applied to other chronic medical disorders such as diabetes (Ali et al. 2014) and hepatitis C (Yehia et al. 2014).

Similar to serologically confirmed undetectable HIV viral load, continuous abstinence from opioids can be objectively monitored with routine urine toxicology and serve as a biomarker for a primary outcome (i.e., opioid-free samples). Patients abstinent from opioids and on maintenance treatment with buprenorphine, methadone, or XR-naltrexone are at minimal risk for opioid overdose. Implementing quality measures within an OUD Treatment Cascade holds great promise to improve treatment outcomes and reduce overdose death. Identifying which patients struggle at which stages of the cascade can help in targeting clinical and policy interventions to help federal and state efforts achieve the greatest impact.

Developing an Opioid Use Disorder Cascade of Care

Building on the evidence base of effective prevention and treatment of OUD, along with existing quality measures, an OUD Cascade of Care model encompasses interrelated stages under a unified framework for all persons with OUD or at risk for developing OUD: prevention, identification, treatment, and recovery. The *OUD Treatment Cascade* refers to stages of treatment among affected individuals, including engagement in care, MAT initiation, retention >6 months on MAT, and recovery.

Figure 14–1 serves as a conceptual model encompassing the relationships between prevention, identification, treatment, and recovery for persons with OUD or at risk for overdose. Importantly, the model as presented emphasizes a distinction between acute presentations (e.g., overdoses, emergency department visits) and routine screening and management for populations based on risk level. This distinction is in-

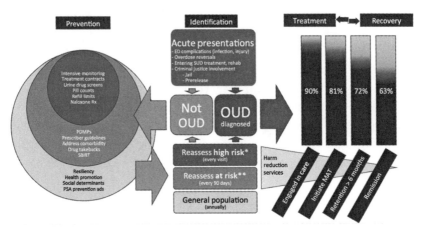

FIGURE 14–1.   OUD cascade of care conceptual model.

Percentages in the columns reflect theoretical targets for success under a 90-90-90 model derived from the global UNAIDS goal for HIV by the year 2020.

ED=emergency department; MAT=medication-assisted treatment; MEQ=morphine-equivalent doses per day; OUD=opioid use disorder; PDMP=prescription drug monitoring program; PSA=public service announcement; SBIRT=Screening, Brief Intervention, and Referral to Treatment; SUD=substance use disorder; UNAIDS=Joint United Nations Programme on HIV/AIDS.

*High-risk population=individuals prescribed >90 mg MEQs daily; individuals with a history of SUD treatment or diagnosis; individuals with unstable psychiatric comorbidity; individuals with acute presentation in prior 5 years.

**At-risk population=individuals receiving long-term opioid therapy; individuals with a family history of SUD; young males (ages 18–35); individuals with active problematic substance use.

tended to emphasize the opportunity that acute presentations offer for inducing patients with OUD onto MAT. As listed within the concentric circles under "Prevention," many touted interventions and services for responding to the epidemic (e.g., PDMPs, prescriber guidelines) address primary prevention but do not necessarily facilitate progression through the treatment end of the cascade for individuals with OUD. This framework can galvanize responses to develop interventions that are tailored to treatment stages to help engage affected individuals in care, initiate a MAT pharmacotherapy, adhere to MAT for a minimum of 6–12 months, and eventually enter long-term recovery (i.e., no longer meeting criteria for OUD).

A key decision for developing any quality measure framework pertains to the primary outcome. Recovery is depicted in Figure 14–1 on a bidirectional continuum with "Treatment" and includes remission (no longer meeting past-year criteria for OUD) as the final stage along the treatment section of the cascade. Because even a single episode of opioid use can carry risk of death, the ideal of continuous abstinence could serve as an organizing principle despite the fact that many patients will receive benefit from OUD treatment even if continuous abstinence has not been achieved or is not the individual patient's treatment goal. The same can be said in other areas of medicine, wherein patients benefit from treatment (e.g., diabetes, hypertension) but do not necessarily meet primary end points continuously (i.e., HbA1c < 6.5%, blood pressure < 140/90 mm Hg). Although stigma, prejudice, and misinformation have historically led to the erroneous and premature discharge of patients from OUD treatment, an impulse to protect patients from these harms should not obscure the importance of continuous abstinence from opioids as the greatest protection against an opioid-related overdose. The following sections discuss candidate measure considerations, data collection, and reporting approaches for measurement development across the OUD Cascade of Care.

Identification

Patients with OUD are difficult to identify, track, and engage in treatment because of their marginalized status and a health care system that is often ill equipped to detect SUDs generally. Many patients in need of addiction treatment lack insight, struggle with ambivalence, or fear stigmatization and prejudiced responses from providers and do not proactively seek treatment (Substance Abuse and Mental Health Services Administration 2012; Williams et al. 2015). Others who are eligible for Medicaid or subsidized private insurance through the Affordable Care Act's health insurance exchanges may have unstable lives that compromise their ability to enroll in health insurance, much less engage in primary care. As a result, active screening and comprehensive assessments that are nonjudgmental are needed to identify patients with risky behaviors or an undiagnosed OUD.

Ideally, surveillance data could be collected in a uniform fashion across all municipalities and reported at the state level to allow for analyses of trends between states over time in comparison with overall national changes. Figure 14–1 delineates three populations at varying risk for developing OUD. Factors that put individuals at high risk include long-term opioid therapy for noncancer pain, taking more than 90 mg morphine equivalents (MEQs) daily, a history of SUDs, unstable psychiatric comorbidity, active problematic substance use (e.g., binge drinking or cocaine use), prior overdose, and prior criminal arrest (Cicero and Ellis 2017; Compton et al. 2016). These risk factors are especially predictive of addiction liability among young males ages 18–35 years (Compton et al. 2016). Among the general population (i.e., those not prescribed long-term opioid therapy and not endorsing past-month recreational opioid use), screenings for OUD should follow guidelines recommended by the framework of Screening, Brief Intervention, and Referral to Treatment (SBIRT), as advocated by SAMHSA, whereby all primary care patients are assessed once annually for SUDs (Babor et al. 2007). Table 14–4 includes candidate quality measure concepts related to identification of individuals with OUD.

Treatment

Figure 14–2 models existing quality measures (see Table 14–3) in relation to the treatment end of the OUD Cascade of Care under an OUD Treatment Cascade (far right side of Figure 14–1). In general, existing quality measures relate to service delivery in the initial stages of referring and engaging patients with OUD in care. However, aside from the recently developed process measure #3715, Continuity of MAT for 180+ days, they fail to reference the evidence base specific to the treatment of OUD.

The HIV cascade of care is an especially useful framework given that patients must progress through a given stage in order to reach a subsequent stage successfully. Adapting the framework to an OUD Treatment Cascade (see far right side of Figure 14–1) includes stages of engagement in care of those who are diagnosed with OUD; MAT initiation among those engaged in care; retention on MAT for a minimum of 180 days among those who initiate MAT; and remission, meaning not meeting (past-year) diagnostic criteria for OUD among those retained in care.

In order to track and improve patient outcomes along the cascade, SUD treatment providers (both publicly funded and private providers) would need to reorient their systems to track all patients who enter care for OUD, especially those who discontinue MAT or stop appearing for appointments. Intensive case management with patient navigators has

TABLE 14–4. Candidate quality measure concepts for the identification of opioid use disorder

Structural	Percentage of medical examiner offices equipped to test for a predefined list of substances (e.g., heroin, fentanyl) among decedents who are suspected of overdose-related mortality
	Percentage of medical examiner offices reporting mortality figures to the state on a quarterly basis
	Percentage of emergency rooms with a specialist clinician who can assess overdose victims for OUD during all operating hours
	Percentage of EHR systems equipped to report OUD cases directly to the state (i.e., through an encrypted, confidential reporting linkage)
Process	Percentage of high-risk patients routinely screened for OUD (e.g., documentation in a clinical note that a patient receiving > 90 mg MEQ has been assessed for OUD)
	Percentage of at-risk patients screened quarterly for OUD
	Percentage of clinical sites reporting prevalence of OUD at least once a quarter
Outcomes	Annual reduction in the prevalence of OUD in a given municipality or treatment system
	Reductions in the percentage of patients on long-term opioid therapy for chronic pain who meet criteria for OUD
	Percentage of insurance plans with identified populations within 10% of estimated prevalence

Note. EHR=electronic health record; MEQ=morphine-equivalent doses; OUD=opioid use disorder.

been developed as models in HIV, tuberculosis, and diabetes care and can be adapted for OUD treatment. Patient navigators and peer counselors can assist patients in accessing long-term, community-based recovery services and improve retention in treatment. State Medicaid offices and Single State Agencies for Substance Abuse Services (i.e., each state's substance abuse services authority that oversees the funding and regulation of specialty addiction facilities) have opportunities under

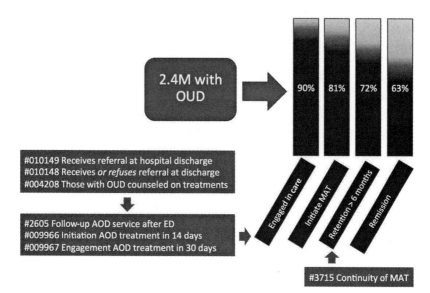

FIGURE 14–2.   Application of existing quality measures to the OUD Treatment Cascade.

Percentages in the columns reflect theoretical targets for success under a 90-90-90 model derived from the global UNAIDS goal for HIV by the year 2020. Quality measures (boxes on left) are identified by their numbers in the NQF and AHRQ quality measure clearinghouses.

AHRQ=Agency for Healthcare Research and Quality; AOD=alcohol and other drug; ED=emergency department; HIV=human immunodeficiency virus; MAT=medication-assisted treatment; NQF=National Quality Forum; OUD=opioid use disorder; UNAIDS=Joint United Nations Programme on HIV/AIDS.

new funding streams (e.g., funding via the 21st Century Cures Act of 2016 [P.L. 114-255]) to reimburse these efforts. Information about individuals who "fall off" the cascade will be key for designing interventions and improving outcomes over time (Chalk and Mark 2017). Table 14–5 includes candidate measure concepts related to stages of an OUD Treatment Cascade.

Recovery

As with the mental health field generally, discourse on the definition of *recovery* has loosened rigid ideologies on what constitutes treatment success. In the past, abstinence was the only outcome deemed acceptable (and this is still preferred by the FDA for medication approval, al-

TABLE 14–5. Candidate quality measure concepts for treatment of opioid use disorder

Structural	Percentage of treatment programs that offer MAT pharmacotherapies
	Percentage of MAT providers with EHR capacity to upload records of MAT provision
Process	Percentage of patients offered MAT during intake for OUD treatment
	Percentage of patients receiving evidence-based (e.g., contingency management, motivational interviewing, cognitive-behavioral therapy) counseling to improve adherence rates
Outcomes	Percentage of patients with OUD who are engaged in care and have an overdose event
	Percentage of patients who have negative urine toxicology in the first month following MAT initiation

Note. EHR = electronic health record; MAT = medication-assisted treatment; OUD = opioid use disorder.

though there have been recent signs of reconsideration); however, increasing attention has emphasized the importance of clinically meaningful reductions in drug use (e.g., the number of heavy drinking days), reductions in high-risk behaviors (e.g., drug injection and needle sharing), and quality of life for persons with SUDs (Bray et al. 2017). Additionally, the benefits of harm reduction approaches (represented by the triangle in the bottom right quadrant of Figure 14–1) such as needle exchange, naloxone distribution, and supervised injection facilities have become more apparent, energizing the message that many service providers embrace "meeting patients where they are" rather than making treatment and service provision contingent on complete abstinence. Chapter 12, "Harm Reduction: Caring for People Who Misuse Opioids," discusses harm reduction strategies in greater depth. Although continuous abstinence may not be achievable or desirable for some patients with OUD, the complete cessation of opioid use confers the greatest protection against opioid-related overdose death. However, this should not be interpreted to suggest that patients do not benefit from treatment and related services if they continue to intermittently use opioids, as indicated in the depiction of treatment and recovery on a continuum in Figure 14–1.

As with their monitoring and reporting on the treatment stages of MAT initiation and retention, OUD service providers could enhance their ability to report on the percentage of patients in treatment who eventually achieve remission from opioid use and related clinical outcomes (e.g., overdose events, all-cause mortality), and states should be incentivized to follow patients who drop out of active treatment longitudinally for surveillance and quality improvement purposes. Table 14–6 includes candidate measure concepts for clinical management of OUD under a long-term recovery model.

Implementation of Quality Measures

Because the addiction treatment system has historically operated outside the traditional health care system and has not been eligible for insurance reimbursement, policy makers face complex administrative challenges integrating quality measures and practice improvement efforts into addiction treatment settings (Friedmann et al. 2003). Single State Agencies for Substance Abuse Services have opportunities to help their states' treatment programs qualify for insurance reimbursement, whether public or commercial (Buck 2011). Currently, many drug treatment programs do not meet insurers' credentialing requirements, and over one-third of publicly funded programs tracked by SAMHSA do not or cannot accept insurance of any kind as a result (Andrews et al. 2015). The development of quality measures will have the most impact if additional resources are allocated for their adoption and tracking and for the development of interventions to improve outcomes in response.

Figure 14–1 encompasses the relationships between prevention, identification, treatment, and recovery and includes examples of interventions and processes for many of the stages. However, it does not currently contain outcome measures that are reliable, feasible, and clinically meaningful for each stage as proposed in the text (see Tables 14–4, 14–5, and 14–6). With adoption of the OUD Cascade of Care, quality measures can be developed and tested in a more systematic fashion and iteratively refined in order to maximize care outcomes. For the time being, the candidate quality measure concepts at the structural, process, and outcome levels are given here as possible starting points for researchers, clinicians, and policy makers.

TABLE 14–6. Candidate quality measure concepts for recovery among persons with opioid use disorder

Structural	Percentage of states with a central office and reporting system with the capacity to track patients who drop out of care
	Percentage of programs with a staff member who can do wellness visits for no-show patients
Process	Percentage of visits with urine toxicology results documented
	Percentage of patients at 12 months (from intake) routinely tested for opioids (e.g., twice monthly or intermittently)
	Percentage of patients on MAT who receive concomitant opioid prescriptions from outside providers
	Percentage of patients in long-term recovery whose care can be transferred to primary care providers
Outcomes	Percentage of patients who initiate MAT who are opioid abstinent at 12 months according to urine toxicology
	Percentage of patients retained on MAT with clinically meaningful reduction in opioid use
	Percentage of patients with an overdose event following 12+ months of MAT maintenance

Note. MAT=medication-assisted treatment.

Resources for the Clinician

There is no simple solution for resolving an epidemic as complex as the current opioid crisis. However, all clinicians throughout the health system have an opportunity to contribute to improving rates of identifying and effectively treating patients with OUD to reduce risk of overdose and death. There are extensive and freely available trainings and resource materials online to help clinicians learn more about MAT pharmacotherapy and how to improve their evidence-based practice. Several are listed below.

Provider's Clinical Support System for Medication-Assisted Treatment (PCSS-MAT) is a robust online training and mentorship initiative funded by SAMHSA and spearheaded by the American Academy of Addiction Psychiatry (AAAP). Many modules are posted at https://pcssnow.org/education-training/.

National Institute on Drug Abuse (NIDA) has a website that is dedicated to updates on evidence-based treatment for OUD: https://www.drugabuse.gov/publications/effective-treatments-opioid-addiction/effective-treatments-opioid-addiction.

Substance Abuse and Mental Health Services Administration (SAMHSA) has published an extensive Treatment Improvement Protocol (TIP 42) on treating patients with comorbid SUDs and mental illness: https://store.samhsa.gov/product/TIP-42-Substance-Abuse-Treatment-for-Persons-With-Co-Occurring-Disorders/SMA13-3992.

Key Chapter Points

▶ Despite a strong evidence base for the use of U.S. Food and Drug Administration–approved medications (methadone, buprenorphine, and extended-release naltrexone) to effectively treat OUD, few patients receive medication-assisted treatment.

▶ There is a tremendous need to strengthen accreditation standards for programs purporting to treat OUD and address the many barriers impeding patient access to quality care.

▶ Few existing quality measures in health care can be applied specifically to the treatment of OUD.

▶ Among those quality measures currently in use, all are process measures that reflect patterns of service delivery rather than specifically incorporating the evidence base for the treatment of OUD and related patient-level outcomes.

▶ Other fields of medicine offer an opportunity to develop a unified framework of measure development, such as an OUD Cascade of Care, to identify critical gaps in care and improve patient outcomes.

▶ To maximize impact, coordinated measures are needed at the following levels: structural (i.e., program accreditation requirements), process (i.e., service delivery and standards of care), and outcome (i.e., clinical improvement).

▶ The use of quality measures requires systems for data collection and reporting, but many addiction treatment providers in the United States are currently ill equipped to meet these requirements.

References

Ali MK, Bullard KM, Gregg EW, et al: A cascade of care for diabetes in the United States: visualizing the gaps. Ann Intern Med 161(10):681–689, 2014 25402511

American Society of Addiction Medicine: Advancing Access to Addiction Medications: Implications for Opioid Addiction Treatment. Chevy Chase, MD, American Society of Addiction Medicine, 2013

American Society of Addiction Medicine: The ASAM Standards of Care for the Addiction Specialist Physician. Chevy Chase, MD, American Society of Addiction Medicine, 2014

Andrews C, Abraham A, Grogan CM, et al: Despite resources from the ACA, most states do little to help addiction treatment programs implement care reform. Health Aff (Millwood) 34(5):828–835, 2015 25941285

Babor TF, McRee BG, Kassebaum PA, et al: Screening, Brief Intervention, and Referral to Treatment (SBIRT): toward a public health approach to the management of substance abuse. Subst Abus 28(3):7–30, 2007 18077300

Bray JW, Aden B, Eggman AA, et al: Quality of life as an outcome of opioid use disorder treatment: a systematic review. J Subst Abuse Treat 76:88–93, 2017 28190543

Buck JA: The looming expansion and transformation of public substance abuse treatment under the Affordable Care Act. Health Aff (Millwood) 30(8):1402–1410, 2011 21821557

Chalk M, Mark T: Deploying the cascade of care framework to address the opioid epidemic means taking a closer look at quality measures. Health Affairs Blog, Health Policy Lab, June 21, 2017. Available at: https://www.healthaffairs.org/do/10.1377/hblog20170621.060677/full/. Accessed April 5, 2018.

Cicero TJ, Ellis MS: Understanding the demand side of the prescription opioid epidemic: does the initial source of opioids matter? Drug Alcohol Depend 173 (suppl 1):S4–S10, 2017 28363319

Cicero TJ, Dart RC, Inciardi JA, et al: The development of a comprehensive risk-management program for prescription opioid analgesics: researched abuse, diversion and addiction-related surveillance (RADARS). Pain Med 8(2):157–170, 2007 17305687

Cicero TJ, Ellis MS, Kasper ZA: Increased use of heroin as an initiating opioid of abuse. Addict Behav 74:63–66, 2017 28582659

Compton WM, Thomas YF, Stinson FS, Grant BF: Prevalence, correlates, disability, and comorbidity of DSM-IV drug abuse and dependence in the United States: results from the National Epidemiologic Survey on Alcohol and Related Conditions. Arch Gen Psychiatry 64(5):566–576, 2007 17485608

Compton WM, Dawson D, Duffy SQ, et al: The effect of inmate populations on estimates of DSM-IV alcohol and drug use disorders in the United States. Am J Psychiatry 167(4):473–474, 2010 20360330

Compton WM, Jones CM, Baldwin GT: Relationship between nonmedical prescription-opioid use and heroin use. N Engl J Med 374(2):154–163, 2016 26760086

Curtis BL, Lookatch SJ, Ramo DE, et al: Meta-analysis of the association of alcohol-related social media use with alcohol consumption and alcohol-related problems in adolescents and young adult. Alcohol Clin Exp Res 42(6):978–986, 2018 29786874

Degenhardt L, Bucello C, Mathers B, et al: Mortality among regular or dependent users of heroin and other opioids: a systematic review and meta-analysis of cohort studies. Addiction 106(1):32–51, 2011 21054613

Donabedian A: The quality of care: how can it be assessed? JAMA 260(12):1743–1748, 1988 3045356

Friedmann PD, Saitz R, Samet JH: Linking addiction treatment with other medical and psychiatric treatment systems, in Principles of Addiction Medicine. Chevy Chase, MD, American Society of Addiction Medicine, 2003, pp 497–507

Gardner EM, McLees MP, Steiner JF, et al: The spectrum of engagement in HIV care and its relevance to test-and-treat strategies for prevention of HIV infection. Clin Infect Dis 52(6):793–800, 2011 21367734

Garnick DW, Horgan CM, Chalk M: Performance measures for alcohol and other drug services. Alcohol Res Health 29(1):19–26, 2006 16767849

Garnick DW, Lee MT, Horgan CM, et al; Washington Circle Public Sector Workgroup: Adapting Washington Circle performance measures for public sector substance abuse treatment systems. J Subst Abuse Treat 36(3):265–277, 2009 18722075

Ghitza UE, Tai B: Challenges and opportunities for integrating preventive substance-use-care services in primary care through the Affordable Care Act. J Health Care Poor Underserved 25(1 suppl):36–45, 2014 24583486

Gordon AJ, Lo-Ciganic WH, Cochran G, et al: Patterns and quality of buprenorphine opioid agonist treatment in a large Medicaid program. J Addict Med 9(6):470–477, 2015 26517324

Haffajee RL, Jena AB, Weiner SG: Mandatory use of prescription drug monitoring programs. JAMA 313(9):891–892, 2015 25622279

Han B, Compton WM, Jones CM, et al: Nonmedical prescription opioid use and use disorders among adults aged 18 through 64 years in the United States, 2003–2013. JAMA 314(14):1468–1478, 2015 26461997

Hanson CL, Cannon B, Burton S, et al: An exploration of social circles and prescription drug abuse through Twitter. J Med Internet Res 15(9):e189, 2013 24014109

Harris AHS, Humphreys K, Finney JW: Veterans Affairs facility performance on Washington Circle indicators and casemix-adjusted effectiveness. J Subst Abuse Treat 33(4):333–339, 2007 17400416

Horberg MA, Hurley LB, Klein DB, et al: The HIV care cascade measured over time and by age, sex, and race in large national integrated care system. AIDS Patient Care STDS 29(11):582–590, 2015 26505968

Hser YI, Evans E, Grella C, et al: Long-term course of opioid addiction. Harv Rev Psychiatry 23(2):76–89, 2015 25747921

Hunter S, Feder M, Granger B, et al: Reliability study pretest analysis, in Section 18, National Survey on Drug Use and Health: Methodological Resource Book. Prepared for the Substance Abuse and Mental Health Services Administration, Office of Applied Studies, under Contract No 283-2004-00022, RTI/0209009. Research Triangle Park, NC, RTI International, 2005

Jarvis BP, Holtyn AF, Subramaniam S, et al: Extended-release injectable naltrexone for opioid use disorder: a systematic review. Addiction 113(7):1188–1209, 2018 29396985

Kampman K, Jarvis M: American Society of Addiction Medicine (ASAM) national practice guideline for the use of medications in the treatment of addiction involving opioid use. J Addict Med 9(5):358–367, 2015 26406300

Kazemi DM, Borsari B, Levine MJ, et al: Systematic review of surveillance by social media platforms for illicit drug use. J Public Health (Oxf) 39(4):763–776, 2017 28334848

Kolodny A, Courtwright DT, Hwang CS, et al: The prescription opioid and heroin crisis: a public health approach to an epidemic of addiction. Annu Rev Public Health 36:559–574, 2015 25581144

Lee JD, Friedmann PD, Kinlock TW, et al: Extended-release naltrexone to prevent opioid relapse in criminal justice offenders. N Engl J Med 374(13):1232–1242, 2016 27028913

Lee JD, Nunes EV, Novo P, et al: Comparative effectiveness of extended release naltrexone versus buprenorphine-naloxone for opioid relapse prevention (X:BOT): a multicentre, open label, randomised controlled trial. Lancet 391(10118):309–318, 2018 29150198

McLellan AT, Lewis DC, O'Brien CP, et al: Drug dependence, a chronic medical illness: implications for treatment, insurance, and outcomes evaluation. JAMA 284(13):1689–1695, 2000 11015800

Mugavero MJ, Amico KR, Horn T, et al: The state of engagement in HIV care in the United States: from cascade to continuum to control. Clin Infect Dis 57(8):1164–1171, 2013 23797289

National Center for Health Statistics: Provisional counts of drug overdose deaths, as of 8/6/2017. National Center for Health Statistics, Centers for Disease Control and Prevention, 2017. Available at: https://www.wabe.org/ga-doctors-required-get-opioid-prescription-training/. Accessed April 5, 2018.

National Committee for Quality Assurance: Proposed Changes to Existing Measures for HEDIS 2018: Initiation and Engagement of Alcohol and Other Drug Dependence Treatment (IET) and Identification of Alcohol and Other Drug Services (IAD). Washington, DC, National Committee for Quality Assurance, 2017

National Consensus Development Panel on Effective Medical Treatment of Opiate Addiction: Effective medical treatment of opiate addiction. JAMA 280(22):1936–1943, 1998 9851480

National Quality Forum: Behavioral Health 2016–2017. 2017. Available at: https://www.wabe.org/ga-doctors-required-get-opioid-prescription-training/. Accessed April 5, 2018.

Rudd RA, Seth P, David F, et al: Increases in drug and opioid-involved overdose deaths—United States, 2010–2015. MMWR Morb Mortal Wkly Rep 65(5051):1445–1452, 2016 28033313

Ruhm CJ: Geographic variation in opioid and heroin involved drug mortality rates. Am J Prev Med 53(6):745–753, 2017 28797652

Rutkow L, Turner L, Lucas E, et al: Most primary care physicians are aware of prescription drug monitoring programs, but many find the data difficult to access. Health Aff (Millwood) 34(3):484–492, 2015 25732500

Saloner B, Karthikeyan S: Changes in substance abuse treatment use among individuals with opioid use disorders in the United States, 2004–2013. JAMA 314(14):1515–1517, 2015 26462001

Socías ME, Volkow N, Wood E: Adopting the 'cascade of care' framework: an opportunity to close the implementation gap in addiction care? Addiction 111(12):2079–2081, 2016 27412876

Sordo L, Barrio G, Bravo MJ, et al: Mortality risk during and after opioid substitution treatment: systematic review and meta-analysis of cohort studies. BMJ 357:j1550, 2017 28446428

Stein BD, Sorbero M, Dick AW, et al: Physician capacity to treat opioid use disorder with buprenorphine-assisted treatment. JAMA 316(11):1211–1212, 2016 27654608

Strang J, McCambridge J, Best D, et al: Loss of tolerance and overdose mortality after inpatient opiate detoxification: follow up study. BMJ 326(7396):959–960, 2003 12727768

Substance Abuse and Mental Health Services Administration: Results from the 2011 National Survey on Drug Use and Health (HHS Publ No SMA 12-4713). Rockville, MD, Substance Abuse and Mental Health Services Administration, 2012. Available at: https://www.samhsa.gov/data/sites/default/files/Revised2k11NSDUHSummNatFindings/Revised2k11NSDUH SummNatFindings/NSDUHresults2011.htm. Accessed April 5, 2018.

Substance Abuse and Mental Health Services Administration: National Survey of Substance Abuse Treatment Services (N-SSATS): 2015: Data on Substance Abuse Treatment Facilities (BHSIS Series S-88, HHS Publ No SMA-17-5031). Rockville, MD, Substance Abuse and Mental Health Services Administration, 2017a. Available at: https://www.samhsa.gov/data/sites/default/files/2015_National_Survey_of_Substance_Abuse_Treatment_Services.pdf. Accessed April 5, 2018.

Substance Abuse and Mental Health Services Administration: Results from the 2016 National Survey on Drug Use and Health (HHS SMA17-5044), Rockville, MD, Substance Abuse and Mental Health Services Administration, 2017b

Timko C, Schultz NR, Cucciare MA, et al: Retention in medication-assisted treatment for opiate dependence: a systematic review. J Addict Dis 35(1):22–35, 2016 26467975

U.S. Department of Health and Human Services, Office of the Surgeon General: Facing addiction in America: the Surgeon General's report on alcohol, drugs, and health. Chapter 4, p 21. November 2016. Available at: https://addiction.surgeongeneral.gov/sites/default/files/chapter-4-treatment.pdf. Accessed April 5, 2018.

Volkow ND, Frieden TR, Hyde PS, et al: Medication-assisted therapies—tackling the opioid-overdose epidemic. N Engl J Med 370(22):2063–2066, 2014 24758595

Weiss RD, Potter JS, Griffin ML, et al: Long-term outcomes from the National Drug Abuse Treatment Clinical Trials Network Prescription Opioid Addiction Treatment Study. Drug Alcohol Depend 150:112–119, 2015 25818060

Williams AR: Opioid overdose epidemic: quality improvement. Oral presentation to the Substance Abuse and Mental Health Services Administration, Center for Substance Abuse Treatment, Council of Directors, August 10, 2017

Williams AR, Bisaga A: From AIDS to opioids—how to respond to an epidemic. N Engl J Med 375(9):813–815, 2016 27579632

Williams AR, Olfson M, Galanter M: Assessing and improving clinical insight among patients "in denial." JAMA Psychiatry 72(4):303–304, 2015 25651391

Williams AR, Nunes EV, Olfson M: To battle the opioid overdose epidemic, deploy the "cascade of care" model. Health Affairs Blog, Health Policy Lab, March 13, 2017. Available at: https://www.healthaffairs.org/do/10.1377/hblog20170313.059163/full/. Accessed April 5, 2018.

Williams AR, Nunes EV, Bisaga A, et al: Developing an opioid use disorder treatment cascade: a review of quality measures. J Subst Abuse Treat 91:57–68, 2018 29910015

Wu LT, Zhu H, Swartz MS: Treatment utilization among persons with opioid use disorder in the United States. Drug Alcohol Depend 169:117–127, 2016 27810654

Yehia BR, Schranz AJ, Umscheid CA, et al: The treatment cascade for chronic hepatitis C virus infection in the United States: a systematic review and meta-analysis. PLoS One 9(7):e101554, 2014 24988388

Zanoni BC, Mayer KH: The adolescent and young adult HIV cascade of care in the United States: exaggerated health disparities. AIDS Patient Care STDS 28(3):128–135, 2014 24601734

Index

Page numbers printed in **boldface** type refer to tables and figures.